76.00

D1557924

More Than Ramps

LISA I. IEZZONI
BONNIE L. O'DAY

More Than Ramps

A Guide to Improving
Health Care Quality and Access
for People with Disabilities

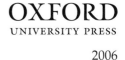

OXFORD
UNIVERSITY PRESS

2006

OXFORD
UNIVERSITY PRESS

Oxford University Press, Inc., publishes works that further
Oxford University's objective of excellence
in research, scholarship, and education.

Oxford   New York
Auckland   Cape Town   Dar es Salaam   Hong Kong   Karachi
Kuala Lumpur   Madrid   Melbourne   Mexico City   Nairobi
New Delhi   Shanghai   Taipei   Toronto

With offices in
Argentina   Austria   Brazil   Chile   Czech Republic   France   Greece
Guatemala   Hungary   Italy   Japan   Poland   Portugal   Singapore
South Korea   Switzerland   Thailand   Turkey   Ukraine   Vietnam

Copyright © 2006 by Oxford University Press, Inc.

Published by Oxford University Press, Inc.
198 Madison Avenue, New York, New York 10016

www.oup.com

Oxford is a registered trademark of Oxford University Press

Library of Congress Cataloging-in-Publication Data
Iezzoni, Lisa I.
   More than ramps : a guide to improving health care quality and access for people with
disabilites / Lisa I. Iezzoni and Bonnie L. O'Day.
      p.   ; cm.
   Includes bibliographical references and index.
   ISBN-13: 978-0-19-517276-8
   ISBN-10: 0-19-517276-0
   1. People with disabilities—Services for—United States.   2. People with disabilities—Medical care—
United States.   3.   Insurance, Health—United States.   4.   Patient advocacy—United States.   I. O'Day,
Bonnie.   II. Title.

HV1553.I42   2005
362.4—dc22   2005040876

9 8 7 6 5 4 3 2 1

Printed in the United States of America
on acid-free paper

To Reed
—L. I. I.

In loving memory of my father, Michael O'Day,
and in deep appreciation of my husband, Bob Hartt
—B. L. O.

Preface

Many people likely notice Bonnie and me, even if by sidelong glances, when we go out together in public. Bonnie, who was born blind, uses a white cane. I, who have had multiple sclerosis for almost thirty years, roll in my battered but generally trustworthy motorized scooter. Most passersby give us a wide berth. Others—engrossed by private thoughts or wireless phones and oblivious to their surroundings—pose imminent dangers. Bonnie and I must remain constantly vigilant to avoid collisions with those insentient pedestrians hurtling toward us.

When out in the world, persons with disabilities spend much of their time anticipating and circumventing innumerable barriers, animate and inanimate, impeding or endangering their way. For more than thirty years, federal and state statutes have aimed to remove or mitigate the environmental, institutional, and societal barriers that have historically prevented people with disabilities from participating fully in daily life in homes, communities, and workplaces. Important progress has occurred, largely motivated by visionary and tireless disability rights advocates. New technologies, such as Bonnie's computer that reads texts out loud and my power scooter, increasingly compensate for functional impairments.

But numerous challenges persist. Speaking broadly, persons with disabilities are much more likely than others to be poor, uneducated, and unemployed and to live alone. Assistive technologies and other supportive items and services often fall beyond their financial reach. Many communities remain physically inaccessible. Although public and private mass transportation must now accommodate wheelchairs, the lifts on buses frequently malfunction, and drivers sometimes refuse to pick up passengers using wheelchairs. Although legislating physical access is feasible, mandating public attitudes is not. While societal perceptions of some persons with disabilities are now accepting and even welcoming, persistent negative views pose more intractable hurdles. Fully opening communities to people with disabilities still requires considerable work.

Our book concentrates on health care. This might seem counterintuitive. Given its humanistic intent, certainly health care should offer unobstructed safe havens, a welcoming and accessible source of compassionate care, a place where patients are kept front and center—regardless of their abilities and disabilities. As elsewhere, however, barriers intrude, arising from such diverse sources as the so-called "built environment" (i.e., any setting constructed by humans), medical equipment, institutional policies and procedures, long-held professional assumptions, clinicians' technical knowledge, interpersonal communication, and awareness of and attitudes toward disability. Therefore, many persons with disabilities do not receive the high-quality health care that they should.

Purpose and Organization

Our overall purpose is twofold: to describe the experiences of adult Americans with physical and sensory disabilities as they seek primary health care services, and to suggest ways to overcome or circumvent barriers to high-quality care. We have organized the book into three parts. Part I sets the stage by describing the population, defining disability, and sketching the overarching health care environment in the United States. Part II examines health care experiences of persons with disabilities along several dimensions, including physical and financial access to care and interpersonal and technical communication. Part III parallels part II, offering specific suggestions and resources for improving health care access and experiences of persons with disabilities.

These topics are broad, and disabilities are diverse. To make our task manageable, we needed to focus. We did so along two dimensions: our target population of persons with disabilities, and the aspects of the health care system that we address. Even so, we acknowledge that this book provides a whirlwind tour, touching only briefly on complex topics. Especially in part III, we merely introduce potential solutions, while directing readers to resources that offer more in-depth information.

Although critical concerns (e.g., civil rights protections) transcend particular disabilities, specific practical needs and clinical issues vary by the nature of the sensory or physical impairment. Realizing that we could not encompass all potentially disabling conditions, we decided to focus on sensory (specifically vision and hearing) and physical disabilities among adults. This population includes millions of elderly persons with sensory and physical impairments related to aging and chronic disease, as well as younger persons with conditions since birth or early in life. Some people have multiple impairments. For example, persons with diabetes can develop blindness from retinopathy, as well as mobility difficulties when gangrene leads to amputation of toes or legs.

Our choice excludes many persons, such as individuals with developmental, psychiatric, and cognitive disabilities, many of whom experience difficulties obtaining high-quality health care. (Intractable barriers are often embedded within the health care payment system, such as "carve outs" of mental health care from other services.) It also excludes children, whose vulnerability is frequently exacerbated by poverty and shortfalls in sectors beyond health care, such as day care, education, nutrition, and housing.

To refine our task further, we decided to limit what aspects of health care we consider. This is not a clinical textbook; we do not describe specific clinical entities, evaluations, or interventions. Instead, we examine aspects of health care delivery and clinician-patient communication where practical and feasible changes could enhance patients' experiences and perhaps outcomes of care. Although we have written this book for all clinical professionals and health care managers, our data sources, including federal surveys (see below), focus primarily on services provided by physicians. We recognize that the best quality care for persons with disabilities generally involves teams of clinicians representing diverse professional perspectives.

In part I, we describe the global context of health care financing, offering an overview of the implications of health insurance and reimbursement policies for persons with disabilities in the United States. This overall context frames health care experiences. Delineating solutions for overarching financing problems—remedies that have eluded policy-makers for decades—is beyond our scope. We believe that long-term solutions must include health insurance for *all* Americans.

We concentrate largely on community-based outpatient care, including preventive and primary care and items and services (e.g., assistive technologies, rehabilitation therapies) relating specifically to functional impairments. Hence, we do not address the crucial complexities of institutional long-term, nursing home, and community-based home care—critical services for younger and older persons with severe functional deficits or profound frailty. We also exclude detailed discussions of personal assistance services, home health aides, and other supportive services that interact closely with health care and carry important implications for health. Nonetheless, we strongly endorse the goals embedded within the U.S. Supreme Court's landmark 1999 decision in *Olmstead v. L.C.*, which held that states must ensure that persons of all ages with disabilities receive the services necessary to reside in communities in the least restrictive settings possible.[1]

---

1. In *Olmstead v. L.C.*, decided six to three on June 22, 1999, the U.S. Supreme Court ruled that, under Title II of the Americans with Disabilities Act, states must place persons with mental disabilities in community rather than institutional settings if (a) the state's treatment professionals determine that community placement is appropriate; (b) the affected individuals do not object to being transferred from an institution to the community; and (c) the community placement can be reasonably accommodated, given the state's resources and needs of other residents with mental disabilities. The plaintiffs, two women with mental retardation and psychiatric conditions who had been voluntarily institutionalized by Georgia officials, sued the state for transfer to the community after their clinicians determined that community-based treatment programs were appropriate. Five years after *Olmstead*, progress in building social service and other systems to support persons with disabilities living in communities is evident but slow: much remains to be done (Rosenbaum and Teitelbaum, 2004).

Information Sources

We present our points using both narratives and numbers. Between us, Bonnie and I have accumulated decades of experiences within the health care system—some good, others not so good. However, this book relies primarily upon the observations and experiences of other persons with disabilities, as well as analyses of nationally representative surveys and the published literature. Most of our information, including the survey analyses, comes from a study on quality of care for persons with disabilities conducted by Bonnie and me from 1999 to 2003 and funded by the federal Agency for Healthcare Research and Quality (AHRQ). A few points come from a project I conducted from 1997 to 2000 funded by The Robert Wood Johnson Foundation, during which I interviewed persons with walking difficulties, primary care physicians, physical and occupational therapists, and assorted others. Findings from that study are documented extensively in the book *When Walking Fails* (Iezzoni, 2003; the associated Web site, www.ucpress. edu/books/pages/9456.html, details the study's methods).

To quantify the health care experiences of persons with sensory and physical disabilities, we analyzed three nationally representative surveys. When surveys included both persons living in institutions (e.g., nursing homes, residential care facilities) and in homes and apartments throughout communities, we focused exclusively on community-dwelling respondents. All numbers presented throughout this book used weights from the survey sampling schemes to produce national estimates. Briefly, the surveys include the following:

- *2001 Medical Expenditure Panel Survey (MEPS).* This survey, conducted by the AHRQ, interviewed roughly 22,650 adults representing civilian, community-dwelling, U.S. residents. In addition to gathering self-reported information about health and functional abilities, the survey asked numerous questions about the use and costs of health care services and insurance coverage.[2]

---

2. The MEPS selects respondents using the same sampling frame as the National Health Interview Survey, conducted by the National Center for Health Statistics. The MEPS uses a panel design, interviewing selected household respondents periodically over two years. It involves four component surveys: a household component—a sample of families and individuals living in communities nationwide; a nursing home component—a sample of nursing homes and persons residing in nursing homes nationwide; a provider component—surveys of hospitals, physicians, and home care providers of respondents from the household survey; and an insurance component—including questions of employers and union officials about health insurance provided to household respondents. Some survey questions change from year to year. In several instances, we use MEPS 2000 data to make specific points; in 2000, the MEPS surveyed roughly 16,700 adults living in the community. More information about the MEPS is available at www.meps.ahrq.gov/whatis.htm.

- *1996 Medicare Current Beneficiary Survey (MCBS).* This survey, conducted by the Health Care Financing Administration (renamed the Centers for Medicare and Medicaid Services in 2001), interviewed approximately 16,400 Medicare beneficiaries living in communities throughout the United States. The survey oversampled persons under sixty-five years of age (eligible for Medicare because of disability), as well as persons ages eighty-five years and older. The survey gathered self-reported information about functional abilities and asked twenty questions about various aspects of health care experiences.[3]
- *1994–1995 National Health Interview Survey (NHIS) disability supplement.* This survey, conducted by the National Center for Health Statistics, contains the most detailed questions about self-reported functional abilities, use of assistive technologies, and perceptions of disability of any recent federal survey. Roughly 145,000 community-dwelling adult civilians living throughout the United States answered this survey.[4]

As shown in tables 1–3 in appendix 4, we used responses from these surveys to identify persons with difficulties with vision, hearing, and leg, arm, and hand functioning. We noted all sensory and physical difficulties identified by each survey respondent.

The survey data offer important benefits, notably their national scope. However, such surveys inevitably have important drawbacks. First, they rely exclusively on self-reports of the survey respondents or their proxies (Iezzoni et al., 2000b).[5] The accuracy of self- and proxy-reports, especially

---

3. We replicated the analyses presented in this book using the 2001 MCBS, which interviewed roughly 15,050 community-dwelling Medicare beneficiaries. The 1996 and 2001 surveys generated comparable results, although the magnitudes of the findings differed somewhat. We present the 1996 results here because the complete methods and findings are described in readily available publications (Iezzoni et al., 2002, 2003). More information about the MCBS is available at www.cms.hhs.gov/MCBS/default.asp.

4. The National Center for Health Statistics continuously conducts the NHIS to collect basic information about the health of U.S. residents; detailed information on disabilities was gathered in the 1994 and 1995 disability supplements (so-called NHIS-D). In the currently ongoing NHIS, a limited set of questions addresses activities of daily living and selected functional abilities. More information on the NHIS-D is available at www.cdc.gov/nchs/about/major/nhis_dis/nhis_dis.htm.

5. Some surveys have proxies respond when the targeted respondent is a child or is unable to respond because of physical, cognitive, or emotional concerns or absence from the home. In the NHIS, proxies provided about one third of the responses (Iezzoni et al., 2000a). The mean age of self-respondents was forty-six years, compared with forty-one for persons with proxies; men were less likely to respond themselves (45 percent) than women (67 percent). Self-respondents were more likely to report lower extremity mobility problems (13 percent) than those with proxy respondents (7 percent). One possibility is that self-respondents were at home explicitly because of mobility problems, while those without mobility difficulties were out and unable to respond in person. Determining the true effect of proxy responses on survey findings requires further study.

about the presence of functional impairments, can be suspect. For instance, persons may hesitate to admit that they have trouble seeing, hearing, or walking. In addition, errors in survey responses may result when respondents do not understand the question or interpret the question in unintended ways. Second, although these surveys interviewed thousands of persons, the numbers of individuals with specific impairments was often too small for us to produce reliable national estimates.[6] In some tables, therefore, we collapsed our disability categories (e.g., considered all persons with vision difficulties rather than separating those who are blind from persons with some vision difficulties). We noted situations where, because of relatively few survey respondents, our estimates may be unreliable. Collapsing disability categories can mask important differences, such as those between deaf persons and those who are hard of hearing; because the hard of hearing group is perhaps ten times larger than the deaf population, findings relating specifically to deafness may be lost.

Finally, although the surveys asked many important questions, none collected every piece of information we could want. For example, the 2001 MEPS did not gather age of onset of specific impairments, information about whether conditions are bilateral (e.g., vision or hearing loss in one eye or ear has different implications than bilateral losses), or data about specific assistive technologies used by respondents. Age of onset is especially important for persons who are deaf: did they become deaf before or after the age at which persons learn speech (prelingually versus postlingually, typically viewed as before or after three years of age)? As noted throughout the book, persons with congenital or early childhood conditions can have different attitudes toward their disabilities than do adults who experience progressive impairments later in life. Without this and other critical information, we were unable to explore important issues using the survey data alone.

The stories and insights offered by interviewees filled this void. We took quotations from verbatim transcripts of thirteen group interviews with 106 adults with disabling conditions. We conducted the interviews in 2000 and 2001 in metropolitan Boston, metropolitan Washington, DC, rural Massachusetts, and rural Virginia (Iezzoni and O'Day, 2003; Iezzoni et al., 2004;

---

6. Experts in MEPS at the AHRQ, along with their computing contractor, generously conducted the analyses using the 2001 MEPS database. Our presentation of MEPS findings therefore conforms with certain statistical standards applied by the AHRQ MEPS team, specifically involving the sample sizes required to produce reliable and stable national estimates. For each estimate, we reviewed the relative standard error (RSE), a measure of an estimate's reliability. RSEs are computed by dividing the standard error of an estimate by the estimate itself; analysts then express RSEs as a percentage of the estimate. RSEs of 30 or greater are considered unreliable. To reduce the RSEs, we sometimes collapsed the disability categories. In analyses where only isolated RSEs exceeded 30, we flagged those results as potentially unreliable. For more about the definition of RSE, see the National Center for Health Statistics Web site at www.cdc.gov/nchs/datawh/nchsdefs/relativestandarderror.htm.

O'Day, Killeen, and Iezzoni, 2004). We recruited participants from the community, not from specific health care providers; we asked centers for independent living, self-help groups, condition-specific advocacy groups, and athletic organizations to help solicit interviewees. We made no attempt to identify specific local clinicians or hospitals mentioned by interviewees.

All interviewees provided written informed consent and are referred to in the text by pseudonyms. Nine focus groups (all except the four in rural areas) involved either men or women with specific disabling conditions (blindness, deafness, hardness of hearing, and significant mobility impairments). In the rural areas, which have relatively small and dispersed populations, we separated men and women but interviewed persons across disabilities. For background, we also conducted interviews with experts in health care and policy issues regarding specific disabling conditions (Iezzoni, 2003; Iezzoni et al., 2004; O'Day, Killeen, and Iezzoni, 2004).

Although I claim the first-person voice throughout this book, that choice is simply for convenience. All words come from Bonnie and me. This has truly been a productive and enjoyable collaboration, from which we have each learned tremendously.

Bonnie and I hope that someday people won't particularly notice us when we venture out together. Now, we likely attract attention because we are not typical passersby. But we are hardly unique. According to the 2000 decennial census, almost 8.9 million adult Americans report sensory disabilities, and nearly 20.7 million report physical disabilities (see chapter 1). Disabling conditions are especially common after age sixty-five. Thus, as "baby boomers" age, considerably more persons with disabilities will live throughout communities. Given the proclivities of our generation, we suspect that these "boomers" will not retreat behind closed doors. People like Bonnie and me will no longer be unusual on neighborhood or city sidewalks.

—*Lisa I. Iezzoni*

Acknowledgments

Many individuals and organizations contributed generously to our work. In particular, about one hundred persons with sensory and physical disabilities allowed us to interview them and responded with eloquence and insight. This book uses their own words to describe their journeys through the American health care system.

Organizing and conducting these interviews required considerable planning. Numerous individuals and organizations—including centers for independent living, self-help and advocacy groups, and sporting clubs for persons with disabilities—helped us recruit interviewees and provided invaluable other assistance. Melissa Wachterman, then my stellar research assistant in Boston and now a physician-in-training, gave tirelessly to these efforts. Marcie Goldstein assisted Bonnie with organizing two focus groups.

Our research was funded by a grant from the federal Agency for Healthcare Research and Quality (AHRQ), led by Carolyn M. Clancy, who—whenever she saw me—always wanted to know what we were finding and what it meant for ways to improve the American health care system. Dr. Clancy and Helen R. Burstin, her AHRQ colleague, offered boundless enthusiasm and encouragement for our work, always pushing us to articulate practical solutions to address any quality shortfalls we identified.

Other AHRQ staff members also contributed significantly to this project. Janet L. Valluzzi spent many hours generating information for us from AHRQ's Medical Expenditure Panel Survey, ably assisted by data analysts Linda Andrews and Matt Ellenburg. David Meyers worked thoughtfully to organize peer review of our draft manuscript, culminating in a meeting with the reviewers at AHRQ in September 2004. We are deeply grateful to these reviewers for their helpful critiques and incredible gift of time: Steven Barnett, Helen Burstin, R. Speed Davis, Rhonda G. Hughes, Kristi L. Kirschner, David Meyers, Laurie Ringaert, Lorraine Rovig, Carolyn Stern, and Peter W. Thomas. Work colleagues also provided helpful reviews, especially Suzanne Leveille and Jaye Hefner. Jane Soukup, an expert data analyst, performed computer programming and assisted me in deciphering reams of data output. Mary Killeen spent hours combing the texts of the interviews to help Bonnie and me better focus our analysis.

During manuscript preparation, three individuals provided special assistance to our understanding of Deaf culture. David Ebert guided me through a sample teletypewriter conversation, and Steven Barnett and Danielle Suzanne Ross advised our description of linguistic and grammatic features of American Sign Language.

Believing that pictures convey volumes—especially as we aim to highlight barriers that still block access for persons with disabilities, as well as potential solutions—we are enormously grateful to three wonderful photographers who contributed to this project, as well as to the persons who agreed to be portrayed. All individuals in these photographs are persons with disabilities, although we recreated some situations from typical occurrences to depict specific points. Mark L. Rosenberg took photographs in his native Georgia, and Bruce Wahl, often ably assisted by Asa Jane Bell, photographed persons in greater Boston.

Crafting the right title poses a daunting challenge. Our main title borrows three words from a sister work, *It Takes More Than Ramps to Solve the Crisis in Healthcare for People with Disabilities* (2004), written by Judy Panko Reis, Mary Lou Breslin, Kristi L. Kirschner, and me, and funded by an award from The Robert Wood Johnson Community Health Leadership Program to the Rehabilitation Institute of Chicago's Women with Disabilities Center. That report uses the conceptual and legal framework of the Americans with Disabilities Act to examine barriers to health care for persons with disabilities and to highlight "best practices" around the country that attempt to overcome these barriers. Those three words—"more than ramps"—succinctly and forcefully remind us that improving health care access and quality for *all* persons with disabilities requires comprehensive changes that go well beyond removing only physical barriers.

Finally, Bonnie and I express our deepest thanks to our family, friends, and colleagues for their steadfast support as we wrote this book and in countless other ways.

—*Lisa I. Iezzoni*

Contents

I

SETTING THE STAGE: DISABILITY AND ACCESS TO HEALTH CARE IN THE UNITED STATES

1

Roots of the Problem

Eleanor Peters likes her physician and social worker, but she has trouble getting into and out of their clinic—the large plate glass door with its gleaming chrome handle does not open automatically (figure 1.1). Opening the door from her power wheelchair requires strength and dexterity that Eleanor, who contracted polio in early childhood and is now in her late-forties, does not have. "The doors are beautiful, shiny," concedes Eleanor, "but I can't get into the clinic. I have to sit outside and wait until somebody comes and opens the door." Eleanor, who works as a vocational rehabilitation counselor, wonders why the people who designed the clinic did not think about patients like her and her clients. She has a clear message for those designers: "Everyone becomes disabled sooner or later. The older they get, the more disabled they'll become, whether it's wearing glasses or not hearing well or arthritis or whatever it is. They could fall off the sidewalk and break their hip. People might as well get on the bandwagon and be on our side, so when they become disabled or they need things to help *them* out, those things'll be there."

The plate glass doors to Eleanor Peters's clinic offer a convenient metaphor for the countless barriers people with disabling conditions face when seeking health care. Often these obstacles are as transparent as glass: people can easily see beyond the barriers to the access and services they need. Nevertheless, such barriers can prove virtually shatterproof, especially when multilayered with intertwining financial, organizational, geographic, sociodemographic, interpersonal, and attitudinal impediments.

This book builds upon a basic premise: that the health care delivery system in the United States is not structured to care effectively for persons with disabilities. We use the word "structure" as did the late Avedis Donabedian who, almost thirty years ago, articulated an enduring three-part framework for assessing health care quality. In Donabedian's structure-process-outcome triad, the last two concepts—"process," or what clinicians do for patients, and "outcomes," or the results of care—generally attract the most attention. "Structure," or the environment in which care occurs, typically is relegated

3

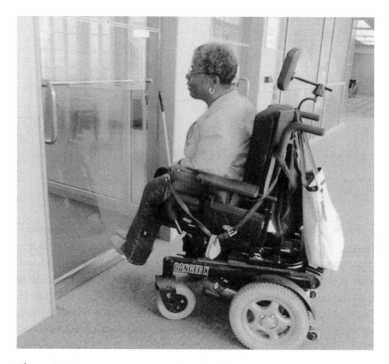

Figure 1.1. Glass barrier. Because she cannot open the heavy glass door that has no automatic opener, Eleanor Peters must wait for someone to let her inside the clinic.

to the "bricks and mortar" realms of fire codes and public health regulations. However, in Donabedian's mind, "structure" meant much more:

> The relatively stable characteristics of the providers of care, of the tools and resources they have at their disposal, and of the physical and organizational settings in which they work. [It] includes the human, physical, and financial resources that are needed to provide medical care . . . [and] the number, distribution, size, equipment, and geographic disposition of hospitals and other facilities. But the concept also goes beyond the factors of production to include the ways in which the financing and delivery of health services are organized, both formally and informally. (1980, p. 81)

Thus, Donabedian's structure encompasses such issues as health insurance coverage and the training of clinicians, as well as technologic capabilities and physical settings.

Given this foundation, this book has two goals: to describe the experiences of adults with sensory and physical disabilities as they seek basic health care services (part II); and to suggest ways to overcome, circumvent, or remove the barriers they confront (part III). Two factors underscore the importance of this topic—the large and growing numbers of persons with disabling conditions and the compelling evidence that they receive substandard health care.

Demographic Demands

Almost one fifth of U.S. residents—19.3 percent of persons age five and older or 49.7 million persons—report disabilities (U.S. Census Bureau, 2003a). These numbers represent persons living in communities, not in institutions like nursing homes. As described in chapter 2, definitions of disability differ widely depending on the context, complicating efforts to obtain exact estimates of how many persons have disabling conditions. The 2000 decennial census asked several questions to quantify disability from various perspectives.[1] Table 1.1 shows estimated numbers and percentages of persons with disabilities, overall and using different definitions, for men and women within two broad age groups. At younger ages, males report higher overall rates of disability than females, while the reverse occurs over age sixty-four. People report physical disabilities more often than sensory or mental health disabilities.

The 2000 census figures provide an important snapshot, but more compelling numbers come from looking ahead. Overall, persons age sixty-five and older report disabilities much more frequently than do younger persons—41.9 percent compared with 18.6 percent (table 1.1)—and the numbers of older persons will grow substantially in coming decades. By 2030, the number of persons age sixty-five and older will rise to 69.4 million (20 percent of the population) from 34.7 million (12.6 percent) in 2000 (Day, 1996, pp. 9–10). Over the next fifty years, the numbers of persons age eighty-five and older will grow more rapidly than any other segment of the population, rising from 4.26 million (1.6 percent) in 2000 to 18.22 million (4.6 percent) in 2050.

This growth reflects lengthening life expectancies. The average male born in the United States in 1900 could anticipate living roughly forty-eight years; one century later, his life expectancy extends to seventy-four years (Arias, 2004, p. 3). Life expectancies for females rose from slightly less than fifty-one years in 1900 to almost eighty in 2002.[2] Even in the past thirty years, decreasing death rates from heart disease have substantially prolonged longevity, increasing the numbers of persons living with chronic, nonfatal, but disabling conditions. Aging is the leading cause of vision and hearing loss.

Persons with significant physical disabilities in early life also live longer than in prior years largely because of medical breakthroughs, notably antibiotics. Enhancing healthy aging with disability is clinically imperative, as persons with conditions such as cerebral palsy, polio, and spina bifida in-

Table 1.1. Estimates from the 2000 U.S. Census

Age and Type of Disability	Population in Millions (Percent)		
	Total	Males	Females
Total (age 5+ years)	257.2 (100.0)	124.6 (100.0)	132.5 (100.0)
With any disability	49.7 (19.3)	24.4 (19.6)	25.3 (19.1)
Age 16 to 64 years	178.7 (100.0)	87.6 (100.0)	91.1 (100.0)
With any disability	33.2 (18.6)	17.1 (19.6)	16.0 (17.6)
Sensory	4.1 (2.3)	2.4 (2.7)	1.7 (1.9)
Physical	11.2 (6.2)	5.3 (6.0)	5.9 (6.4)
Mental	6.8 (3.8)	3.4 (3.9)	3.3 (3.7)
Self-care	3.1 (1.8)	1.5 (1.7)	1.7 (1.9)
Going outside the home	11.4 (6.4)	5.6 (6.4)	5.8 (6.4)
Employment disability	21.3 (11.9)	11.4 (13.0)	9.9 (10.9)
Age 65+ years	33.3 (100.0)	13.9 (100.0)	19.4 (100.0)
With any disability	14.0 (41.9)	5.6 (40.4)	8.3 (43.0)
Sensory	4.7 (14.2)	2.2 (15.6)	2.6 (13.2)
Physical	9.5 (28.6)	3.6 (25.8)	6.0 (30.7)
Mental	3.6 (10.8)	1.4 (9.9)	2.2 (11.4)
Self-care	3.2 (9.5)	1.0 (7.5)	2.1 (11.0)
Going outside the home	6.8 (20.4)	2.3 (16.8)	4.5 (23.0)

Adapted from: U.S. Census Bureau (2003a).

creasingly live into their seventh decade and beyond. For instance, persons who become paraplegic at age forty and survive one year following spinal cord injury can expect to live another twenty-nine years, compared with thirty-eight years for persons without injuries (National Spinal Cord Injury Statistical Center, 2001).[3] During much of these twenty-nine years, many persons with spinal cord injury will live healthy, productive, and active lives.

Aging does not invariably produce disability, until perhaps the very end of life. Centenarians frequently remain reasonably healthy until shortly before death. Patterns of functional declines prior to death vary depending on the nature of underlying diseases and overall health. Researchers have mapped four patterns of functional declines organized around causes of death (figure 1.2): sudden, unexpected deaths, with no preceding functional debility; deaths from terminal diseases such as cancer, where functioning falls sharply just before death; failing organs, such as heart, lung, and kidneys, with fluctuating functional status; and frailty, where functioning declines unchecked as patients near death (Lunney, Lynn, and Hogan, 2002; Lunney et al., 2003). These four trajectories hold varied implications for the type and timing of health care interventions required to maximize quality of life.[4]

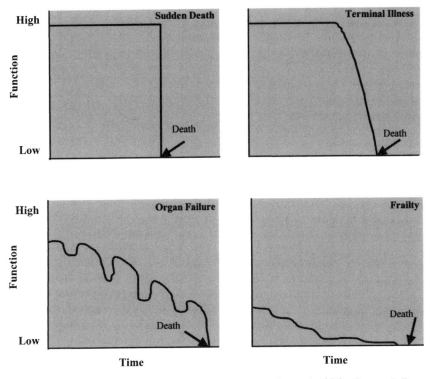

Figure 1.2. Patterns of declines in functioning at the end of life. *Source:* J. R. Lunney et al., 2003, Patterns of Functional Decline at the End of Life, *Journal of the American Medical Association,* 289(18):2388.

Recent reports suggest that rates of disability among older individuals fell substantially during the 1990s (Freedman, Martin, and Schoeni, 2002). Multiple factors likely produced improved functional abilities among older persons, including new medical therapies and healthier lifestyles, such as decreased smoking. However, questions remain about whether rates of very severe disabilities have decreased over time. With the aging population, the absolute number of Americans with functional limitations will rise by over 300 percent by 2049 if the age-specific prevalence of major chronic conditions remains unchanged (Boult et al., 1996, p. 1391; see chapter 16).

As stated in the preface, to make our task manageable, we focused on adults with sensory and physical disabilities. These conditions are common (table 1.2), affecting an estimated 39.5 million (18.9 percent) persons living in the community (e.g., not in nursing homes) in 2001.[5] Lower extremity mobility difficulties are the most prevalent problem (10.0 percent of adults), with hearing losses next in frequency (7.2 percent). Except for hearing loss, women report higher rates of sensory and physical disabilities than men, and percentages increase substantially between younger and older ages.

Table 1.2. Estimates of Sensory and Physical Impairments among Adults

Impairment	Estimated Millions	Percent	Age and Sex (Percent[a])			
			Age 18–64	Age 65+	Men	Women
Vision impairments						
Some	9.9	4.7	4.2	7.7	3.9	5.4
Blind or major	3.3	1.6	0.9	4.8	1.2	1.8
Hearing impairments						
Some	12.8	6.1	3.8	17.9	8.3	4.2
Deaf or major	2.2	1.1	0.6	3.2	1.5	0.7
Lower extremity mobility difficulty						
Minor	7.2	3.4	2.4	8.6	2.9	4.0
Moderate	5.7	2.8	1.9	7.0	2.4	3.1
Major	7.8	3.8	1.7	13.8	2.8	4.4
Upper extremity mobility difficulty						
Some	6.7	3.2	2.0	9.3	2.4	3.8
Major	5.2	2.5	1.2	8.5	1.6	3.0
Difficulties using hands						
Some	5.3	2.5	1.5	7.4	1.9	3.0
Major	2.2	1.0	0.6	3.5	0.8	1.2
Any impairment[b]	39.5	18.9	13.4	46.4	18.3	19.3
Any major	14.1	6.7	3.8	21.4	5.8	7.4

Data source: 2001 Medical Expenditure Panel Survey.

[a]Figures by sex account for age category; figures by age account for sex.

[b]Any of the sensory or physical impairments identified in this table.

While 13.4 percent of persons age eighteen to sixty-four report any disability, 46.4 percent of persons age sixty-five and older note at least one impairment.

One further demographic issue demands emphasis. Disability frequently tracks with personal attributes, including minority race and ethnicity, low educational attainment, and poverty, that portend social disadvantage in the United States, even within the health care delivery system. Overall, because of very high rates of hearing problems among white men, white persons are more likely than individuals of black, Hispanic, or other races to report any sensory or physical disability (table 1.3).[6] Especially for the three physical disabilities, blacks report higher rates than whites, while relative rates for Hispanics vary.

Persons with physical or sensory disabilities are also much more likely than others to have never completed high school, to be currently unemployed, and to live in poverty (table 1.4). Only 45.4 percent of working-age individuals reporting any major disability work, compared with 78.7 per-

Table 1.3. Race and Ethnicity

	Race and Ethnicity (Percent[a])			
Impairment	White	Black	Hispanic	Other
Vision impairments	6.5	6.3	5.6	5.1
Hearing impairments	7.9	3.8	4.9	5.0
Lower extremity mobility difficulty	9.9	12.0	9.5	7.4
Upper extremity mobility difficulty	5.4	7.1	7.0	5.7
Difficulties using hands	3.3	5.2	4.1	4.6
Any impairment[b]	19.6	17.7	17.1	13.8
Any major impairment	6.6	7.7	7.3	5.8

Data source: 2001 Medical Expenditure Panel Survey.
[a]Figures account for age category and sex.
[b]Any of the impairments listed above.

cent of those without disabilities. Not surprisingly, persons with disabilities live in poverty much more often than do others: 22.7 percent of individuals with any major physical or sensory disability, compared with 8.9 percent of those without.

Despite these sobering statistics, many individuals with disabilities do not fit those sociodemographic stereotypes. For instance, high-profile celebrities have rolled in their wheelchairs before the public eye: the late Christopher Reeve, who once portrayed a comic book superhero, became a leading albeit controversial advocate of medical research; John Hockenberry, a broadcast journalist, reports from around the world; Stephen Hawking, an astrophysicist, spins theories of the universe; and Barbara Jordan, the late congresswoman from Texas, spoke with, as some said, the voice of God. In other words, persons with disabilities demonstrate the same wide range of core human abilities and achievements as do their counterparts without disabilities.

Questions about Health Care Quality

Widespread and growing alarm about the quality of health care provides the second impetus for this book. In its seminal report *Crossing the Quality Chasm,* the Institute of Medicine (Committee on Quality, 2001, p. 2) noted the irony of these worries:

At no time in the history of medicine has the growth in knowledge and technology been so profound. . . . Genomics and other new technologies on the horizon offer the promise of further increasing longevity, improving health and functioning, and alleviating pain

Table 1.4. Education, Employment, and Poverty-Level Household Income

	Percent[a]			
Impairment	Less Than High School	College Graduate	Currently Employed	Lives in Poverty
No impairment	17.4	26.9	78.7	8.9
Vision impairments				
Some	20.4	18.7	70.9	17.1
Blind or major	30.6	14.6	52.7	27.5
Hearing impairments				
Some	16.5	22.4	72.4	14.1
Deaf or major	23.2	17.8	79.0	19.2
Lower extremity mobility difficulty				
Minor	18.0	17.1	64.3	15.4
Moderate	28.4	10.3	39.7	27.6
Major	38.6	7.2	24.2	26.3
Upper extremity mobility difficulty				
Some	27.8	13.8	46.6	25.2
Major	36.9	7.4[b]	16.3	18.7
Difficulties using hands				
Some	31.0	8.5	35.7	24.3
Major	23.8	4.4	37.0	27.0
Any impairment	21.5	17.8	64.5	16.8
Any major impairment	29.6	11.7	45.4	22.7

Data source: 2001 Medical Expenditure Panel Survey.

[a]Figures account for age category and sex; "currently employed" considers only persons 18 to 64 years of age.

[b]Because of small number of respondents, this estimate may be unreliable.

and suffering. Advances in rehabilitation, cell restoration, and prosthetic devices hold potential for improving the health and functioning of many with disabilities. . . .

As medical science and technology have advanced at a rapid pace, however, the health care delivery system has floundered in its ability to provide consistently high-quality care to all Americans.

The role of health care varies across different disabilities. Certain fixed or constant conditions, such as congenital blindness or deafness, may not require explicit medical interventions. Instead, these conditions shape needs for communication and other accommodations in many aspects of daily life, including accessing health care. When, with aging, these individuals develop such chronic disorders as hypertension or diabetes, vision or hearing impairments could affect strategies for their management. In contrast, other disabling conditions require that persons themselves actively and continually manage basic bodily needs. For instance, persons with spinal cord injury or neurological conditions affecting bladder or bowel function must attend closely to these processes to avoid dangerous acute complications. In such situations, patients often know much more than their clinicians about how best to handle these basic concerns. Other sensory and physical disabilities arise from medical conditions that progress or change over time, sometimes influenced by clinical interventions and patients' own behaviors. For instance, diabetes, heart disease, and emphysema demand explicit medical treatments (e.g., medications), but each can also respond to patients' lifestyle (e.g., exercise, diet). In these various situations, collaboration between patients and clinicians—with a true patient-centered focus—offers the best opportunity for maximizing health and minimizing complications and functional declines.

Regardless of the specific disability, however, persons with sensory and physical impairments are particularly susceptible to substandard health care in the United States. Sources of quality shortfalls run the gamut, from absent or inadequate health insurance, to faulty communication between clinicians and patients, to inaccessible buildings and equipment. Persons with chronic medical conditions and disabilities often slip through the fault lines crisscrossing health care delivery systems, partly because these individuals can have extensive health-related needs and partly because delivery systems still focus primarily on acute short-term treatments. Even persons with common chronic conditions frequently do not receive routine, recommended health care services. One study found that Americans receive, on average, roughly half of recommended health care services: for example, only 57.3 percent of persons with osteoarthritis get recommended care, as do 45.4 percent and 22.8 percent of persons with diabetes and hip fractures, respectively (McGlynn et al., 2003, p. 2643).

Taking a public health perspective, *Healthy People 2010* (U.S. Department of Health and Human Services, 2000), which sets national health priorities, explicitly notes that persons with disabilities often get left behind. Misconceptions about people with disabilities contribute to troubling disparities in the services they receive, especially an "underemphasis on health promotion and disease prevention activities" (p. 6-3). Persons with substantial difficulty walking receive significantly fewer screening and preventive services, such as mammograms, Pap smears, and tobacco queries than do other individuals (Iezzoni et al., 2000a). Less than 1 percent of persons with arthritis receive public health interventions, such as community-based exercise programs, that could improve or maintain their physical functioning (Centers for Disease Control and Prevention, 2003d, p. 490). Thus, "as a potentially underserved group, people with disabilities would be expected to experience disadvantages in health and well-being compared with the general population" (U.S. Department of Health and Human Services, 2000, p. 6-5).

The Institute of Medicine asserts that only fundamental restructuring can rectify the myriad shortfalls of today's health care delivery system. Major changes should ensure that health care is

- Safe—avoids injuring patients
- Effective—based on scientific evidence of benefit
- Patient-centered—respectful of patients' preferences, needs, and values
- Timely—reduces waits and harmful delays
- Efficient—avoids waste of equipment, supplies, ideas, and energy
- Equitable—equal quality regardless of patients' personal characteristics (Institute of Medicine, Committee on Quality, 2001, pp. 41–42)

As noted throughout this book, each of these aims holds special resonance for persons with disabilities, especially patient centeredness. By definition, patient centeredness—respect for and responsiveness to individual patients' preferences, needs, and values—asserts the primacy of the views and perspectives of the patient. To create health care systems that can accommodate each individual patient's values and preferences requires anticipating the physical, sensory, cognitive, emotional, and spiritual needs of all persons, regardless of their abilities or disabilities. This inclusive mindset reflects an approach called "universal design," which strives to create systems, products, and environments that meet the needs of all potential users (see chapter 10). In other words, universal design strives to accommodate everyone.

In this book, we describe the experiences of adults with disabilities as they seek basic health care services (part II) and use universal design principles to suggest ways to overcome or circumvent identified barriers to good quality care (part III). Drawing upon Donabedian's triad, we focus on those processes and structures of care where practical and feasible improvements could ultimately enhance patients' outcomes, including quality of life and satisfaction with care. Many problems with obtaining high-quality or even adequate care pertain to all persons, such as limited health insurance coverage especially for prescription drugs, poorly coordinated services, and medical errors. However, as noted throughout this book, aspects of disabilities can magnify the consequences of problems endemic across the U.S. health care system.

Although individuals with sensory and physical impairments share important global concerns, specific practical needs and solutions do vary across disabling conditions as described in later chapters. For example, while Eleanor Peters cannot open the door to her clinic, a physically robust, walking person who happens to be deaf would breeze through. In contrast, while

Eleanor communicates effectively with her clinicians using spoken English, effective communication when the patient is deaf might require the services of a sign language interpreter.

Most persons with disabilities fall into one of two broad subgroups: persons who were either born with their condition or developed disability relatively early in life; and those who became progressively disabled in later years due to common chronic conditions, such as arthritis, diabetes, and cardiovascular disease, as well as aging-related vision and hearing losses. Persons within these two subgroups often express fundamentally different attitudes toward disability and its symbols. Eleanor Peters, for example, had polio when she was two years old. Now, more than four decades later, she happily uses her power wheelchair:

> I wouldn't trade my life for anything. I wouldn't trade having my disability. I love my chair. The only thing that gets me upset is sometimes when I can't get in and out of a door or there aren't curb cuts in the sidewalk or the lifts on the buses don't work—things that have to do with the system and the city. But I wouldn't trade my wheelchair in to anybody. This is my transportation. This is my feet.

Eleanor's attitudes contrast starkly with those of Tom Norton, a retired business executive in his early seventies who had developed motor neuron disease—a neurological condition that profoundly weakened his left lower leg and foot—thirty years ago. Tom spent years exercising, unsuccessfully "trying to beat it" and frustrating his wife, who accused Tom of being "in denial." Although he started falling frequently, Tom wouldn't consider using mobility aids, not even a cane. Tom worried that a cane would "interfere" with his image: "Company presidents don't use canes."

Although Eleanor Peters and Tom Norton could both benefit from an automatic door to the clinic, their approaches for confronting this barrier probably differ significantly. Eleanor Peters states her needs forthrightly, occasionally kicking the bottom of the door to attract the attention of clinic staff since she cannot extend her arms to knock. Tom Norton likely struggles silently to open the heavy door, eschewing any offer of help. The former decries this barrier to access, while the latter would never utter a critical word. Universal design principles, exemplified by an automatic door opener, consider the needs and perspectives of both Eleanor and Tom—as well as parents pushing strollers, persons carrying armloads of packages, and anyone else who cannot easily pull open a heavy plate glass door.

When addressing needs related to disability, boundaries inevitably blur between health care and other services necessary to maintain and enhance health. Casting a wide net, virtually all sectors within communities become relevant, including housing, employment, income maintenance, social services, transportation, public safety, education, and civil rights. We address some of these topics briefly: adequate transportation, for example, is crucial for obtaining health care services (see chapter 9). Virtually all sectors, including housing and community development, would benefit from adopting universal design principles in their future planning (see chapter 16).

We focus here, however, on health care as traditionally defined. This in itself is a tall order. "The purpose of the health care system must be to continuously reduce the impact and burden of illness, injury, and disability and to improve the health and functioning of the people of the United States" (President's Advisory Commission, 1998, p. 2). Ample evidence suggests that the health care system must do a better job for persons with disabilities.

Defining Disability

Kate Cather moved to town only a few months ago but is already well connected within the local Deaf community.[1] Now in her late twenties, Kate has always used American Sign Language (ASL): "I was born to a Deaf family— I'm third generation deaf. So I've been signing since day one. I grew up attending a Deaf school." Kate earned college and graduate degrees and works in the hearing world as a research assistant at a large university. She does not view herself as disabled, but she thinks that most clinicians do: "The medical community has a pathologic view of deaf people. There's a cultural view of Deaf people that these providers do not hold. They don't see us as a linguistic minority. I don't identify myself as a disabled person. There's a certain kind of pity on us as deaf people."

These attitudes and inadequate communication (see chapter 6) make Kate unwilling to seek health care services: "Thank God I'm healthy, and I don't need to go very much." Nevertheless, Kate needs routine screening and preventive care to maintain her excellent health. She does not have a primary care clinician.

Kate Cather's perceptions highlight the complexities of defining disability and introduce potential pitfalls for ensuring high-quality health care. The anatomic and acoustic acts of hearing are irrelevant to Kate. She has never heard, and since she does not use hearing aids, she does not need hearing-related health care services, like audiology evaluations. Within her family and the Deaf community, she communicates as naturally and fully in ASL as speakers of other languages do in their own native tongues. When visiting the hearing world as she daily must, Kate views herself as a linguistic minority, subject to the vicissitudes confronting other foreigners. She emphatically does not feel disabled. Any problems lie with a majority culture that fails to understand her.

Yet the first thing that many clinicians probably notice about Kate is her deafness. Federal law—the Americans with Disabilities Act (ADA)— requires clinicians not only to notice Kate's deafness but also to make explicit accommodations to ensure effective communication with her; for example, by hiring and paying for an ASL interpreter (see chapter 4). Thus, law requires clinicians to view Kate as disabled to ensure that she receives good care, although the ADA certainly does not ask them to pity Kate. In fact, the law's advocates held the diametrically opposite intent.

Thus, differences in underlying concepts of disability between clinicians and patients can fundamentally affect communication, relationships, and even perhaps the nature and quality of health care services that patients receive. As noted in chapter 1, many people with disabling conditions—certainly Kate Cather—have "normal" life expectancies or live for decades beyond the onset of their disability. Although disability can arise from disease or anatomical, physiological, or other organic processes that deviate from "norms,"

disability ≠ sickness

Persons with disabilities do not necessarily feel ill or need acute medical attention to preserve their lives. Furthermore, they may not view their conditions in terms of illness even if they clearly have a diagnosed disease. As one woman with multiple sclerosis told me, "I'm not sick. I just can't stand up."

Although individual circumstances vary widely, many people with disabling conditions want clinicians to see them as "whole" persons, interested in maximizing their physical, mental, emotional, and reproductive health and wellness. Specific clinical interventions and health promotion strategies do differ depending on a person's underlying medical conditions and functional impairments. Health care for persons with disabilities should reflect each individual's preferences and values—patient-centered care, just as for other persons.

As suggested earlier, however, society, professions, governments, and laws also weigh in, identifying individuals as disabled for specific purposes (e.g., civil rights protections, income support). Scholars have spent decades trying to define disability and the disablement process—the interrelated chain of events and personal or environmental circumstances that produce disability (Albrecht, Seelman, and Bury, 2001; Institute of Medicine, Committee to Review, 2002). Dozens of formal definitions of disability exist, embedded within federal and state laws and regulations. Many appoint clinicians, primarily physicians, as arbiters, to determine whether individuals meet some established criterion for disability and thus deserve a benefit like income support, health insurance, or accessibility ("handicapped") license plates or parking placards. Thus, an uneasy dance ensues, where opinions and perceptions of clinicians and patients can diverge.

This chapter introduces different definitions of disability, setting the stage for our later observations. The contradictions raised by defining disability have long historical roots, with varying models holding sway during different eras. These definitional threads ultimately lead down two major paths—medical and social—each carrying important but distinct implications. When considering health care access and quality, we ultimately link these two definitions.

Historical Roots of Disability Definitions

Reaching back millennia, societal views of disabilities juxtaposed perceptions of meritorious needs against concerns about moral worthiness. Ancient hunter-gatherer societies recognized that some members could neither hunt nor gather nor tend fields and therefore needed help simply to survive. Yet, from early on, questions about moral worth and culpability arose. In the Old Testament, Leviticus (21:16) listed "blemishes" that precluded persons from "drawing near" religious ceremonies: "a man blind or lame, or one who has a mutilated face or a limb too long, or a man who has an injured foot or an injured hand, or a hunchback, or a dwarf. . . ." Throughout the Middle Ages, clergy admonished parishioners that infirmities represented visitations from a judgmental God.

As societies developed, practical secular concerns pressed, with communities striving to identify individuals meriting assistance. New social orders depended on persons working to support themselves and their families while contributing to communal coffers, including funds to assist needy people. Officials dispensing charity easily identified and verified certain worthy persons, such as widows, elderly people, and orphans. But determining meritorious persons with disabilities posed a problem. For centuries, societal leaders had assumed a lazy citizenry, anxious to avoid work by exaggerating debilities.[2] According to political scientist Deborah Stone, disability

> has always been more problematic, both because no single condition of "disability" is universally recognized, and because physical and mental incapacity are conditions that can be feigned for secondary gain. Hence, the concept of disability has always been based on perceived need to detect deception. . . . Therefore, the validating device must rely on information that cannot be manipulated by the individual claimants. (1984, p. 23)

Starting in the early nineteenth century, physicians with newly invented diagnostic tools entered as "objective" validators of disability. The 1819 invention of the stethoscope by French physician René Laënnec, who claimed his instrument freed physicians from patients' reports inevitably tainted by prejudice or ignorance, offered the initial breakthrough. Other technologies soon followed, including the microscope, radiograph, spirometer, and ophthalmoscope. With each invention, "the proponents of the new technology emphasized its ability to free the physician from the information and judgments of the patients. . . . They were also quick to advertise the usefulness of the new technologies for disability certification" (Stone, 1984, p. 105). In 1862, for example, advocates urged ophthalmoscopic examinations to detect feigned nearsightedness among potential shirkers of military service.

As new diagnostic tools emerged, along with dawning appreciation of biological causes of diseases, society began fundamentally rethinking the nature of disability. Beliefs shifted from supernatural to biological explanations (Linton, 1998; Byrom, 2001). This thinking led logically to medical and other professional involvement, such as state schools and asylums for persons who were blind, deaf, or mentally retarded. Proponents believed that institutionalization offered progressive, humanitarian custody grounded in science. Nevertheless, "modernist ideals mean the society would not tolerate being bogged down by those who can't keep up, who are thought to drain resources, or who remind us in any way of the limitations of our scientific capabilities" (Linton, 1998, p. 46). Institutionalization solved that problem by hiding people away.

Many institutions persisted well into twentieth-century America, sometimes polarizing concerned constituencies. Residential schools for deaf children, for example, generated vigorous debates between two opposing factions: persons who supported sign language communication and employed Deaf teachers, and those advocating "oralism" or the "auditory-verbal approach" by banning sign language, requiring that deaf students learn to speak and read lips, and hiring only hearing teachers (Burch, 2001). Many members of the Deaf community fought oralism, viewing residential schools as the cradle of Deaf culture. In the 1920s, the invention of the audiometer, which measures hearing, helped clarify how speaking ability relates to the timing and extent of deafness.[3] Although these apparently objective findings bolstered the Deaf community's arguments, the oralists refused to cede. Detailing this and other fascinating disability histories is beyond our scope here (informative sources include Groce, 1985; Gallagher, 1994, 1998; Shapiro, 1994; Byrom, 2001; Fleischer and Zames, 2001; Longmore and Umansky, 2001). Suffice it to say that medical approaches reached beyond "validating" disability into other critical aspects of community life, including education, housing, and employment.

A medical model of disability thus became firmly entrenched. "The *medical model* views disability as a problem of the person, directly caused by disease, trauma or other health condition, which requires medical care. . . . Management of the disability is aimed at cure or the individual's adjustment and behaviour change. Medical care is viewed as the main issue . . ." (World Health Organization [WHO], 2001, p. 20). The medical model builds on two assumptions: that individual persons should strive, largely alone, to overcome disabilities; and that clinicians know what is best for their patients.

The aftermaths of World Wars I and II introduced yet another dimension to the disability discourse—rehabilitation. Massive influxes of otherwise fit young men, injured in their prime through service to their country, catapulted widespread efforts to restore functional abilities. Here, organized medicine initially trailed behind occupational and physical therapy, which pursued training in daily living and vocational skills.[4] Goals of rehabilitation professionals went beyond treating physical impairments to comprehensive restoration of mental, emotional, vocational, and social abilities (Institute of Medicine, Committee on Assessing, 1997, p. 31). Even makers of prosthetic limbs emphasized restoring the "whole person" and considering patients' personalities and the "attitudes of the general public, and particularly of close friends, toward visible injury and toward the prosthesis" (Klopsteg and Wilson, 1954, p. 153). In 1954, Detley W. Bronk, president of the National Academy of Sciences, lauded rehabilitation specialists for healing "psychological trauma, which is no less grievous than the bodily loss itself. . . . This furtherance of spiritual well-being is the greatest contribution" (Klopsteg and Wilson, 1954, p. vi). Many rehabilitation professionals nevertheless retained standard medical perspectives, assuming they knew what was best for their patients.

Despite general support of veterans with debilitating war injuries, stigmatization of other persons with disabilities persisted into the mid-twentieth century. The late sociologist Erving Goffman (1963, p. 19) termed stigma the "spoiled social identity"—being "discredited . . . facing an unaccepting world" because one is, for instance, blind, "crippled," "multiple sclerotic," or hard of hearing.[5] A "good adjustment," according to Goffman (1963, p. 121), requires that "the stigmatized individual cheerfully and unselfconsciously accept himself as essentially the same as normals, while at the same time he voluntarily withholds himself from those situations in which normals would find it difficult to give lip service to their similar acceptance of him."[6] The experiences of the late Hugh Gregory Gallagher, who contracted polio in 1952 at age twenty, exemplify the potentially toxic consequences of Goffman's observation. For twenty years, Gallagher soared in the world of "normals," attracting numerous professional accolades, assuring those who asked that he never thought about his paralyzed body. Yet, as Gallagher (1998, p. 157) wrote in the third person:

> The price he paid to live in the world of the fit was to keep his burdens and his bitterness to himself. He tried—whether with friends, employees, or strangers—to be cheerful, healthy, interested, and never dependent or vulnerable. This makeup he assumed, like the movie star, but time was eating away at it.

Gallagher's ultimate price was deep and desperate depression. He eventually emerged to speak eloquently about disability, dying in 2004 at age seventy-one.

A revolution began in the 1970s for Gallagher and many others that turned notions of disability upside down and swept away exhortations to cheerfully and wordlessly fit in. Instead, the new thinking held that "problems lie not within the persons with disabilities but in the environment that fails to accommodate persons with disabilities and in the negative attitude of people without disabilities" (Olkin, 1999, p. 26). Disability is "imposed on top of our impairments by the way we are unnecessarily isolated and excluded from full participation in society" (Oliver, 1996, p. 22).

This revolution traces back through multiple wellsprings that ultimately became a powerful, albeit sometimes untidy, force. Early hints of the impending shift include the productive labors of newly employed persons with disabilities, alongside women, on the home front while able-bodied men fought in World War II (Linton, 1998). Employees with disabilities, like women, nonetheless faced layoffs when the soldiers returned. For World War II veterans with disabilities, a grateful nation made accommodations to allow them to obtain college educations and work (Fleischer and Zames, 2001). In some instances, these precedents offered others with disabilities similar access.

Over the next two decades, additional forces joined to motivate broad societal changes, including the independent living movement, the rise of consumerism, a growing interest in self-help rather than professional interventions, large-scale deinstitutionalization of persons with disabilities, and nationwide campaigns for civil rights and equal opportunity for racial minorities and women. On the disability front, arguments coalesced around a "social" model:

> The *social model* . . . sees the issue mainly as a socially created problem, and basically as a matter of the full integration of individuals into society. Disability is not an attribute of an individual, but rather a complex collection of conditions, many of which are created by the social environment. . . . The issue is therefore an attitudinal or ideological one requiring social change, which at the political level becomes a question of human rights. (WHO, 2001, p. 20)

Other authors have chronicled in detail the compelling history of the disability rights movement (including West, 1991; Shapiro, 1994; Pelka, 1997; Young, 1997; Francis and Silvers, 2000; Fleischer and Zames, 2001; Longmore and Umansky, 2001). The outcome is obvious today. Persons with disabilities now participate actively at all levels—throughout communities, businesses, governments, and cultural and educational institutions. Although much remains to be done, enormous strides have been made.

Nonetheless, a definitional divide persists. Champions of the medical and social models often seem at loggerheads, erecting a "sterile and rather contrived distinction" between the two viewpoints (Williams, 2001, p. 125). Other disability scholars, advocates, researchers, and clinicians increasingly concede the value of both perspectives, albeit with more nuanced language. Over two decades, WHO efforts to categorize and classify disabilities typify these shifts. In its 1980 nomenclature, the *International Classification of Impairments, Disabilities, and Handicaps* (ICIDH), WHO (p. 28) asserted, "In the context of health experience, a disability is any restriction or lack (resulting from an impairment) of ability to perform an activity in the manner or within the range considered normal for a human being." This language locates disability firmly within individual persons, alongside the parallel concept of "handicap": "a disadvantage for a given individual, resulting from an impairment or disability, that limits or prevents the fulfillment of a role that is normal" (WHO, 1980, p. 29).

Throughout the 1990s, definitional complexities dogged WHO efforts to revise ICIDH. One revision dropped the word "disability" altogether, noting it caused "misunderstanding between health care professionals and people who experience disablement" (WHO, 1997, p. 24). The final version, the *International Classification of Functioning, Disability and Health* (ICF), which was unanimously approved in May 2001 by 190 member countries, integrates the medical and social models, creating a "biopsychosocial" approach that "attempts to achieve a synthesis, in order to provide a coherent view of different perspectives of health, from a biological, individual and social perspective" (WHO, 2001, p. 20).

To organize its classification, the ICF identifies three interrelated concepts: (a) impairments, or significant deviations or losses involving body functions or structures; (b) activities, the execution of tasks or actions by an individual; and (c) participation, individuals' involvement in life situations (WHO, 2001, p. 10).[7] Taking a global view, ICF then defines disability as an "umbrella term for impairments, activity limitations or participation restrictions" (p. 3), conceiving "a person's functioning and disability . . . as a dynamic interaction between health conditions (diseases, disorders, injuries, traumas, etc.) and contextual factors" (p. 8), including environmental and personal attributes. Introducing environmental factors that "interact with all the components of functioning and disability" represents a signal contribution of the ICF, clearly recognizing the role of external forces in precipitating or mitigating disability: "The basic construct of the Environmental Factors component is the facilitating or hindering impact of features of the physical, social, and attitudinal world" (p. 8). Ultimately, the ICF aims to shift the disability paradigm to universality, encompassing everyone.

> Heretofore, disability has been construed as an all or none phenomenon: a distinct category to which an individual either belonged or not. The ICF, on the other hand, presents disability as a continuum, relevant to the lives of all people to different degrees and at different times in their lives. Disability is not something that happens only to a minority of humanity, it is a common (indeed natural) feature of the human condition. . . . Over the lifespan, [disability is] a universal phenomena. (Üstün et al., 2003, p. 82)

Practical Realities and Determining Disability

Despite centuries spent trying to define disability, complexities persist. Semantic distinctions among definitions remain elusive, especially across clinical, social science, political, and legal disciplines. "It is often difficult to communicate conceptual constructs within the same discipline, let alone across . . . professional fields, which may account for some of the misinterpretations that have been plaguing this area" (Institute of Medicine, Committee on a National Agenda, 1991, p. 321). Some view shifting definitions, like the ICF's conceptual leap, as of scholarly significance only. "While each of these models suggests a theoretical definition of disability, none offers a detailed operational definition. . . . Once the definitions are applied under real-world conditions, they necessarily operate under constraints of one sort or another" (Institute of Medicine, Committee to Review, 2002, p. 54).

Practical realities thus remain. As in hunter-gatherer societies from earlier times, someone still needs to decide whether an individual qualifies for assistance or some other public benefit because of disability. Today in the United States, that someone is typically a physician.

Health care financing and much of the delivery system remain firmly rooted in classic medical thinking about disability. This means that items and services that might address environmental barriers—like power wheelchairs to allow persons who cannot walk to move easily around their communities—often fall outside the boundaries of insurance coverage (see chapter 9). The origins of many structural impediments to meeting the needs of persons with disabilities arise directly from continued exclusive focus on traditional medical precepts.

Governmental agencies and legal precedents retain many distinct definitions of disabilities. Two hold special relevance for Americans: that used by Social Security, which focuses on work disability to determine eligibility for Medicare and Medicaid coverage for millions of individuals; and evolving interpretations of the ADA's disability definition, which identifies persons meriting accommodations by public and private entities, including health care professionals and institutions. Social Security relies exclusively on medical definitions, while the ADA aims—at least in principle—to cast a broader net.

Social Security Disability Determinations

The Social Security Act authorizes two programs providing cash benefits and health insurance eligibility to persons with disabilities: Social Security Disability Insurance (SSDI) under Title II, and Supplemental Security Income (SSI) under Title XVI. SSDI gives benefits to persons who are "insured" by virtue of having worked and contributed to the Social Security trust fund

---

Box 2.1.   Social Security Administration (SSA) Disability Definitions

---

Definition of Disability

"For all individuals applying for disability benefits under Title II, and for adults applying under Title XVI, the definition of disability is the same. The law defines disability as the inability to engage in any substantial gainful activity by reason of any medically determinable physical or mental impairment(s) which can be expected to result in death or which has lasted or can be expected to last for a continuous period of not less than 12 months." (SSA, 2003, p. 4)

Medically Determinable Impairment

"An impairment that results from anatomical, physiological, or psychological abnormalities which can be shown by medically acceptable clinical and laboratory diagnostic techniques. A physical or mental impairment must be established by medical evidence consisting of signs, symptoms, and laboratory findings—not only by the individual's statement of symptoms." (SSA, 2003, p. 4)

---

through withholdings on their earnings. SSDI also covers certain disabled dependents of insured persons. The 1972 Social Security Act amendments granted eligibility for Medicare to people who have received SSDI cash benefits for two years.[8] Title XVI provides SSI payments to persons, including children, who are disabled, blind, or elderly and have passed a means test documenting limited income and resources. Persons qualifying for SSI immediately receive Medicaid coverage, and some states supplement the federal income benefit with additional cash payments. Poor persons receiving SSDI can also obtain SSI benefits after passing the means test.

The United States was the last major industrial nation to enact social insurance (Stone, 1984). While the Social Security Act of 1935 covered elderly people, federal disability insurance arrived more than two decades later, with various provisions coming in spurts.[9] Anxious to prevent abuses, Congress structured Social Security as the "last resort" for people who absolutely could not work because of long-term impairments.

SSDI and SSI use identical definitions of disability for adult participants (box 2.1). To qualify, working-age persons must meet a yes/no standard: either they can or cannot engage in "substantial gainful activity" because of medically proven physical or mental impairments.[10] The Social Security Administration (SSA) contracts with each state's Disability Determination

Service (DDS) to assess applicants. Briefly, the disability claims process involves four steps: (a) initial applications and preliminary screening at SSA district offices; (b) disability determinations by state DDSs using federal regulations and SSA guidelines and procedures; (c) reviews by state DDSs of applicants denied disability eligibility at Step B; and (d) reviews by SSA administrative law judges for applicants denied at Step C who submit appeals (Institute of Medicine, Committee to Review, 2002, p. 21).

As codified by 1968 regulations, the SSA requires state DDSs to start with its Listings of Impairments (the so-called "List," SSA, 2003) to determine disability. The List itemizes impairments, grouped by body system, that should be sufficiently severe to preclude substantial gainful employment among adults (or to indicate disability among children).[11] The List stipulates specific tests (e.g., audiometers, radiographs) and physical examination findings required to validate each condition. For instance, the List includes impaired central visual acuity (corrected vision in the better eye of 20/200 or less); hearing impairment (meeting specified decibel levels) not restorable by a hearing aid; and multiple sclerosis, with "significant and persistent disorganization of motor function" or "significant, reproducible fatigue of motor function with substantial muscle weakness" (SSA, 2003, pp. 25, 26, 63). If people do not qualify based on the List, they receive in-depth evaluations of their functional abilities.[12]

The Social Security disability determination process deserves several comments. First, Kate Cather, Bonnie, and I would likely qualify as disabled by List standards. Nonetheless, all three of us are substantially gainfully employed. We have made the necessary accommodations, as have our employers. Bonnie could not work without her screen reader, which converts texts on her computer screen to audible information, and I could not work without my motorized scooter and the flexibility to work some days at home. Bonnie and I, however, qualify as "privileged." We hold doctoral degrees and have good financial resources and social supports. We have the knowledge and wherewithal to identify and obtain necessary assistive technologies and workplace accommodations. Many people with sensory and physical impairments do not have these advantages (see chapter 3), and neither Social Security nor other governmental programs consistently and systematically pays for job accommodations or work-related assistive devices.[13]

The second point relates to the SSA's explicit preference that an individual's own physician, the so-called "treating source," perform disability evaluations. According to the SSA (2003, p. 10), these physicians are "likely to be the medical professionals most able to provide a detailed longitudinal picture of the claimant's impairments and may bring a unique perspective to the medical evidence that cannot be obtained from the medical findings alone or from reports of individual examinations or brief hospitalizations." This role, however, makes some "treating sources" nervous, especially if they believe—as does happen—that their patients could still work.

"People come to us with a form," Johnny Baker, a primary care physician, told me. "Doctors hate that—most doctors do—because they're confused about their role. Usually the doctor is the advocate for the patient, and the doctor counts on patients to be open and honest. With these disability forms, all of a sudden, you're not the patient's doctor. You're the doctor for Social Security. Patients want the form filled out a certain way and might not give the exact same history as they would otherwise. So the rug is pulled out from under the usual doctor-patient interaction."

Outright confrontations can erupt when doctors believe patients are bilking the system. Dr. Doris Weiner, another primary care physician, called to ask my opinion about a patient. "She's in her late forties," said Dr. Weiner, "and the first thing I noticed was her anger. She's angry about her hypertension, her diabetes, and now she has this problem with her left leg. It's something neurological that I don't really understand. She still walks without a cane, but now she wants to stop working, get Social Security disability." Dr. Weiner didn't think that the patient's current impairments warranted SSDI, and she wanted her to continue working. In the end, though, Dr. Weiner admitted she'd called me primarily to vent her frustrations. To maintain her relationship with the patient, Dr. Weiner realized she couldn't contest the patient's decision.

This scenario with Dr. Weiner's patient underscores the third point to be made about Social Security disability determinations: despite the apparent objectivity of the List and extensive regulations and procedures, disability determinations often remain subjective and highly variable. With a nonspecific disorder of her left leg, Dr. Weiner's patient may not qualify for SSDI, although the patient has sought advice from an advocate to strategize about ways to maximize her chances. For many reasons (including labor market and demographic trends, regulatory changes, court decisions, and cost shifting by states), rates of Social Security disability applications and the percentage of applicants who qualify fluctuate, sometimes widely, over time. In 1960, 49.6 percent of applicants obtained awards; the percentage fell to 31.4 percent in 1980 but rose to 46.7 percent in 2000 (Institute of Medicine, Committee to Review, 2002, p. 36). Underlying medical conditions leading to disability eligibility have also changed. Between 1981 and 2000, the percentage of SSDI awards based on circulatory conditions (the top ranked condition in 1981) declined by 52 percent, as musculoskeletal conditions increased by 41 percent, becoming the largest single cause of disability eligibility (Institute of Medicine, Committee to Review, 2002, p. 46).

Finally, although perceptions of what constitutes disability have changed dramatically in the past forty years, basic SSA disability determinations have altered little. With its explicitly medical model, the SSA still locates work disability squarely within individuals and their physical, sensory, cognitive, and mental abilities, without considering the implications of their work environments or potential accommodations, like assistive technology. During the mid-1990s, the SSA briefly considered fundamentally redesigning the disability determination process to introduce new concepts about disability and work (Institute of Medicine, Committee to Review, 2002). The complexities of doing so proved overwhelming, so in 1999, the SSA decided to focus instead on updating the List and streamlining review procedures. Thus, as enshrined in statute, Social Security will continue to dispense disability benefits based primarily on applicants' physical, sensory, cognitive, and mental diseases and disorders.

Americans with Disabilities Act

According to its opening statement, the Americans with Disabilities Act (ADA, P.L. 101-336) aims "to provide a clear and comprehensive national mandate for the elimination of discrimination against individuals with disabilities." Title I of the ADA charges the Equal Employment Opportunity Commission, established initially with the Civil Rights Act of 1964, with ensuring that employers do not discriminate because of disability against otherwise qualified individuals "in regard to job application procedures, the hiring, advancement, or discharge of employees, employee compensation, job training, and other terms, conditions, and privileges of employment" [Sec. 102(a)].[14] Discrimination includes "not making reasonable accommodations to the known physical or mental limitations" [Sec. 102(b)(5)(A)]). Title II prohibits discrimination or denial of services provided by public entities, while Title III prohibits discrimination involving public accommodations and services operated by private entities, including the "professional office of a health care provider, hospital, or other service establishment" [Sec. 301(7)(F)]. Box 2.2 shows how Title III defines "discrimination."

When President George H. W. Bush signed the ADA on July 26, 1990, people with disabilities assumed the right, in Bush's words, to "pass through once-closed doors into a bright new era of equality, independence and freedom" (Young, 1997, p. 231). Unlike the civil rights movements for racial minorities and women, the disability rights movement "had never filled the streets with tens of thousands of protestors" but was instead "largely invisible, almost underground" (Shapiro, 1994, p. 117). Strong opposition from powerful business interests and fractious arguments among diverse disability constituencies nearly derailed the legislation. Ultimately, however, sheer numbers ensured the ADA's passage. Most people—presidents, members of Congress, government officials, private citizens—either have a disability or know someone who does. The cause seemed universal.

The universality of the ADA derives largely from the law's expansive definition of disability (box 2.3). With its three-pronged approach and language, the ADA's disability definition "is amenable to an infinite array of interpretations" (Illingworth and Parmet, 2000, p. 3). Importantly, however, un-

---

Box 2.2.   Definition of Discrimination: Americans with
Disabilities Act Title III, Sec. 302(b)(2)(A)

Discrimination includes:

(i) The imposition or application of eligibility criteria that screen out
or tend to screen out an individual with a disability . . . from fully
and equally enjoying any goods, services, facilities, privileges, advantages, or accommodations, unless such criteria can be shown to
be necessary for the provision of these [items];

(ii) A failure to make reasonable modifications in policies, practices, or
procedures, when such modifications are necessary to afford such
goods, services, facilities, . . . or accommodations to individuals
with disabilities, unless the entity can demonstrate that making
such modifications would fundamentally alter the nature of such
[items];

(iii) A failure to take such steps as may be necessary to ensure that no
individual with a disability is excluded, denied services, segregated or otherwise treated differently than other individuals because of the absence of auxiliary aids and services, unless the entity can demonstrate that taking such steps would fundamentally
alter the nature of the [items] being offered or would result in an
undue burden;

(iv) A failure to remove architectural barriers, and communication
barriers that are structural in nature, in existing facilities . . .
where such removal is readily achievable; and

(v) Where an entity can demonstrate that the removal of a barrier under clause (iv) is not readily achievable, a failure to make such
goods, services, facilities, . . . accommodations available through
alternative methods if such methods are readily achievable.

---

like Title VII of the Civil Rights Act of 1964, "the ADA generally prohibits
discrimination only against 'an individual with a disability,' rather than anyone who is discriminated against on the basis of disability. The statute thus
usually requires that an individual who brings a claim show that he or she
falls within the protected class" (Illingworth and Parmet, 2000, p. 3). Liti-
gants therefore must first prove, sometimes to a skeptical judiciary, that they
are disabled before they can broach questions about discrimination.

The ADA's definition of disability parallels, almost word for word, the
definition contained in amendments to the Rehabilitation Act of 1973. Since
1918, prompted initially by waves of wounded veterans and youthful sur-

ADA Congressional Findings

Sec. 2(7) "Individuals with disabilities are a discrete and insular minority who have been faced with restrictions and limitations, subjected to a history of purposeful unequal treatment, and relegated to a position of political powerlessness in our society, based on characteristics that are beyond the control of such individuals and resulting from stereotypic assumptions not truly indicative of the individual ability of such individuals to participate in, and contribute to, society; . . ."

ADA Definitions

Sec. 3(2) "The term 'disability' means, with respect to an individual—(A) a physical or mental impairment that substantially limits one or more of the major life activities of such individual; (B) a record of such an impairment; or (C) being regarded as having such an impairment."

Sec. 101(8) "The term 'qualified individual with a disability' means an individual with a disability who, with or without reasonable accommodation, can perform the essential functions of the employment position . . ."

Definitions in ADA Regulations: 28 CFR Part 36, Sec. 36.104

"It is not possible to include a list of all the specific conditions . . . that would constitute physical or mental impairments. . . . However, [examples include]: Orthopedic, visual, speech and hearing impairments; cerebral palsy; epilepsy, muscular dystrophy, multiple sclerosis, cancer, heart disease, diabetes, mental retardation, emotional illness, specific learning disabilities, HIV [human immunodeficiency virus] disease (symptomatic or asymptomatic), tuberculosis, drug addiction, and alcoholism."

"Major life activities include such things as caring for one's self, performing manual tasks, walking, seeing, hearing, speaking, breathing, learning, and working."

To be substantially limited, an individual's important life activities must be "restricted as to the conditions, manner, or duration under which they can be performed in comparison to most people."

vivors of industrial accidents, Congress had passed various laws establishing federally funded vocational rehabilitation and jobs training programs. Following these precedents, the 1973 law guaranteed federal support for vocational rehabilitation of "handicapped persons." But with little debate or appreciation of the far-reaching consequences, amendments to the act added antidiscrimination provisions. Specifically, Section 504 prohibited all entities receiving federal funds from discriminating against "otherwise qualified" persons " 'solely by reason of . . . handicap'. . . . The wording clearly was copied straight out of the Civil Rights Act of 1964, which ruled out discrimination in federal programs on the basis of race, color, or national origin" (Shapiro, 1994, p. 65).

Section 504 thus took a huge leap from the primary intent of prior rehabilitation legislation. Previous laws had created programs specifically for persons who could not work without vocational rehabilitation. Section 504 gave a new broad "right" to all "handicapped persons," regardless of whether they sought or could benefit from vocational training. "The original entitlement statute required a definition of disability that was narrow and applied only to those who otherwise could not work. The new antidiscrimination provision which was aimed at ensuring the right to work and study for those who could not work and study required a far broader, less exceptional definition of disability" (Illingworth and Parmet, 2000, p. 12). Recognizing the need to expand the definition, Congress amended the Rehabilitation Act in 1974, providing the new three-pronged definition: "Handicapped persons means any person who (i) has a physical or mental impairment which substantially limits one or more major life activities, (ii) has a record of such an impairment, or (iii) is regarded as having such an impairment."

Delays in promulgating Section 504 regulations proved the crucible of the disability rights movement. As successive administrations, under Presidents Ford and Carter, postponed issuing Section 504 regulations because of worries about potentially high costs, disability rights activists girded for a fight. Sit-ins and vocal public demonstrations eventually compelled governmental action (Shapiro, 1994; Fleischer and Zames, 2001). However, neither the activists nor federal officials paid much attention to the definition of disability.

Over the years, specific wording did evolve. Section 103(d) of the Rehabilitation Act Amendments of 1986 changed "handicapped persons" to "individuals with handicaps," using the plural "handicaps" but nonetheless explicitly including persons with "only one handicap" (U.S. Department of Health and Human Services, 1988). The updated regulations adopted the "person first" language—"individuals with handicaps" rather than "handicapped individuals"—preferred by many disability rights advocates.

Section 504's definition also introduced the notion of "major life activities," defined somewhat cryptically as "caring for one's self, performing manual tasks, walking, seeing, hearing, speaking, breathing, learning, and working." Obviously, these actions carry vastly different implications. For example, "breathing" is highly specific, inherently physiological, and easily quantified, whereas "working" could mean almost anything. In its regulations, Section 504 identified specific conditions that qualify as physical or mental impairments, thus reverting to an explicitly medical approach.

However, Section 504's disability definition generated little confusion or discussion. "For the most part, courts construing the Rehabilitation Act simply assumed that individuals who claimed to have a handicap within the meaning of the statute did indeed have one" (Illingworth and Parmet, 2000, p. 12). Lawsuits focused instead on "what disability advocates have referred to as the comparatively 'easy' issues—for example, architectural and transportation accessibility" (Fleischer and Zames, 2001, p. 94). Many cases targeted inaccessible buildings and public transportation systems.

Litigation under Section 504 helped refine the law's pioneering concept of "reasonable accommodations"—the notion that the actions required to provide access to persons with disabilities should not generate prohibitive expense or extraordinarily demanding effort. As a bottom line, courts at all levels found that disabilities and potential accommodations are too diverse to yield a single standard for reasonableness across all settings. Individual solutions are necessary: a practical framework adopted by the ADA. Questions about *reasonable* accommodations within health care delivery settings wend throughout this book.

With implementation of the ADA, questions about defining disability immediately leapt to the fore, especially around employment discrimination.[15] By encompassing both private and public sectors, the ADA generated much more heat and complicated emotions than did Section 504 (Francis and Silvers, 2000; Fleischer and Zames, 2001). Anti-ADA sentiments arose quickly. Unlike other civil rights legislation, the ADA requires businesses to make accommodations, which businesses assume cost substantial dollars, for persons with disabilities. Some accommodations cost nothing, as when the Supreme Court compelled the Professional Golfers Association to allow Casey Martin, who has painful swelling of his right leg, to ride a cart while competing in golf tournaments.[16] Over 70 percent of workplace accommodations cost less than $500 (Olkin, 1999, p. 147).

A flurry of ADA lawsuits aimed straight at the heart of defining disability:[17]

> The definition of disability that previously had presented a relatively low hurdle for plaintiffs began to appear insurmountable. Case after case began to question whether an individual who brought a claim under the ADA was "truly disabled." More often than not, plaintiffs who were found to meet the statutory definition were also found to be too limited to be qualified to work. (Illingworth and Parmet, 2000, p. 12)

Two Supreme Court decisions in 1999 demonstrate instances where the Court clearly struggled with defining disability. In *Sutton et al. v. United Air Lines, Inc.*, twin sisters with uncorrected vision of 20/200 who see normally with glasses sued the airlines for refusing to hire them as commercial pilots. In *Murphy v. United Parcel Service, Inc.*, a mechanic with hypertension controlled by medication sued after being fired from his job. During oral arguments on April 28, 1999, Justice Stephen G. Breyer worried openly about the consequences of finding the twin sisters in *Sutton* "disabled," wondering, "Is it then necessary to say that everyone who uses false teeth or glasses is disabled, or is there a way of drawing a line?" (Greenhouse, 1999). The sisters and the mechanic both lost their cases by votes of seven to two.

More troubling for many disability rights advocates was the *Toyota Motor Manufacturing Inc. v. Williams* decision on January 8, 2002. A unanimous Supreme Court ruled against Ella Williams, who claimed that her carpal tunnel syndrome prevented her from performing her job at a Toyota manufacturing plant. The justices decided that Williams was not "disabled" because she could still perform routine tasks at home, such as brushing her teeth and gardening—in other words, that her condition did not limit "major life activities." This ruling seemingly views employment-related tasks as outside "major life activities," the standard used by the ADA to identify disability.

Definitions of disability under the ADA will likely evolve further as courts adjudicate individual cases. However, fallout from prior rulings continues to percolate. The *Sutton* and *Murphy* cases gave employers the right to determine when potential employees qualify for jobs. Furthermore:

> Although it may seem a simple and unsurprising result that people with myopia are not entitled to claim "disability," the Court's reasoning has profound implications for many people who face persistent discrimination and whom Congress meant to protect. The ruling that the term "disability" in the ADA is determined by examining the individual claiming discrimination in their "corrected" state, even if the employer's reason for not hiring or firing was the underlying uncorrected condition, leads to the perverse result that a person with a disability who avails him- or herself of the benefits of technological and medical advances thereby risks losing protection from job discrimination. . . .
>
> The crabbed interpretation delivered by the Supreme Court puts a rejected applicant with a disability in the untenable position of emphasizing all the things he or she cannot do in order to claim ADA protection, and then, once through the courthouse door, downplaying limitations in order to prove he or she is qualified for the job. . . . By attempting to limit the ADA to the "truly disabled," the Supreme Court continues to look at disability as a matter for pity rather than equality. In essence, the Supreme Court condones exactly the behav-

ior Congress sought to eradicate. (Mayerson and Diller, 2000, pp. 124–125)

With other ADA cases pending, debates over legal definitions of disability—and their implications—are far from over.

How We Define Disability

As noted in chapter 1, we focus here on improving health care quality for adults with sensory and physical impairments—potentially disabling conditions. By targeting sensory and physical conditions, we connect with the ICF's categorization of impairments, which falls under the ICF's linguistic "umbrella" defining disability (WHO, 2001, p. 3).[18] Our interest extends from persons born with these conditions to those who develop impairments over time, with aging or progressive chronic disease. Thus, we embrace the ICF's concept of universality: that disability "is a common (indeed natural) feature of the human condition. . . . Over the lifespan, [disability is] a universal phenomena" (Üstün et al., 2003, p. 82).

We must underscore two points. First, we make no presumptions that individuals with sensory or physical impairments are, in fact, disabled, how-

Table 2.1. Perceptions of Disability

Impairment	Perceived as Disabled by (Percent)[a]	
	Self	Others
Blind or major difficulty with vision	42.3	40.7
Deaf or major difficulty with hearing	27.4	24.8
Major difficulty with lower extremity mobility	71.6	65.9
Uses mobility aid:		
Cane or crutches	59.9	54.2
Walker	68.4	65.4
Manual wheelchair	79.9	79.3
Power wheelchair	84.5	76.5
Scooter	88.3	86.1
Major difficulty with upper extremity mobility	75.3	68.9
Major difficulty using hands and fingers	68.8	67.3

Data source: 1994–1995 National Health Interview Survey disability supplement.

[a]The percentage of persons who answered "yes" to two questions: "Do you consider yourself to have a disability?" and "Would other people consider you to have a disability?" Population estimates based on 81,840 (56.4 percent) adults who responded themselves rather than using a proxy respondent; figures account for age category and sex.

ever they choose to define the word. We fully recognize Kate Cather's identification as a linguistic minority rather than as someone with a disability, regardless of how societal programs or mandates like Social Security and the ADA would categorize her. According to the 1994–1995 National Health Interview Survey disability supplement, which asked respondents if they saw themselves as disabled, only 27.4 percent of persons who report being deaf or having major difficulty hearing view themselves as disabled (table 2.1). Just 42.3 percent of persons who report blindness or major vision difficulties and 79.9 percent of those using manual wheelchairs say they are disabled. Table 2.1 also shows respondents' perceptions of whether other people view them as disabled; percentages are roughly comparable to those for self-perceived disability.

Most of the problems we identify with the health care delivery system represent structural problems, including training and communication skills of clinicians and health insurance policies, thus reflecting a "social model" perspective. In other words, problems arise from an unaccommodating, barrier-strewn health care system rather than from patients who might have disabling conditions. But to make care accessible—to remove those impediments—patients might need to accept a disability identity, for example, by invoking their rights under the ADA. We fully acknowledge the ironies and implications of our arguments, but we are practical. Rather than striving for definitional purity, we want to improve health care delivery for populations who have historically lived on the margins.

Health Insurance and Accessing
the Health Care System

Fred Bender lives in Distant Dunes (the fictional name we've given a real rural community on the mid-Atlantic shore), which has several primary care practices and a small hospital. Although Fred has a local doctor, he must travel three hours to a large city to get the specialized care he sometimes needs. He usually drives but has trouble affording the gasoline: Fred never completed high school, and he stopped working because of failing health. "To get gas, I have to wait till somebody comes along with money they can loan me," Fred admitted. "But I can't pay them back."

Now in his early sixties, Fred has had diabetes for years, which is affecting his heart and sapping his endurance and strength: "I could walk across the street, and when I get over there, I'd stand and puff and pant a while." He had qualified for Social Security Disability Insurance (SSDI), receiving Medicare coverage after two years. But the monthly SSDI check does not cover his living expenses, let alone the costs of his medications. Although Fred receives assistance from two local programs for indigent persons, he can't pay for his many drugs.

"I take needles three times a day," Fred reported. "90 units of insulin in the morning, 40 at noon, and 80 at night, plus two other diabetes medicines. My medication runs $714.78 a month. That's way more than my disability check." When asked if he can get all these medications every month, Fred replied, "No, because I'm not able. I don't get all the medicine I really need."

At the outset of each focus group, we asked participants their overall impression of the quality of health care in the United States. Almost universally, respondents immediately mentioned cost—not the technical proficiency of clinicians, their bedside manner, or clinical acumen. Instead, having financial access to care was the number one quality concern. As one man who is blind stated, "It all boils down to money. If you've got money, you're going to get treated rich. I'm poor, so I'm going to get treated poor."

Getting health care in the United States often requires resources that many persons with disabilities do not have. Like Fred Bender, persons with disabilities are more likely than others to be poorly educated, unemployed, and impoverished (see table 1.4). Disability and sometimes poverty can make persons eligible for critical social "safety net" programs like Medicare (through SSDI) or Medicaid. Nevertheless, as with Fred's expensive drug regimen, needs can outstrip the benefits allowed. Unable to pay for uncompensated items or services, persons with disabilities do without, perhaps further compromising their health and functional abilities.

Many persons confront financial barriers to care, regardless of disability. However, specific health insurance policies—notably limited coverage of long-term rehabilitation services and assistive technologies—pose particular problems for some persons with disabilities. In addition, difficulties experienced by many people, such as paying for prescription drugs, happen more often among persons with disabilities. A survey of Medicare beneficiaries conducted in 2004 found that 48 percent of persons under age sixty-five (those who qualify for Medicare because of disability) reported significant difficulties paying for prescription drugs, compared with 17 percent of older beneficiaries (Kaiser Family Foundation/Harvard School of Public Health, 2004). Furthermore, 42 percent of disabled beneficiaries (compared with 16 percent of seniors) said they have not filled a prescription in the past year because of cost, and 46 percent (compared with 17 percent of seniors) have cut pills in half or skipped doses to make medications last longer.

To close part I, this chapter briefly reviews health insurance, focusing on several issues especially relevant to persons with disabilities. Nationwide, worries about health insurance—its dramatically escalating costs and shrinking benefits—loom large, extending across populations and political persuasions. An estimated 45.0 million persons, 15.6 percent of the population, had no health insurance during 2003, up from 15.2 percent in 2002 (DeNavas-Walt, Proctor, and Mills, 2004, p. 14). Declining employment-based health insurance exacerbates the growing number of uninsured. As annual insurance premiums keep rising, employment-based coverage will likely continue to drop.

No innovation, such as health maintenance organizations (HMOs) or managed care, has yet solved health care's deepening financial crisis. Purchasers and insurers continually experiment with new ways to finance care. Therefore, we do not describe particular health insurance approaches but instead cover basic issues, drawing upon Medicare for our primary examples. Often, private health plans follow Medicare's lead. Medicaid coverage policies particularly pertinent to persons with disabilities (e.g., for prescription drugs, personal assistant services, rehabilitation therapies, and assistive technologies) differ widely across states and change over time as state revenues fluctuate.

Having Health Insurance Matters

Regardless of disability, having health insurance matters, not only to individuals but also to their families and communities. "Health insurance pools the risks and resources of a large group of people so that each is protected from financially disruptive medical expenses resulting from an illness, accident, or disability" (Institute of Medicine, Committee on the Consequences, 2001, p. 20). Yet, as noted earlier, more than 15 percent of U.S. residents— almost 44 million persons—lack health insurance.

Although the majority of Americans believe that uninsured individuals get necessary medical services, they do not. Their chronic conditions are often neglected or poorly managed medically, further worsening disease and disability (Institute of Medicine, Committee on the Consequences, 2001, p. 22). For instance, the Centers for Disease Control and Prevention (2003b, p. 833) estimates that diabetes affects 29 million (14.4 percent) Americans over twenty years of age, like Fred Bender. But 29 percent of diabetes remains undiagnosed. Certainly, uninsured persons are much less likely than others to seek care, be diagnosed, and receive possibly life-prolonging treatments. Quality of life can suffer. Uninsured people who cannot walk are 40 percent less likely to have wheelchairs or walkers than insured persons (Iezzoni, 2003, pp. 225–226). Being uninsured for only one to four years can decrease overall health and, over the long term, heighten risks of premature death (Institute of Medicine, Committee on the Consequences, 2002a, p. 4).

Negative consequences of lacking health insurance extend beyond individuals. "The health of one member of the family can affect the health of the other members and of the unit as a whole" (Institute of Medicine, Committee on the Consequences, 2002b, p. 8). If being uninsured worsens one family member's health, this could lessen the well-being of other members, especially children. Lacking insurance coverage can also precipitate considerable emotional stress, further eroding the physical and mental health of family members. Indeed, high levels of uninsurance may compromise population health throughout communities: "The sheer number of uninsured persons in an area contributes disproportionately to the community's burden of disease and disability, because of the poorer health of uninsured community members and from spillover effects on other residents" (Institute of Medicine, Committee on the Consequences, 2003b, p. 12). After studying uninsurance for several years, the Institute of Medicine concluded:

> The aggregate, annualized cost of the diminished health and shorter life span of Americans who lack health insurance is between $65 and $130 billion for each year of health insurance foregone. These are the benefits that could be realized if extension of coverage reduced the morbidity and mortality of uninsured Americans to the levels for individuals who are comparable on measured characteristics and who have private health insurance. . . .
>
> Providing all members of American society with health insurance coverage would contribute to the realization of democratic ideals of equality of opportunity and mutual concern and respect. By tolerat-

ing a society in which a significant minority lacks the health care and coverage that most Americans enjoy, we are missing opportunities to become more fully the nation we claim to be. (Institute of Medicine, Committee on the Consequences, 2003a, pp. 4, 119)

Being uninsured primarily affects younger persons, since nearly all elderly people have Medicare. Most persons under age sixty-five receive voluntary, employer-based, private health insurance—a benefit that burgeoned initially among industrial workers during World War II. Since 1954, the Internal Revenue Service has exempted the employers' shares of health insurance premiums from their taxable incomes; this and other tax benefits yielded a $125.6 billion federal subsidy for employment-based health insurance in 2000 (Institute of Medicine, Committee on the Consequences, 2001, p. 45). However, rates of employer-based health insurance have fallen since the 1970s. In 2003, 60.4 percent of persons (174.0 million) had insurance through employers, down from 61.3 percent in 2002 (DeNavas-Walt, Proctor, and Mills, 2004, p. 14). About 80 percent of uninsured persons belong to families with at least one wage earner, and roughly 60 percent of uninsured individuals are employed, typically in low-paying jobs (Institute of Medicine, Committee on the Consequences, 2001, p. 60).

Fearing higher health insurance premiums, some employers avoid hiring workers with disabilities (Batavia, 2000). The Americans with Disabilities Act (ADA) does not specifically address employment-based health insurance, although it prohibits employers from discriminating against employees in "terms, conditions, and privileges of employment" [Sec. 102(a)]. Such "terms" presumably encompass health insurance, among other benefits. The ADA's legislative history suggests that employers and health insurers can offer health plans with restricted coverage if the exclusions or limitations rely "on sound actuarial principles" (Feldblum, 1991, p. 102).[1] Thus, employees with disabilities may find that their health insurance fails to cover care for conditions that predate their employment.

Health Insurance and Persons with Disabilities

The social safety net clearly rescues many persons with disabilities from being uninsured. In 2004, Medicare, a federal program, insured roughly 41.7 million persons, including 6.4 million individuals under age sixty-five with disabilities (Centers for Medicare and Medicaid Services [CMS], 2004). The joint federal and state program Medicaid covered 42.4 million persons in 2004, including 7.9 million who are blind or disabled. Of an estimated $242.4 billion expenditure in 2001, Medicare spent $31.9 billion on beneficiaries with disabilities (CMS, 2002, p. 26). Blind and disabled recipients consumed 37.8 percent of Medicaid's resources in 2001 (CMS, 2002, p. 29).[2]

Table 3.1. Health Insurance Coverage for Working-Age Persons

Impairment	Insurance Status (Percent[b])[a]		
	Any Private Insurance	Public Insurance Only	Uninsured
No impairment	79.1	5.9	15.0
Vision impairments			
Some	68.9	13.8	17.2
Blind or major	51.5	27.2	21.4
Hearing impairments			
Some	71.5	14.4	14.0
Deaf or major	76.1	6.8	17.1
Lower extremity mobility difficulty			
Minor	75.2	14.0	10.8
Moderate	49.1	39.1	11.9
Major	41.4	47.3	11.3
Upper extremity mobility difficulty			
Some	52.9	27.9	19.2
Major	48.6	39.8	11.6
Difficulties using hands			
Some	46.7	35.1	18.2
Major	39.5	47.5	13.0
Any impairment	67.4	17.3	15.3
Any major impairment	53.2	29.8	16.9

Data source: 2001 Medical Expenditure Panel Survey.
[a]Public insurance = Medicare, Medicaid, or Medicare and Medicaid. Uninsured = lacking insurance for entire prior year.
[b]Figures account for age category and sex.

Despite Medicare and Medicaid, working-age adults with any sensory or physical disability have slightly higher rates of being uninsured in the past year than do persons without these conditions (15.3 percent compared with 15.0 percent, table 3.1). Persons with disabilities are much more likely than others to have only public insurance: 29.8 percent for persons with any major disability, compared with 5.9 percent of those without any disability. Rates of Medicaid coverage alone exceed the percentage with either Medicare alone or Medicare plus Medicaid (table 3.2).

Persons with disabilities who have health insurance still may not get services they need. According to a 2000 survey, 28 percent of insured people with disabilities reported having special needs that insurance does not cover—for particular therapies, equipment, and medications—compared with 7 percent of those without disabilities (Harris Interactive, 2000). Among

Table 3.2. Public Health Insurance for Working-Age Persons

Impairment	Type of Public Insurance (Percent[a])		
	Medicare Only	Medicaid Only	Medicare and Medicaid
No impairment	0.7	5.8	0.6
Any vision impairment	3.5	12.2	3.5
Any hearing impairment	3.3	10.4	1.4
Lower extremity mobility difficulty			
Moderate	7.6	29.4	7.5
Major	18.7	30.9	7.8
Major upper extremity mobility difficulty	22.2	35.0	4.3
Major difficulties using hands	15.3	32.1	8.7
Any impairment	4.6	14.0	3.2
Any major impairment	10.7	19.7	5.7

Data source: 2001 Medical Expenditure Panel Survey.

[a]Figures for persons eighteen to sixty-four years old account for age category and sex.

persons with very severe disabilities, 40 percent reported this gap. Cost problems cause substantial barriers to care, as suggested by a survey (late 2002–early 2003) of working age persons with disabilities, 95 percent of whom had health insurance:

> Overall, prescription drug and dental care are the services or benefits most commonly named as causing problems, cited as a serious problem by 32 percent and 29 percent of the sample, respectively. In addition, 21 percent of those who use equipment to manage their disabilities said they had serious difficulties paying for such equipment. . . . Sizeable shares of this sample reported having postponed care (37 percent) or gone without necessary items such as equipment and eyeglasses (46 percent) because of cost. In addition, 36 percent . . . reported having skipped medication doses, split pills, or gone without filling a prescription altogether to save money. (Hanson et al., 2003, p. W3-560)

Persons with disabilities blamed lack of affordability for 33.9 percent of failures to comply with prescription medication regimens (Kennedy and Erb, 2002, p. 1121).[3]

The Twenty-Nine-Month Gap

By statute, one group of persons with disabilities explicitly falls through the social safety net, at least for twenty-nine months: individuals who newly qualify for SSDI but not Supplemental Security Income (SSI). P.L. 92-603, signed by President Richard Nixon on July 1, 1972, set a five-month wait- ing period between qualifying for SSDI and receiving cash payments. The law then granted Medicare coverage to persons who have received SSDI cash benefits for twenty-four months [42 U.S.C. Sec. 226(b)(2)(A)].[4] Thus a total of twenty-nine months must elapse between SSDI determination and Medicare eligibility. (On July 1, 2001, Congress rescinded the twenty-four- month wait for Medicare coverage, but only for persons who qualify for SSDI because of amyotrophic lateral sclerosis—a profoundly debilitating neurologic condition that often progresses rapidly to death.)

Separating Medicare coverage from disability determination makes little sense. The prevailing political rationale was that waiting periods would limit Medicare costs. Nonetheless, to get SSDI, applicants must prove that they have medically verified physical or mental conditions that prevent them from working and will cause death or continue for at least a year (see chap- ter 2). If applicants face imminent death or cannot work because of debili- tating medical conditions, surely they need health insurance. Persons who qualify for SSI, which uses the same disability criteria as SSDI, immediately get Medicaid coverage.

Being without employment and health insurance clearly places new SSDI recipients into an intractable bind. Jimmy Howard is in his late forties with arthritis and diabetes (Iezzoni, 2003). He has a high school education and had worked lifting heavy boxes in ManuCo's warehouse for years before being fired because of walking problems. Mr. Howard strides slowly but firmly with an aluminum cane, although he sometimes falls unexpectedly. After ManuCo fired him, he applied to Social Security for disability bene- fits. He has incapacitating stiffness each morning and meets the specified objective medical criteria for arthritis of a major weight-bearing joint.

Five months following his disability determination, Mr. Howard started receiving cash SSDI benefits. He must wait another two years to get Medicare coverage. Mr. Howard, however, needs health insurance now. He must keep his diabetes under control and treat his arthritis. Mr. Howard pays $400 per month for private health insurance under COBRA (Consolidated Omnibus Budget Reconciliation Act) provisions.[5] But sometimes he and his wife, who also doesn't work, can barely make this payment.

Beyond 1972's prevailing political justification, today's continuing ra- tionale for this waiting period remains murky. Vladeck and colleagues (1997) offer six "stories" that might explain these policies, such as

> ambivalence about the meaning of disability itself. . . . The truly dis- abled—those who have a clear right to protection—cannot be easily identified in the modern social context in which disability is a matter of degree. . . . Disability consists of a hard physical core with an ex- panding penumbra of mental and psychosocial nuance not generally

as visible (or acceptable) to society. As a result, gaps in services betray a deeply rooted ambivalence toward certain classes of the disabled. Most especially, a fundamental skepticism of those who are disabled because of a mental illness, alcoholism, or drug addiction seems ingrained in the culture. (Vladeck et al., 1997, p. 87)

In earlier years, the plurality of new SSDI recipients qualified because of clinical diagnoses that obviously warranted active medical interventions. In 1981, circulatory conditions accounted for 25 percent of disability determinations, followed by other systemic diseases (19 percent); musculoskeletal conditions contributed 17 percent and mental disorders 11 percent (Institute of Medicine, Committee to Review, 2002, p. 47). By 2003, the diagnostic mix had changed considerably: musculoskeletal conditions contributed the largest single percentage (26.3 percent) of all new disabled workers, with mental disorders in second place at 22.8 percent (SSA, 2004, p. 92). Circulatory disorders had fallen to 11.4 percent.

Relatively little is known about the health and health care of SSDI beneficiaries during the waiting period. Among those newly entitled to SSDI in 1995, 11.8 percent died during the waiting period, while 2.1 percent recovered; 61.8 percent of those who qualified as disabled because of cancer died, compared to 1.0 percent for musculoskeletal disabilities (Riley, 2004, p. 390). Dale and Verdier (2003) estimate this population at 1.26 million individuals in 2002. Approximately one third (400,000 persons) lacked health insurance during the waiting period, while roughly 40 percent (504,000 adults) enrolled in Medicaid, costing federal and state governments $7.6 billion in 2002.[6]

Questions remain about what SSDI recipients do for health care services during the wait for Medicare. Having financial access to health care services is essential to "fostering early interventions to prevent diseases or impairments from becoming permanent work disabilities" (Mashaw and Reno, 1996, p. 135). However, while awaiting Medicare coverage, new SSDI beneficiaries without health insurance might skimp on care that could prevent or slow progression of debilitating conditions. Delays or reductions in treatment and preventive care could decrease longevity, hasten functional declines, and increase eventual health care costs. One study interviewed twenty-one persons with disabilities during the waiting period or shortly afterward and confirmed these fears:

Nearly all say they are forced to pay out-of-pocket for most services and almost all prescription medications; put off doctor's visits, or visit much less frequently, or not at all (some opting to use the emergency room instead); and in many cases, forego necessary medications, tests, and rehabilitation therapy. Because of lack of coverage . . . inconsistent care is taking a toll on their health. (Williams et al., 2004, p. 7)

Adding new SSDI beneficiaries to the Medicare rolls would increase to-tal programmatic costs. Eliminating the waiting period would add about $8.7 billion (3.4 percent) to Medicare costs at 2002 spending levels, but re-ductions in state and federal Medicaid expenditures would offset roughly 30 percent of the Medicare rise (Dale and Verdier, 2003).[7] The unanswered question is whether longer-term savings from potentially improved health and functioning might further reduce these costs. Jimmy Howard's primary care doctor told me two years later that his diabetes had become poorly con-trolled and he risked losing toes to gangrene—a costly consequence to both Mr. Howard and the health care system. Medicare coverage may not have prevented or slowed that progression, but it could have given Mr. Howard better access to services that might have helped.[8]

As Fred Bender found, having health insurance does not guarantee cover-age, especially for all medications, assistive technologies, and other items and services needed by many persons with disabilities. Enrollees must ex-amine the fine print: what benefits does their insurance cover? Individuals with "health care insurance are rarely covered for (and have access to) ad-equate preventive care and long-term medical care, rehabilitation, and as-sistive technologies. These factors demonstrably contribute to the incidence, prevalence, and severity of primary and secondary disabling conditions and, tragically, avoidable disability" (Institute of Medicine, Committee on a National Agenda, 1991, p. 280).

Public and private health insurers typically make reimbursement decisions in stages: first, organization-wide decisions about what services particular plans will "cover"; and second, case-by-case decisions about the "medical necessity" of covered services for individual persons (Singer and Bergthold, 2001). A third-order decision, potentially critical for persons with disabilities, involves the set-ting of care: whether persons can receive services at home. For items and serv-ices relating to disability, private and public health insurers generally consider two major factors in making coverage decisions:

- How long will individuals need the services?
- Will the services measurably improve physical or sensory deficits caused by medical illness or injury?

Neither question portends especially well for persons with disabilities who need items and services for the long term and are unlikely to improve. In-surers generally balk at covering long-term needs, especially when impair-ments will probably persist—even if these items and services help maintain a person's functioning and independence.

Designing Benefits Packages

All health care purchasers, including the federal government for Medicare, choose which types of items and services they will reimburse or cover under health insurance—the so-called "benefits package." Health insurance plans that cover more services typically cost more. Coverage policies reflect their historical roots. Private health insurance, which first appeared during the Great Depression, aimed to make acute hospital care affordable to low- and moderate-income families and to ensure the financial survival of these increasingly expensive institutions. With extraordinary but costly advances in hospital-based interventions over ensuing decades, most health insurance plans concentrated on reimbursing expensive but time-limited hospital care, along with associated physician fees.

Thus, from the start, benefits packages neglected daily health- and function-related needs of persons with chronic medical conditions, including many persons with disabilities. Historically, such individuals received care in homes, generally from female relatives or nurses with little formal training who were overseen occasionally by physicians making house calls. Even after recovering from acute events, like poliomyelitis infections, many persons rarely left their homes, remaining hidden from view (Gallagher, 1994). Therefore, paying for technologies, devices, and therapeutic interventions to maintain, restore, or maximize independent function never emerged as a pressing public issue.

Years of political maneuvering, compromises, and retrenchment of expectations were required to achieve passage of Medicare and Medicaid in 1965. Congress feared opening the door to runaway costs.[9] Medicare *did* cover more nonacute care, such as limited skilled nursing home stays and home health care visits including rehabilitation services, than any other governmental, nonprofit, or commercial insurer at the time (Fox, 1993). Nonetheless, in the end, "left out were provisions that addressed the particular problems of the chronically sick elderly: medical conditions that would not dramatically improve and the need to maintain independent function rather than triumph over discrete illness and injury" (Marmor, 2000, p. 153). Policy-makers strayed occasionally, such as adding coverage for selected screening tests and palliative care, but little changed for forty years until George W. Bush signed the Medicare Prescription Drug, Improvement, and Modernization Act (MMA, P.L. 108-173) of 2003 on December 8. In addition to the prescription drug benefit that will start in 2006, the MMA altered many nuances of coverage policy. "The full details of the changes will take time to become evident" (Medicare Payment Advisory Commission, 2004a, p. xv).[10]

By statute, Medicare explicitly covers only services that are "reasonable and necessary for the diagnosis or treatment of illness or injury or to improve the functioning of a malformed body member" (42 C.F.R. Sec. 402.3). Medicare explicitly does not cover "services related to activities for the general physical welfare of beneficiaries (for example, exercises to promote overall fitness)" [42 C.F.R. Sec. 409.44(c)(1)].[11] Other specific exclusions include routine physical checkups, routine foot or dental care, hearing aids, eyeglasses, white canes, wheelchairs for use outside the home, and so-called "personal comfort" items, such as grab bars (42 C.F.R. Sec. 411.15; see also chapter 9).

Individuals themselves pay for uncovered items and services, although most Medicare beneficiaries purchase private supplemental insurance to reimburse some uncovered costs, including deductibles and coinsurance.[12] These insurance supplements also vary in coverage, with broader packages costing more. Nineteen percent of Medicare beneficiaries with disabilities lack supplemental insurance; these persons have much lower annual incomes ($13,400 after out-of-pocket medical expenses, which consume almost 25 percent of their total incomes) than disabled beneficiaries with supplemental insurance (Medicare Payment Advisory Commission, 2004b, 209).

In designing Medicaid, Congress recognized that low-income persons have little money to spend on care, so it adopted broader benefits than for Medicare. All states must cover core services, like inpatient hospitalizations, skilled nursing facility stays, and home health care. In addition, states can offer various optional services, including prescription drugs, physical and occupational therapy, personal assistant services (PAS), prosthetic devices, prescription eyeglasses, and durable medical equipment. Medicaid often fills in the gap for poor and near-poor Medicare beneficiaries, for example, by paying Medicare premiums and cost sharing and reimbursing needs not covered by Medicare (Crowley and Elias, 2003).

When facing substantial budget shortfalls, states frequently cut Medicaid benefits, eliminating or reducing payments for optional items and services. "Spending on drugs in all Medicaid programs increased, on average, by more than 16 percent annually between 1990 and 2000, from an estimated $4.8 billion to $210 billion per year" (Iglehart, 2003, p. 2143), making medication benefits especially ripe for cost cutting. In 2003, 45 states implemented cost controls on prescription drugs and 25 reduced Medicaid benefits, including limiting vision care; dental services; physical, occupational, and speech therapy; and home oxygen (Smith et al., 2003, pp. 9, 11). PAS, offered by most states, may not receive outright cuts, but states can ratchet back the hours they cover. Persons with substantial disabilities who rely on PAS to live independently in their own homes worry that, if Medicaid cuts their PAS hours, they will have to enter nursing homes (Perry, Dulio, and Hanson, 2003, p. 9). Reimbursing nursing homes may, in short order, cost Medicaid more than additional PAS hours. Nonetheless, with continuing budget deficits, state legislatures will likely continue chipping away at Medicaid's covered benefits.

Thus, federal and state governments, like businesses and other private purchasers, "buy" only those health insurance benefits packages that they can afford. The health insurer then administers the plan, paying claims only for covered items and services. Especially in the private sector, health plan enrollees often do not distinguish between the purchaser that selects the benefits and the health insurer that pays the claims. "I don't think that patients really understand the distinction between the people who design their benefits and the people who pay the claims," said the medical director of a private BlueCross/BlueShield plan (Iezzoni, 2003, p. 231). "It's the employers who choose the benefit packages . . . but it's the insurance company that gets the blame when there's a discordance in expectations." This problem dogs Medicare, too, with an aging public and Congress at loggerheads over the benefits package and who will pay.

Determining Medical Necessity

Before reimbursing covered services, insurers often review each case to establish that specific items or services are "medically necessary" for the individual patient. Medical necessity determinations extend across health care settings, from hospital-based acute services to assistive technologies. Insurers generally make yes/no decisions: Is the item or service medically necessary or is it primarily desired for convenience? As noted earlier, Medicare explicitly covers only interventions that are "reasonable and necessary" to diagnose or treat illnesses or injuries or "to improve the functioning of a malformed body member" (42 C.F.R. Sec. 402.3). Local Medicare carriers use this framework to determine whether individual beneficiaries receive requested items or services, like assistive technologies and physical and occupational therapy.[13]

In its pamphlet, "Your Medicare Benefits," the Centers for Medicare and Medicaid Services (2003a, p. 9), which oversees Medicare, informs beneficiaries that "original" or traditional Medicare covers services or supplies that are "medically necessary" or that

- Are proper and needed for the diagnosis or treatment of your medical condition,
- Are provided for the diagnosis, direct care, and treatment of your medical condition,
- Meet the standards of good medical practice in the local area, and
- Are not mainly for the convenience of you or your doctor. (2003a, p. 9)

Long-term physical, occupational, or speech-language therapy to maintain function or prevent further declines often fails these tests. "Treatment" usually assumes recovery or improvement. The prohibition against "convenience" items frequently dooms requests for assistive technologies, as in the case of Erna Dodd, who requested a motorized scooter-type wheelchair.

"I can't keep up with this walker," Ms. Dodd said, moving slowly and laboriously, breathing oxygen from a canister dangling from her walker's handlebars (Iezzoni, 1999, 2003). In her mid-fifties, she had many medical problems, including emphysema, diabetes requiring insulin, congestive heart failure, seizures, obesity, and debilitating arthritis. Nonetheless, she refused our offer to transport her by wheelchair to the clinic. As she said,

Ms. Dodd didn't "want people pushing me in a wheelchair. My nurse put in to get me a [motorized] scooter. He had my doctor fill out some paper for it. This was a letter they sent, telling me they wouldn't give it to me." Reaching into her handbag, she retrieved a legal-size envelope containing a single sheet of paper.

"Medicare sent this to you?" I asked, looking at the letterhead, and then read aloud, "'We have received a prior authorization request for the above named beneficiary for a power-operated vehicle. This request has been denied because the information did not support the medical necessity of the equipment. If you do not agree with this decision, you may request a review in writing within six months of the date indicated in this letter. Submit any additional documentation to the review department.' Did your doctor appeal this?"

"I don't know. I was going to call my doctor and talk to him about it. It would help me a lot." Her primary care physician did contest Medicare's denial, but Erna Dodd died during the appeals process.

Medical necessity decisions frequently appear idiosyncratic and subjective. As for Ms. Dodd, "denial letters rarely explain who made the decision, the reason for the decision, what sources of evidence were considered, what coverage policies were applied, or anything else about the process of making the decision" (Singer and Bergthold, 2001, p. 204). The paucity of scientific evidence demonstrating the effectiveness of disability-related items and services poses particular problems. Few clinical trials examine the effectiveness of long-term physical or occupational therapy in preserving functional abilities or preventing declines. Even less research has rigorously addressed the relative merits of various assistive technologies. The scarcity of research evidence about the effectiveness and clinical outcomes of therapy and assistive technology impedes efforts to make objective medical necessity decisions about the merit of these items and services.

The Institute of Medicine's Committee on a National Agenda for the Prevention of Disabilities lauded the potential for rehabilitation services, assistive technologies, and even modest items like grab bars to improve safety and quality of life for persons with disabilities They noted that the failure of health insurance to pay for these items and services generally blocked their use and was therefore counterproductive:

> Denial of reimbursement for technology that assists in the performance of daily activities and reduces risk of secondary conditions is likely to result in long-term costs that exceed initial savings. For example, Medicare regards grab bars for bathrooms as convenience items, even though falls in the bathroom are a leading cause of hip fractures and other injuries among the elderly. The health care costs associated with hip fractures alone are large and growing. This shortsightedness is also reflected in the inadequate coverage that

most insurers provide for long-term maintenance and replacement of the few assistive technologies they do fund. (Institute of Medicine, Committee on a National Agenda, 1991, p. 227)

Thus, according to the Committee, payment policies impede people from acquiring devices that could not only improve their lives but also could save health care dollars downstream.

Medical necessity decisions sit at an uncomfortable nexus, balancing personal needs against overall programmatic costs. However, Medicare's current medical necessity provisions deny the realities of a large fraction, if not the majority, of its beneficiaries—persons with chronic debilitating conditions that will not improve. With appropriate technological or rehabilitative support, many of these individuals could continue living independently within communities and postpone the overwhelming expense of long-term institutionalization. Admittedly, funding such services would require significant expenditures over many years.

Nevertheless, the process for medical necessity decisions does not engender confidence. "It's pretty loose," replied the medical director of a Blue-Cross plan when I asked him to define medical necessity (Iezzoni, 2003, p. 234). "It means what a reasonable physician thinks is needed for his patient. It has to be a skilled service." Wheelchairs, like Erna Dodd's scooter, can fit this definition, but not "something that's just being done for convenience."

Getting Home Care

To qualify for home-based services, Medicare regulations stipulate that beneficiaries be "homebound," defined as "a normal inability to leave home, that leaving the home requires a considerable and taxing effort by the individual." While Medicare allows absences for medical care, adult day care, and attending religious services, other absences must be "infrequent or of relatively short duration" [42 C.F.R. Sec. 1814(a) and Sec. 1835(a)]. This policy poses a major dilemma for people like Mary Jo, a friend of a colleague who lives in a small mountain town (Iezzoni, 2003).

"She lives three blocks from us. She's thirty-nine or forty, and she has diabetes. She's had one leg amputated, and the other leg is constantly in danger. She lives in a low-income apartment, one of those little places like a motel room. Some friends raised the money and gave her an electric wheelchair—a real cheap one, but it allowed her to get out the door and up to a small park. On a nice spring day, she can go out and sit under a tree and come back in. That's all she ever did with it." Mary Jo's friends had rightly assumed that Medicare would deny her a power wheelchair since she does not need it within her tiny apartment. Just like Erna Dodd's situation, it would not have passed "medical necessity" muster.

But her friends' generosity had unintended consequences. Mary Jo has a home health nurse to treat her ulcerated leg, among other things. "One day, the home health nurse saw the electric wheelchair sitting in the apartment, and she said, 'You know what? I can't come anymore.' Mary Jo is disabled under Medicare, and Medicare won't pay for home health unless the person is homebound. So the wheelchair has now been folded up and is gathering dust in the corner. It's been retired from use, and every time a home health aide comes, she tries not to see it."

The independence conveyed by the power wheelchair risked Mary Jo's eligibility for home-based nursing care for her remaining leg ulcerated by diabetes. Clearly, Medicare's homebound policy makes little sense for Mary Jo. To qualify for nursing care in her home, Mary Jo first needed to demonstrate that skilled services were "medically necessary." With diabetic ulcerations on her remaining leg needing constant clinical attention, meeting the medically necessary criterion was relatively easy. For Mary Jo, traveling daily to a clinic or hospital for this care is infeasible.

For years, concerns about increasing home care costs have stalled efforts to broaden the homebound definition. Home care costs had soared—from 1989 to 1996, Medicare Part A home health care spending grew from $2.8 to $11.3 billion (U.S. General Accounting Office, 1997, 5). To stop this trend, the Balanced Budget Act of 1997 (P.L. 105-33) significantly changed Medicare home health care payment policies. According to the Medicare Payment Advisory Commission (MedPAC, 2003b, p. 75), between 1996 and 2001, total home care expenditures fell by 50 percent, and the average number of days on home care fell 28 percent, from 60 to 43 days. Have these cuts gone too far, especially for persons who are frail, disabled, or medically vulnerable? MedPAC (2003b, p. 79) found "that for beneficiaries with certain clinical conditions, SNF [skilled nursing facility] use may be partly replacing home health use."[14] Furthermore, "a number of home health agencies reported changing the way they operated, being more careful about accepting long-term, chronic, or higher-cost beneficiaries" (MedPAC, 2003b, p. 77). Someone like Mary Jo might have difficulty getting Medicare home care.

The case of David Jayne exemplifies the consequences of Medicare's homebound definition. Jayne, a Georgia resident, developed amyotrophic lateral sclerosis (ALS) in 1987 at age twenty-seven and later became totally physically incapacitated (Byzek, 2003). Medicare paid for skilled nursing care in his home. In 2000, Jayne traveled out of town with a college friend to watch a Georgia Bulldogs football game. An Atlanta newspaper chronicled the trip, and shortly thereafter Jayne's home health agency discharged him for violating the homebound definition.[15] His congressman arranged for Medicare to reinstate the services, and Jayne began campaigning to reform the homebound definition. He founded the National Coalition to Amend the Medicare Homebound Restriction for Americans with Significant Illness (www.amendhomeboundpolicy.homestead.com) and proved an exceptional lobbyist, speaking through a computer. Largely because of his efforts, Section 702 of the 2003 Medicare Prescription Drug, Improvement, and Modernization Act requires that CMS conduct a demonstration project to explore the consequences of changing the homebound rule. The two-year demonstration starts in fall 2004 in Colorado, Massachusetts, and Missouri.

Mismatch of Needs and Payment Policies

This sketch of the financial context for seeking health care highlights the monetary barriers that many persons with disabilities confront, day in and day out. Medicare payment policies often do not match basic needs of persons with disabilities for items and services to maintain, restore, or maximize their functioning. Deep state budget cuts are fraying even Medicaid's safety net. Benefits packages offered by private insurers grow increasingly constrained as costs rise.

Expanding coverage to include more function-related services has always proved politically unpalatable: "The cost implications of disability-related services are so inherently unpredictable as to frighten policy-makers away from contemplating all but the narrowest of expansions. What looks like a half-empty glass when benefits are being designed may be a bottomless pit once the payments begin to flow" (Vladeck et al., 1997, p. 88).

Nevertheless, rethinking fundamental coverage policies relating to chronic conditions and disability is overdue and pressing—the "baby boomers" start turning age sixty-five in 2011 (see chapter 16). Many problems experienced by persons with disabilities and described in part II trace back to inadequate payments, counterproductive insurance policies, or inappropriate financial incentives. Although financial barriers confront many persons trying to enter the health care delivery system, persons with disabilities seem especially at risk.

II

HEALTH CARE EXPERIENCES
OF PEOPLE WITH DISABILITIES

Finding Care

Except for emergencies, most people enter the health care system through a private physician's office, health center, or clinic. Regardless of what persons ultimately need—routine preventive care, specialty care, physical or occupational therapy, home-based nursing care, assistive technologies, or other services—physicians generally must perform, approve, prescribe, or oversee its provision to merit health insurance coverage and meet legal liability requirements. Important exceptions to physician oversight do exist, like certain services provided by nurse practitioners, physician assistants, and physical and occupational therapists. In many settings, clinicians from diverse disciplines work together in teams. Nonetheless, finding care generally starts with finding a specific primary care clinician, almost always a physician.[1]

Persons with disabilities and significant health care needs consider many factors in choosing physicians, ranging from costs and health insurance requirements to physical location and accessibility to physicians' technical knowledge, attitudes, and communication approaches. The experiences of Davey Sutton, in his late thirties, highlight these complexities. "I have a hearing disability, glaucoma, major depression, and severe knee problems," noted Mr. Sutton, who resides in rural Blustery Bluffs (another fictitious name) on the northern Atlantic coast. He walks with a white cane, and since he is poor and unemployed, he has "Mass Health"—Massachusetts Medicaid.

> When I moved out to Blustery Bluffs ten years ago, it took me about five years to find a primary care physician who I liked and trusted. I spent lots of time on the computer looking up doctors. I went to three or four and didn't like their attitudes toward me.
>
> I have to find one that takes Mass Health. A lot of doctors who take Mass Health patients can only have so many of them. Then I had to find a primary care physician who was willing to work with me, someone who would give me referrals to see specialists. A lot of doctors don't like to give referrals to eye or ear specialists.

Table 4.1. Persons without a Usual Source of Care

	Age Group (Percent[a])		
Impairment	18–44 Years	45–64 Years	65+ Years
No impairments	21.6	15.5	7.6
Vision impairments	26.2	13.7	7.8
Hearing impairments	20.7	12.6	4.9
Lower extremity mobility difficulty	19.6	8.8	3.8
Upper extremity mobility difficulty	17.4	9.9	4.4
Difficulties using hands	16.4	8.5	3.6
Any impairment	23.4	12.1	5.2
Any major impairment	20.5	10.6	5.4

Data Source: 2001 Medical Expenditure Panel Survey.
[a]Figures account for age category and sex.

Now I have a wonderful physician. She's very understanding, maybe 'cause she's a woman—I seem to get on much better with women doctors. . . . She's like a friend to me; we talk about everything. Am I eating healthy? She talks about my weight concerns. I always tell her, "You're a gift from God. Don't ever leave me." I don't know if I'll ever find another one like her.

Davey Sutton believes that searching for physicians involves two steps: "First off, you must find a doctor who'll take Mass Health," which typically pays lower fees than other insurers. "Then you sit down, explain your situation, what your handicaps are, what your concerns are, what you're looking for in a doctor, and see if they can help you. If they can't, then go out and look for someone else. You have to feel comfortable with a doctor. That's my number one concern—to feel comfortable and hopefully get the right care."

Especially among younger adults, surprisingly large fractions of persons with disabilities report not having a usual source of health care—a particular doctor's office, clinic, health center, or other care setting where they seek care and medical advice (table 4.1). Among persons age eighteen through forty-four with major disabilities, 20.5 percent do not have a usual source of care—neither do 10.6 percent of their counterparts age forty-five to sixty-four. Roughly 36 percent of working-age persons without a usual source of care attribute this absence to high costs, while nearly 10 percent say they do not know where to go to get care.[2] People without usual clinicians may delay or neglect important care that could ameliorate their impairments or prevent further declines. For instance, persons with chronic joint symptoms who do not have a health care provider are 2.1 times more likely than those with providers to have never sought care for their condition (Centers for Disease Control [CDC], 2003a). Among Medicare beneficiaries with a usual source of care, persons with disabilities express more dissatisfaction with the costs and ease of access to care than do nondisabled beneficiaries (table 4.2).

Following Davey Sutton's two-part framework, this chapter examines how persons with disabilities find their primary care provider. We start with financial considerations, building on the discussion of health insurance begun in chapter 3, using Medicare and Medicaid for our examples. We then move to other major factors, including physicians' willingness to accept patients with disabilities, particular concerns for persons with congenital conditions moving from pediatric into adult care settings, and location. Later chapters address topics such as interpersonal communication and attitudes critical to fostering patient-clinician relationships.

Uninsured persons report not having a usual source of care much more often than those with insurance. Among working-age persons with any major sensory or physical impairment, 52.6 percent of uninsured individuals report having no usual source of care, compared with 14.2 percent of those with any private insurance.[3]

Some practitioners turn away individuals with insurance that generally pays lower fees, such as Medicaid. Nationwide, among nearly 156,000 practicing primary care physicians in 2001, 74 percent accepted patients with Medicare, while 68 percent took Medicaid, and 77 percent took noncapitated private insurance (Cherry, Burt, and Woodwell, 2003, p. 37). Given their dependence on Medicaid, many persons with disabilities thus face significant challenges to finding care.

A national telephone survey conducted in late 2002 and early 2003 of working-age persons with disabilities produced troubling results that frame our discussion:

> Although the majority of survey respondents said that they have a regular doctor, one in four reported having had trouble finding a doctor who understands their disability. . . . The uninsured were also more likely than those with health insurance to say they have no regular doctor and to report trouble finding a doctor who understands their disability. When it comes to finding a doctor who accepts their insurance, 17 percent of the sample reported this problem, with higher rates [22 percent] among those covered by Medicaid. (Hanson et al., 2003, p. W3-560)

Thus, Davey Sutton's difficulties reflect reality. Without insurance—or with less generous insurance—prospects for establishing relationships with physicians can be tenuous.

Table 4.2. Medicare Beneficiaries' Concerns about Costs and Obtaining Care (Percent[a])

				Major Difficulties		
Aspect of Care[b]	No DA[c]	Very Low Vision	Deaf/HOH[c]	Walking	Reaching	Grasping
"Out-of-pocket costs paid for medical services"	10.1	22.5	20.5	21.5	21.8	20.7
"Ease and convenience of getting to a doctor from where person lives"	3.0	12.2	11.2	11.5	12.2	13.5
"Getting all medical care needs taken care of at the same location"	3.6	8.6	9.5	8.8	8.8	10.1
"Availability of medical services at night and on weekends"	3.6	10.6	9.9	7.8	8.1	8.1

Adapted from: Iezzoni et al. (2002, p. 375).

[a]Percentage dissatisfied with costs or other aspect of care; figures account for age category and sex.

[b]Exact wording of question.

[c]DA = disability; HOH = hard of hearing; grasping = grasping and writing.

Paying Enough to Ensure Access to Care

Health care delivery in the United States does not represent a pure competitive marketplace. Nonetheless, it follows one accepted economic precept: neither health care professionals nor institutions typically provide services without payment. Furthermore, reimbursement must be sufficiently high to attract providers to actually offer services. Notable exceptions do exist, such as public clinics for indigent persons and requirements for nonprofit institutions to offer free care.

In general, people with substantial impairments cost more to treat than other patients (DeJong et al., 2002). Over time, persons with sensory and physical impairments typically generate much higher median total health care expenditures than do other persons and also pay more out-of-pocket (table 4.3). For instance, working-age persons with major lower extremity mobility difficulties generated $7,389 in median total health expenditures in 2000, compared with $408 for persons with no impairment.

Persons with disabilities also generally visit health care providers more often than do other people. As shown in table 4.4, more persons with disabilities are hospitalized at least once in the previous year, although the vast majority of them have only one stay. They are also much more likely to have at least one physician office, clinic, or physical or occupational therapist visit, and if they have at least one, their mean number of total visits is higher than for persons without disabilities. Specific subpopulations can exhibit different patterns: for example, prelingually deafened individuals visit physicians less often than do others (Barnett and Franks, 2002).[4] However, since persons with disabilities generally consume more health care services, ensuring adequate payment for these services is essential to finding willing providers.

Paying for Individual Services

Even basic services, like routine office visits, can cost more for persons with disabilities because of additional time, personnel, testing, or equipment required. If payments do not cover costs, some clinicians in private-practice settings may refuse to accept patients with disabilities. Such refusals raise complex legal, professional, and moral questions not examined here. Certainly, health professionals carry strong ethical obligations to treat people regardless of their abilities to pay. Persons with life-threatening health emergencies generally get care. But for the preponderance of nonurgent needs, the amount paid can determine access to health care services. In 2001, only 0.4 percent of office visits in the United States were charity or without charge (Cherry, Burt, and Woodwell, 2003, p. 21).[5]

Fees set for individual services do not consider whether patients have special health care needs or require additional assistance to receive the serv-

Table 4.3. Median Total Health Care Expenditures and Out-of-Pocket Payments in 2001[a]

	Age 18–64		Age 65+	
Impairment	Total ($)	Self[b] ($)	Total ($)	Self[b] ($)
No impairment	408	92	1,885	514
Vision impairments				
Some	1,418	330	3,594	987
Blind or major	1,477	308	4,811	971
Hearing impairments				
Some	1,638	357	4,234	812
Deaf or major	1,060	400	4,179	808
Lower extremity mobility difficulty				
Minor	2,993	532	3,760	905
Moderate	4,207	704	4,825	877
Major	7,389	815	6,528	1,226
Upper extremity mobility difficulty				
Some	4,278	723	4,536	936
Major	6,758	733	7,155	1,205
Difficulties using hands				
Some	4,369	758	5,454	1,167
Major	6,915	560	5,489	1,085
Any impairment	2,164	387	4,228	904
Any major impairment	3,826	510	5,317	1,098

Data source: 2001 Medical Expenditure Panel Survey.
[a]Includes payments for office visits, outpatient clinic visits, hospitalizations, home health care, prescription medications, dental care, vision aids, and other medical equipment and supplies.
[b]Self = out-of-pocket.

ice. Joe Alto's observations highlight the problem. Mr. Alto, a former backhoe operator in his late thirties, has multiple sclerosis and uses a wheelchair. His primary care physician does not have an adjustable examining table that automatically lowers to wheelchair height (see chapter 5), so, "Most of the time, he does my physical exam in my wheelchair. I'm not even undressed. All he does is listen to my heart and ask what's wrong." Joe Alto believes that "When they see me coming in the wheelchair, doctors say, 'That's going to be a lot of work.' Insurers don't pay extra for someone like me, so the doctor doesn't want me there." Minute by minute, "the doctor's not getting as much money for a disabled person as he's getting for someone else."

Joe Alto worries about getting short shrift from his physician—inadequate physical examinations might endanger his health. How often this happens

Table 4.4. Visits to Health Care Settings in Previous Year

Impairment	Settings[a] (Percentage with at Least One Visit [Mean Number of Visits][b])			
	Inpatient	MD Office	Clinic	PT/OT
No impairment	6.9	69.2 (4.6)	16.0 (2.9)	2.3 (8.7)
Vision impairments				
Some	14.0	79.8 (6.6)	22.2 (7.6)	3.7 (8.6)
Blind or major	15.8	68.6 (6.1)	22.0 (7.6)	2.3 (13.7)
Hearing impairments				
Some	13.5	79.4 (6.6)	24.4 (5.7)	4.4 (14.1)
Deaf or major	13.2	80.0 (5.4)	22.7 (5.7)	2.9 (9.6)
Lower extremity mobility difficulty				
Minor	19.3	36.9 (7.7)	28.4 (3.6)	9.1 (14.4)
Moderate	22.2	39.6 (9.6)	39.2 (6.7)	5.8 (8.7)
Major	37.9	90.5 (10.9)	40.4 (10.8)	7.0 (16.4)
Upper extremity mobility difficulty				
Some	27.5	87.5 (9.2)	37.3 (6.6)	11.1 (15.6)
Major	29.4	90.8 (10.2)	33.7 (4.6)	5.3 (14.6)
Difficulties using hands				
Some	23.2	84.2 (11.0)	34.6 (4.3)	7.7 (11.9)
Major	37.2	88.0 (12.2)	40.6 (12.6)	7.9 (20.2)
Any impairment	17.5	81.2 (7.2)	26.3 (5.2)	5.1 (12.1)
Any major impairment	25.6	82.5 (9.1)	32.8 (7.5)	5.1 (15.3)

Data source: 2001 Medical Expenditure Panel Survey.

[a]PT/OT = physical therapist or occupational therapist office-based practice.

[b]Mean number of visits calculated only for persons with at least one visit; figures account for age category and sex.

is unclear, and no one knows exactly how much more time or money it costs clinicians to see patients like Joe Alto in their offices. In 2001, almost 880.5 million clinician office visits occurred in the United States, and many visits involved patients who probably have mobility limitations: musculoskeletal conditions prompted more than 90.4 million office visits, with neurological disorders causing over 25.1 million and falls almost 12.6 million visits (Cherry, Burt, and Woodwell, 2003, pp. 22, 28). Average visit lengths were likely too brief to accommodate fully many patients with major mobility difficulties—as well as multiple or complex conditions or disabilities requiring extra time for appropriate accommodation. Almost 62 percent of 2001 office visits lasted fifteen or fewer minutes, with another 32 percent consuming sixteen to thirty minutes.[6] Even for "healthy" persons, fifteen-minute visits leave little time for comprehensive exchanges between patients and clinicians.

To receive fee-for-service payments for individual office visits, Mr. Alto's primary care physician must submit a claim to Medicare or another insurer listing an Evaluation & Management (E&M) code indicating the level (from five possible levels) of the visit. Clinicians chose the E&M code that matches the extent of the clinical history, physical examination, review of body systems, and time spent discussing clinical concerns. However,

> reimbursement for routine primary care visits is insufficient for the care of many with chronic conditions, as care for this population usually takes a considerable amount of time, particularly when self-management and multiple conditions are addressed. . . . These [E&M] codes fail to adequately reflect the additional complexity and time requirements associated with care for many beneficiaries with chronic conditions. (Eichner and Blumenthal, 2003, pp. 30–31)

Arcane aspects of Medicare's physician reimbursement policies pose additional complexities.[7] Throughout the early 2000s, cuts in fees raised questions about whether physicians would continue accepting Medicare patients. Medicaid, which historically paid lower fees than Medicare, already faced this problem: "In 2002, only 39.4 percent of [physicians] were accepting all new Medicaid patients, down from 48.1 percent three years earlier" (Iglehart, 2003, p. 2143). Unfortunately, Davey Sutton's difficulties finding a physician who takes Medicaid are all too common.

Paying for a Year of Care

The primary alternative to fee-for-service involves paying single lump sums per person ("per capita"), generally covering all care within a given year. This approach started with the prepaid group practices of the 1940s, evolving by the 1970s into health maintenance organizations (HMOs) and by the 1990s into managed care organizations (MCOs). In 2001, 15.6 percent of Medicare beneficiaries enrolled in MCOs (Centers for Medicare and Medicaid Services [CMS], 2002, p. 8). By 2002, approximately 40 percent of Medicaid recipients, more than 15 million persons, participated in prepaid health plans, although this practice varied widely by state (Hurley and Somers, 2003, p. 77).

Models of managed care change constantly. Nonetheless, one defining feature of managed care is having "explicit criteria for selecting providers and financial incentives for members to use network providers, who generally must cooperate with some form of utilization management" (Institute of Medicine, Committee on the Consequences, 2001, p. 146). Medicare beneficiaries with disabilities in managed care are significantly happier with their costs than those with fee-for-service Medicare, although elderly disabled managed care enrollees report much lower satisfaction with specialist referrals (Iezzoni et al., 2002, p. 378).

On the positive side, managed care insurers can plan ahead, possibly offering benefits beyond those in fee-for-service. Thus, managed care could theoretically help people with disabilities by improving "continuity and coordination across a continuum of services" (Institute of Medicine, Committee on Assessing, 1997, p. 184). By anticipating health care needs, plans could enhance overall quality and efficiency for people requiring multiple complex services. One study found that Medicare HMO enrollees with disabilities were much more likely than counterparts in traditional fee-for-service to have a usual source of care and less likely to delay seeking care (Beatty and Dhont, 2001).

Persons with disabilities generate higher average costs during the year than do others: Annual average costs for aged Medicare beneficiaries total $10,209, compared with $12,961 for disabled beneficiaries younger than sixty-five (Riley, Lubitz, and Zhang, 2003, p. 78); beneficiaries age sixty-five and older who originally entered Medicare because of disability have 43 percent higher total annual costs than otherwise comparable beneficiaries (Pope et al., 2000, p. 106). Therefore, to entice managed care plans to enroll persons with disabilities, purchasers like Medicare and Medicaid must offer capitated payments that cover these costs. One strategy involves "risk-adjusting" payments—setting capitated payments levels to account for the health of enrollees. The 1997 Balanced Budget Act stipulated that Medicare "risk adjust" capitation payments starting January 1, 2000. Beginning in 2000, however, managed care plans left Medicare in droves, partially driven by fears that risk-adjusted payments would not cover their costs.

When managed care plans depart Medicare, their enrollees must find another insurer, often in increasingly limited marketplaces. Judi Pitt is blind and has Medicare via Social Security Disability Insurance (SSDI). She joined a Medicare MCO, hoping to get prescription drug benefits. Ms. Pitt is the prototypical beneficiary that MCOs, with their broader benefits, would attract. She is also precisely who MCOs would want to avoid without more generous Medicare reimbursement. During recent years, Judi Pitt's MCOs have left Medicare, forcing her to scramble for new coverage and physicians:

> I've had three different insurance plans for three consecutive years.
> Every time I get used to one doctor and let him know my problems,
> then I get another insurance change. And unfortunately, those same
> doctors are not always on that list of doctors for the new health plan.
> So I'm constantly changing doctors. If you're a complicated case,
> once the doctor's read your chart for the first or second time, then
> you're on to another insurance—you're canceled again! Each time
> I'm canceled, I have to go and search out a plan myself and then try
> to find out: (A) is my primary care physician in this plan? (B), is my

eye doctor in this plan? and (C), do I have to find new doctors and start all over?

Judi Pitt's current MCO covers prescription drugs but only for $1,000 per year: "As of today [early September], I've used up the total $1,000. For the rest of the year, I have to pay out-of-pocket for all my medications. Eye medications cost a lot."[8] While changing plans and providers poses problems for everyone, Judi is blind. She must find a physician with offices near her home or public transportation (see below), and one who is comfortable and adept at communicating with blind patients.

Setting annual payment amounts for MCO enrollees like Judi Pitt presents complicated policy and technical questions. As an overall summary, no payment approach yet accounts for functional impairments that are not adequately captured by diagnostic labels. Therefore, current reimbursement policies fail to attract "risk-adverse" health plans to enroll persons whose costs will likely exceed their payments. Getting physicians to accept patients with managed care presents another hurdle. In 2001, only 59 percent of physicians accepted patients in private capitated plans (Cherry, Burt, and Woodwell, 2003, p. 37).

Costs of Accommodating Disabilities

The Americans with Disabilities Act (ADA) requires that clinical services be accessible to persons with disabilities (see chapter 2). However, when physicians make specific accommodations for visits of individual patients with disabilities, they cannot collect additional fees. The ADA prohibits clinicians from charging patients extra for these accommodations, and health insurers do not pay higher amounts to cover them. These legal and financial factors generate competing incentives, sometimes entangling patients and compromising their quality of care. The hiring of American Sign Language (ASL) interpreters is a case in point.

ASL is a linguistically complete language, fundamentally different from English. It is the native language of many Deaf persons in the United States and English-speaking parts of Canada (box 4.1). For many persons educated in Deaf schools, ASL is their first and primary language. Similarly to many of the world's languages, ASL has no written form. In addition to hand shapes, facial expressions and hand and body movements through space are essential elements of ASL vocabulary and grammar for sighted persons.[9] For individuals who are deaf and blind, such as Lettie, sign language is primarily tactile, as speakers make hand shapes and other movements touching her palms and fingers to convey information (figure 4.1).

The ADA requires "public accommodations" to treat persons with and without disabilities similarly, unless doing so poses an undue burden. This

---

Box 4.1. American Sign Language (ASL)

Linguistically Distinct from English

ASL is not English translated into hand signals. ASL is a visual language, in which hand and body movements and facial expressions all help convey grammatical information. While English is a "subject-prominent" language (sentences generally start with the subject), ASL is "topic prominent" (sentences typically start with the topic).

Sign Languages Vary

Sign language is not universal; for instance, British Sign Language differs significantly from ASL. Worldwide, many populations have developed their own native sign languages, and as with other languages, sign languages change and evolve over time. Even within the United States, certain ASL hand shapes and vocabulary terms vary across regions. ASL shares many vocabulary terms with Old French Sign Language because of the legacy of Laurent Clerc, a French Deaf man who brought French Sign Language to the United States in the nineteenth century.

Learning ASL

Learning to communicate easily and effectively in sign language takes as long as one needs to learn other languages. Universities, community colleges, schools for the Deaf, and other educational programs offer ASL courses. Learning directly from Deaf teachers and immersion in the Deaf Community give the most authentic introduction to ASL. People can learn to sign English grammar and word order—so-called SEE (Signed Exact English) or MCE (Manually Coded English)—but these are not natural languages and differ fundamentally from ASL.

Sources: Steven Barnett, personal communication, December 22, 2004; Danielle Suzanne Ross, personal communication, December 22, 2004; National Association of the Deaf, American Sign Language, www.nad.org, accessed December 22, 2004.

---

can require use of "auxiliary aids and services," like sign language interpreters, to ensure "effective communication" (see box 13.1). Although patients' preferences for auxiliary aids or communication strategies should receive primary consideration, physicians and other providers ultimately have the authority to determine what constitutes effective communication. The ADA does not require insurance payments to cover interpreter costs. Fur-

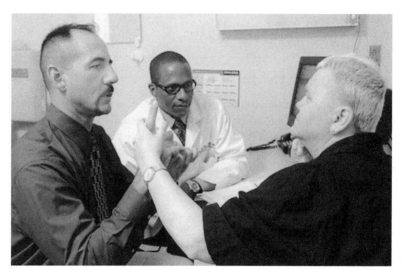

Figure 4.1. Tactile sign language communication. When Lettie, who is deaf and blind, visited her orthopedic surgeon, the sign language interpreter facilitated communication using hand shapes and other movements while touching Lettie's upraised hands, palms, and fingers.

thermore, providers cannot charge individual patients for this expense. In some instances, sign language interpreter fees exceed health insurance reimbursement for the visit. As one physician wrote:

> I can tell you in a nutshell why physicians are not using paid interpreters to see their deaf patients. For a [E&M code] level II visit for a deaf patient who has Medicare, total reimbursement in my geographic area is only $26.46. An interpreter costs $25 per hour with a 1-hour minimum. With an office overhead of a little over 50 percent, I lose money every time I see that patient. (Kulback, 1995, p. 795)

Hiring sign language interpreters for every encounter with deaf patients is neither necessary nor desirable (see chapter 13). Other strategies, like writing notes or typing on a computer or text messaging device, may provide effective and acceptable communication in many instances. Nonetheless, legal experts caution physicians against using communication strategies that their patients perceive as ineffective. Courts have held physicians legally liable for failing to ensure adequate communication, especially when medical injury ensues (e.g., because patients do not understand treatment regimens, potential side effects of therapies, or need for follow-up care). State boards of medicine can discipline physicians for failing to meet ADA requirements.

Several deaf women in our focus group recounted the complex calculus they make when choosing a physician, balancing ease of communication against other factors. Julianne Stone goes "to a certain doctor in Blustery Bluffs with whom I've had a thirteen-year relationship, and I communicate by writing. It's more difficult to do that with someone I don't know. They complain about the cost of having to pay for the interpreter. But it's a private practice. I'd rather not go to a large institution." Julianne knows that, if she travels to a large Boston teaching hospital practice, they would likely provide a medical ASL interpreter, but she fears becoming anonymous in a big facility. "I want to be able to communicate about myself and have someone meet my needs. My doctor does that."[10]

Julianne Stone is satisfied with her trade-off, willingly writing notes with a physician she likes but realizing communication might be better with an interpreter. In contrast, Carmen Valdez wanted an ASL interpreter, but "the doctor refused to get one. I asked them to please call the Massachusetts Commission for the Deaf and Hard of Hearing for the interpreter, and they told me *I* had to do it. I explained to them in a friendly way that the doctor had to pay for the interpreter, and they got angry with me. This happened with my dentist, too. My dentist refused to pay for the interpreter. He said that I had to pay."

When Carmen's physician finally did get the interpreter, waits and delays caused more problems, ultimately increasing costs. "The secretary in the waiting room said I was scheduled last. I say, 'No, you should take me first. The interpreter has to leave for another appointment.' But they wouldn't move me up on the list, so I had to wait." Maybe her physician thought that Carmen's appointment would run over time, delaying other patients. The interpreter did have to leave before her appointment, and since interpreters typically charge by the hour, Carmen's physician paid for unused time. No one compensated Carmen for *her* wasted time.

The ASL interpreter situation provides a clear-cut example of fundamental structural problems within the health care system (see chapter 1) and represents a specific instance of the more general concern voiced by Joe Alto above: that payments do not adequately reimburse accommodations needed by many people with disabilities. Sometimes these accommodations do not require equipment, building renovations, or additional personnel—they can be as simple as additional time. As one man who is hard of hearing said, "Because we're hard of hearing, the first thing we want is to slow things down, take our time. But the doctor tends to go through a checklist real fast." Akysha Nanuet, who is deaf, recounted an excellent experience when her physician hired an ASL interpreter and then took extra time:

> Once we got into the doctor's office, we did introductions, and communication was at the right pace. It was wonderful; it was clear. I could sign whatever I wanted to say, and if the interpreter was confused by medical terms, she stopped me, and I wrote down the medical thing. So often it's "hurry up, get in and get out." This doctor

took the time to explain everything to me, and I was pleasantly amazed.

But in busy practices, as elsewhere, time is money, and insurers do not pay for the extra time, let alone the ASL interpreter.

Finding Willing Clinicians

People often ask me why more practices don't specialize in caring for persons with disabilities. On many levels, such specialty practices make perfect sense. Knowledgeable clinicians, practicing in completely accessible facilities with appropriate equipment and effective communication strategies, seem logical and necessary. However, as suggested above, I can respond in one word: money. Under standard payment policies, practices that see disproportionate numbers of persons with physical and sensory disabilities will almost certainly lose money; likely, lots of money.

Nationwide, a handful of programs have developed specializing in services to persons with disabilities (Blanchard and Hosek, 2003). Common threads linking many of these programs include dedicated clinicians committed to caring for persons with disabilities; effective advocacy by local disability rights organizations; and special funding arrangements, primarily philanthropy (e.g., from foundations, disease-specific advocacy groups, or large health care institutions) as well as partnerships with payers, such as customized contracts with Medicaid. These programs typically rely heavily on nonphysicians, such as nurse practitioners, and providing care in homes, especially to persons with significant physical impairments.

But few such programs exist. Starting new programs requires considerable capital investment to create accessible environments and acquire appropriate equipment. "In addition, many of these programs provide care to an underserved population with needs that have been largely overlooked in the past. Expanding access to such a population will result in initially high costs" (Blanchard and Hosek, 2003, pp. 23–24). Downstream savings may occur as patients receive more preventive services and wellness care that mitigate or stave off costly secondary conditions. Nonetheless, "unless risk-adjusted payments that reflect the higher treatment costs . . . are widely adopted, these programs are likely to remain small" (Blanchard and Hosek, 2003, p. xiv).

Joe Alto speculates that some physicians explicitly avoid wheelchair users, but no statistics exist on whether this actually happens or, if so, how often. One small study in western Pennsylvania found that women with disabilities had difficulties finding physicians who understood their needs or even agreed to provide care. In particular, "some physicians deny them service if they cannot, for example, mount an examination table without assistance, or even refuse to see them solely because of their disability, both of which cases are in violation of the Americans with Disabilities Act" (Blanchard and Hosek, 2003, p. 9).

Refusing to accept or treat persons solely because of their disabilities is clearly illegal, assuming that the physician has adequate technical knowledge and skills to care for such patients. Referring persons with disabilities to other clinicians is certainly appropriate and legal when an individual physician does not have sufficient knowledge about specific clinical issues. The ADA Title III Regulations provide an example pertaining to "medical specialties":

> A health care provider may refer an individual with a disability to another provider, if that individual is seeking, or requires, treatment or services outside of the referring provider's area of specialization, and if the referring provider would make a similar referral for an individual without a disability who seeks or requires the same treatment or services. A physician who specializes in treating only a particular condition cannot refuse to treat an individual with a disability for that condition, but is not required to treat the individual for a different condition. [28 CFR Part 36, Subpart C, Sec. 36.302(b)(2)]

No interviewees reported outright refusal from physicians to care for them because of their disability, with one exception: obstetrical care for pregnant women with major mobility difficulties. The stories of two women with spinal cord injuries suggest that this refusal fits into a broader societal discomfort with women wheelchair users becoming mothers. Marcia McDonough, who is paraplegic and now has a one-year-old daughter, described stinging responses to her pregnancy: "I had one friend who I considered a close friend. She feels I have really burdened my child with my disability. She sees my life as being complicated enough, and how foolish I was to consider such a thing. We really don't speak anymore."

"When I was pregnant, I got some UTIs [urinary tract infections]," stated Caroline Patrick, who is tetraplegic[11] and whose son is now five years old. "UTIs are normal, and I was hospitalized. My obstetrician called a urologist to consult about the best way to treat these infections. When my OB told the urologist that I'm quadriplegic, he said, 'She's what, and she's having a baby? What is she doing? Why is she doing this?'"

Caroline found her obstetrician, Dr. Blackburn, through her father, who is a physician. "Dr. Blackburn is absolutely a wonderful doctor," Caroline said, describing how he called experts around the country to learn what to expect and how to handle potential complications relating to tetraplegia. "He put together an entire team to help with my care."

Marcia McDonough wasn't so lucky. She called six or seven obstetricians without finding one who would accept her into his or her practice. Marcia speculated that their unwillingness perhaps reflected not only personal prejudices but also uncertainty about the technical skills required to care safely for pregnant women with spinal cord injuries, specifically a potential complication called "autonomic dysreflexia."[12]

"I worked the normal sources," Marcia recalled, describing her efforts to find an obstetrician. "I contacted *all* the physiatrists at the major rehab hospitals in Boston and asked them to give me a referral. This went on for almost five or six months: calling, not getting called back, or their saying they would look into it, or they didn't know, or they'll call somebody who might know. And still I came up with zip, nothing. Finally, I found an OB who had delivered a couple of babies to women with spinal cord injuries. That doesn't qualify as an expert, but that was the best I could do." Ultimately, the doctor Marcia found wasn't available for her delivery; nonetheless, Marcia safely had a baby girl (see chapter 11). "I never felt the baby come out," Marcia laughed. "I had to be told she came out. I was clearly thankful for my paralysis!"

Caroline Patrick felt that her example educated at least one doctor—the urologist consulted by Dr. Blackburn for her UTI. "That urologist had the typical perception of disability," Caroline observed, "of people nonfunctioning, not working, staying home. Once he met me, he said, 'This baby is wonderful! It's a great thing.' And now he's my urologist. It's amazing how people's perceptions of disability can change once they get to know you as a person and get rid of their old conceptions."

Moving into the Adult Health Care System

Persons with disabilities from birth or early childhood, especially those with physical disabilities, confront special barriers to finding willing and knowledgeable physicians. Good estimates of how frequently this problem occurs are unavailable. Only about 2 percent of persons reporting major mobility difficulties say these limitations began at birth or early childhood (Iezzoni, 2003, p. 297). Nonetheless, persons with substantial physical impairments who, in the past, often died in infancy or childhood, increasingly live into adulthood and older age. Although exact numbers of adults with cerebral palsy remain unknown, 95 percent of children with diplegia and 75 percent of those with tetraplegia now survive into adulthood, and over the last decades many have moved from institutions into communities (Rapp and Torres, 2000, p. 466). A small survey found that 87 percent of adult women with cerebral palsy living in the community view themselves as healthy, despite their impairments (Turk et al., 1997, p. S-14).

As youths, these individuals typically receive health care from pediatricians, often within specialized clinics or facilities for children with disabilities. As they mature, they need care as adults, but few primary care physicians trained in adult medicine learn about caring for persons with early childhood impairments. Some internists feel they have insufficient knowledge to treat adults with conditions such as cerebral palsy and spina bifida and refuse to accept them as patients. Admittedly, scientific understanding of aging with these conditions has only lately increased:

> There is a growing body of literature about aging issues and secondary conditions among persons with congenital and childhood onset mobility impairments. Systematic studies of secondary conditions have only recently been initiated. . . . Much of the conventional wisdom in this area has been communicated through the network of persons with disabilities. . . . Health care providers and consumers have limited knowledge from which to base decisions regarding adult health issues and anticipated changes in function in these individuals with disabilities. (Turk and Weber, 2005, p. 1519)

Even pediatric facilities where persons with childhood disabilities have had long-term relationships often refuse to treat them once they reach a certain age. This can set adults with childhood disabilities adrift, unsure where to turn for health care services. The experiences and perceptions of Janice Jenkins exemplify this situation. In her late thirties, Janice is an attorney practicing health law in a large city. Given her profession, Janice ruefully acknowledges the irony of her dysfunctional health care situation but feels uncertain how to remedy matters. Born with spina bifida (a neural tube defect in which the bony encasement of the spinal cord does not close properly, producing paralysis[13]), she has long dealt with both disability and the health care system. Nowadays, Janice walks by leaning on two underarm crutches to support her weight while swinging her legs forward together.

"People expect us to constantly sit around pitying ourselves and feeling upset about having a disability, right?" Janice laughed. "I did all that as a small child, four or five years old. I remember being really pissed off and complaining to my mom. And she basically said, 'No, it's not fair, but that's how it is, and you have to learn to live with it. You do the best you can.' So that's really what I did."

Janice feels that perhaps the most important of countless physician encounters during her childhood occurred long before her earliest memory, when pediatricians first talked to her parents about their daughter's condition. "For kids with congenital disabilities, certainly in the old days, the way the doctor talked to your parents could make the difference between being institutionalized or not. Or it could mean life or death if the question was whether or not to treat." Janice's parents, determined that their daughter lead as "normal" a life as possible, kept her home and enrolled her in regular preschool programs. But the public elementary school refused to let her register for first grade.

"They said I was a fire hazard because I couldn't climb stairs. So I had to go to a 'special school' for three years. In terms of socialization, it was great for me. Unfortunately, in the disability world, there's this hierarchy of social acceptability. Being relatively mobile with crutches and cognitively okay, I was at the top of the little hierarchy in this special school. I was the queen bee. So it was quite a shock when I went back to regular school at age nine. I went from the top to the bottom of the totem pole, except that I was smart, which was threatening to people in a different way." (Janice felt that her public school officials never expected disabled children to be smart!)

Janice had multiple surgeries during childhood, including a shunt to prevent further hydrocephalus when she was nine months old, a urostomy to divert her urine to an external bag she empties several times daily, and numerous operations on her hips, ankles, and feet. She lived in a small town, but her parents took her to a nearby city to a special pediatric clinic for children with disabilities. Many of the physicians treated her kindly, trying to minimize her absences from school during her surgeries. Other experiences weren't so positive. "In this one clinic, they lined all us little kids with serious orthopedic problems up on these tables. The doctors would come in and go from table to table, taking five minutes with each of us." Janice felt she was one more cog in the orthopedist's assembly line.

"Through college and even law school, I stuck with the pediatricians back home," Janice admitted. "In real life, I became a grown-up and got a job, then I started looking around for an adult doctor. I don't think I did a very good job despite all my expertise and understanding. To be perfectly honest, just like everyone else in their twenties, even if you have a disability, you think you're going to live forever! Plus, I had trouble finding anyone who had a clue about what to do about my disability."

"What's happening now?" I asked.

"Since I was thirty, I've had aches and pains that you don't usually get until your forties or fifties," Janice laughed. "I've also had chronic UTIs, which are really a big problem. This late onset stuff—the UTIs, the pain—that bothers me a lot partly because I didn't expect it. It's like the dentist not telling you that the fillings aren't permanent in your teeth, and when your teeth start falling apart, you say that's not part of the bargain. I thought that if I made out okay with all my surgeries that I would be set for life. Then at age thirty my body starts to fall apart."

With the exception of one urologist, Janice still hasn't found adult doctors who seem comfortable with her spina bifida and knowledgeable about her specialized needs and clinical options. "One of my pediatricians back home used to tell me I had the ostrich syndrome, which is basically sticking my head in the sand and ignoring it all. There's some truth in that," Janice admitted. "Part of me just didn't want to deal with it." Since her chronic pain and repeated urinary tract infections started at age thirty, however, Janice has actively sought care.

"It takes an enormous investment of time and energy to make sure I get what I need and that it's not fragmented," said Janice. "This takes time away from my career and my personal life." She now sees a urologist who has carved out a niche caring for persons with disabilities within her broader urological practice. Although Janice is well educated and connected within the local health care community, she has not yet found a primary care physician to coordinate her complex care, and she still sees a pediatric orthopedist.

"Location, Location"

For many persons with disabilities, the familiar mantra driving real estate decisions—"location, location"—carries over to health care. When persons cannot drive and must rely on public transportation or their own legs (or wheelchair wheels) for getting around, location can determine selection of a health care provider.[14] Nona Tidewell, who is blind and lives in Washington, DC, depends on the Metro, the local subway system, for traveling around town: "I'm going to a doctor in DC that's accessible to a Metro station, period. So one thing I look at in choosing my insurance plan is where their doctors are."

Interviewees living in rural areas can find primary care clinicians, but often they confront waits and delays. "I called in February to get a physical," said Rick, who lives in Distant Dunes, "and they gave me an appointment for July. So you end up going to doctors in town."

"The quickest thing is to go to the emergency room," suggested Steve, another Distant Dunes resident. "But it'll cost you." This assessment is correct from both personal and societal perspectives. Emergency departments increasingly serve "as a safety net provider for vulnerable populations such as the uninsured, those on Medicaid, and minorities," with numbers of emergency department visits rising 20 percent from 1992 to 2001 (McCraig and Burt, 2003, p. 2).[15] In 2001, 9.1 percent of emergency department visits involved nonurgent conditions. But relying on emergency rooms to get routine or nonurgent care—especially if persons have complicated medical conditions underlying their disabilities—represents an inappropriate use of a costly resource and substandard care.

The largest barrier for rural residents involves gaining access to medical specialists, including dentists. Not surprisingly, few specialists practice in rural areas. Davey Sutton travels from Blustery Bluffs to Boston to see specialists, but the trip exhausts him. "I can't sit for too long because I'm in so much pain. And there aren't many bathrooms along the way that I can use."

Remedying the dearth of specialty care in rural areas will prove difficult. Understandably, specialists typically settle in densely populated areas where they can fill their practices with patients needing specialized care. But the frustrations of persons like Suzy Carlton, who has systemic lupus erythematosus causing debilitating arthritis, are also understandable. "The quality of care in Blustery Bluffs is like a Band-Aid operation. It may be years before you get the proper referral, the proper diagnosis, and the proper tests to make the diagnosis." Like Davey Sutton, she has difficulty traveling to Boston.

Suzy feels that her health problems and disabilities present enough challenges without adding the difficulty of finding doctors. Although she complains that many doctors move to Blustery Bluffs "to retire and go out on yachts," Suzy has had some luck. "My rheumatologist is superb. He opened a practice here that was going to be a part-time retirement practice. He was old when I met him, and he's still old. But we're very in tune with one another."

Getting into and around
Health Care Settings

Eleanor Peters cannot open her clinic's heavy plate glass door, and Joe Alto cannot climb onto his physician's high examining table (chapters 1 and 4). No one knows how often persons with disabilities face such physical barriers within health care facilities. More importantly, no one knows how often these barriers compromise patients' health and safety. Eleanor's heavy door poses an inconvenience but presumably has no lasting consequences. In contrast, Joe's limited physical examination could threaten his well-being, as happened to John Lonberg.

For eighteen years, John Lonberg, in his early sixties and paralyzed below his chest from a spinal cord injury, vainly urged his health care clinic to install an examining table that automatically lowers to wheelchair height. Lonberg belonged to Kaiser Permanente of California, a giant insurer and health care provider serving six million persons statewide, including forty thousand wheelchair users. Without an accessible table, Lonberg thinks his clinicians take "the easy way out and do everything while I sit in the chair. But they miss things"—notably the pressure ulcer developing on his buttocks (Glionna, 2000, p. 3). Detected perhaps a year after it began, the ulcer was infected and required surgery. Poor care seriously injured Lonberg and also made him feel invisible: "You almost feel like you've disappeared. You've fallen off their radar screen. You don't matter."

Lonberg and two other wheelchair users sued Kaiser on July 26, 2000, ten years to the day after the Americans with Disabilities Act (ADA) was signed, alleging that Kaiser failed to provide equal care to persons with disabilities. Kaiser officials responded immediately, settling out of court within nine months and promising to make significant changes throughout their facilities (see chapter 14). Kaiser's California Division president, Richard Pettingill, optimistically predicted "a ripple effect," improving physical accessibility in health care settings nationwide (Glionna, 2001, p. A1). This ripple has not yet materialized.

This chapter examines the physical barriers confronted by people with disabilities upon entering and moving around health care facilities. Before starting, we underscore two points. First, ADA regulations provide minimum standards for ensuring physical access: even when facilities are "ADA compliant," they may remain difficult to navigate. Eleanor Peters's clinic, which opened well after the ADA's passage, did not violate ADA regulations, which do not require health care facilities to install automatic openers on interior clinic doors.

Second, although building and equipping facilities for complete accessibility can cost somewhat more in the short term than ignoring accessibility concerns, long-run benefits likely outweigh these expenditures. Retrofitting doors to add automatic openers costs much more than installing them at the outset. Accessible examining tables cost roughly twice the price of standard tables, but the expense of John Lonberg's pressure ulcer surgery and subsequent rehabilitation—both to Kaiser Permanente and to Lonberg himself—probably far outstripped these differences. Chapter 14 addresses these issues further and proposes strategies for anticipating and removing the barriers described here.

Barriers

Historically, health care institutions were among the first large structures built in growing American cities. Although gleaming new buildings rise and tower above them, the cores of many inner-city hospitals date to the early twentieth century, if not the nineteenth century. Over time, many private physicians' offices, often started in homes, moved to townhouses in urban neighborhoods or small buildings without easy access. Thus, many health care settings, from major medical centers to private offices, predate legal mandates for physical access for persons with disabilities.

Even without removing barriers, altered attitudes of health care personnel can greatly improve physical access. Todd Paulson, in his forties, has witnessed significant improvements in these attitudes and public understanding of disability since his spinal cord injury twenty-two years ago:

> A nurse came by, threw a johnny [hospital gown] in my lap, and said, "Get undressed and get up on the table. I'll be back in five minutes." I didn't say anything. She came back, and I'm just sitting there in my wheelchair with the johnny in my lap. She said, "You're not ready." I said, "I can't undress myself. I need help with that and then getting up on the table." She just looked at me. That's going back at least fifteen years. That's very rare these days. Most offices are able to figure out if you're going to need help, and they're very receptive. It's important to indicate your needs to

them. Ninety-nine times out of a hundred, they're going to go and get the help.

Nevertheless, more accessible equipment would give Todd greater independence, as well as minimize the time and effort required of staff to assist him.

Physical access to health care facilities and services has undoubtedly improved over the past two decades. Despite this, many interviewees describe difficulties—large and small—with entering buildings and offices and safely getting services. In the following sections, we group these observations into categories, summarizing experiences of multiple individuals.[1] This presentation focuses on barriers, because that reflects most of what we have heard. But the good news is that solutions are generally readily at hand, although they may take thought and creativity (see part III).

Getting in the Door and up or down the Stairs

Matt Kerry, who is paraplegic, needed a urologist. "I was in the hospital with a killer urinary tract infection," Matt recalled, "and I had this urologist who helped me come up with some new ideas for urinary care. Great! So I called a few months later and made an appointment to see him. I drove out to his office—it was maybe twenty miles away—and pulled up my car. The office building had five steps, and no other way to get in. I turned right around and went home."

Even though the urologist's office building was old, Matt expected to see some physical access accommodation, most likely a ramp. As described in chapter 14, the ADA requires renovations or retrofitting for physical access but only when "readily achievable"—when required structural changes are not excessively burdensome. However, according to interviewees, efforts to improve physical access do not always succeed. For instance, ramps are sometimes too steep or cramped, without adequate room for persons to easily roll on and off. In tight spaces, sometimes "you're battling the wheelchair which is rolling backward down the ramp [pulled naturally by gravity] and trying to grip the door open."

Another common barrier at front entryways involves a second door being positioned just inside the outside door, presumably to block cold air from rushing in during the winter or hot air in the summer. Although this makes perfect sense to minimize heating and cooling costs, sometimes "there's not enough room between the first and second door for the wheelchair." Wheelchair users can get stuck in tiny vestibules, unable to maneuver to open the door they are facing.

Most wheelchair users confront such physical barriers countless times daily while navigating their communities, and they seem sanguine about anticipating problems. They just don't expect barriers at their clinicians' offices. Some are surprised, shocked, or frustrated that clinicians fail to make their buildings accessible to all potential patients. They feel that efforts to improve exterior access are minimal, at best. As one wheelchair user reported:

> I got a referral to a neurologist, but I can't get in his office. You get to his building, and there's an arrow for access. So you follow the arrow and go down behind the building along a little alleyway. You get to the back door, and there's barely enough room to pull back the door and turn in your wheelchair. Then, once you open the door, which you can barely do, there's a step that's roughly four inches deep inside. That's their idea of accessibility!

Getting around inside Health Care Facilities

Once inside health care facilities, persons with sensory and physical disabilities frequently face additional barriers. For instance, the restroom in Eleanor Peters's clinic is located at the end of an isolated corridor (figure 5.1). Not only does the door not have an automatic opener, but also because of its location and the absence of an intercom or signaling system, front desk staff cannot easily discern when Eleanor needs help getting into the restroom. Furthermore, unless they stay with her while she uses the facilities— a potentially embarrassing breach of Eleanor's privacy—staff are even less likely to know when she wishes to leave.

Myriad barriers block access within facilities, including doors without automatic openers; cumbersome door hardware (e.g., knobs rather than levers or handles); raised door sills that are difficult to roll or walk over; doors without inset windows or "lights" (textured glass), which allow persons to see if anyone is on the other side; cramped spaces and narrow corridors, without easy turning space for larger wheelchairs; inadequate lighting; inaccessible restrooms; slippery and highly polished floors; thick carpeting or flooring that is difficult to roll over; inadequate seating in waiting areas; elevators that are small or difficult to operate; and inaccessible signage. "You go into hospitals and professional medical buildings downtown, and in 2000 they still don't have room numbers in braille or raised letters," observed a woman who is blind. "You just hope you run into somebody in the hall who can assist you."

Some strategies to improve access within facilities can cost little. For instance, posting braille or raised print signage is relatively inexpensive and easy. As described in part III, training both office staff and clinicians about procedures and policies for accommodating physical access can improve access even within spaces that are not optimal.

Persons who are blind or have low vision use several strategies to assist ambulation, including white canes, sighted guides, and guide dogs (see fig-

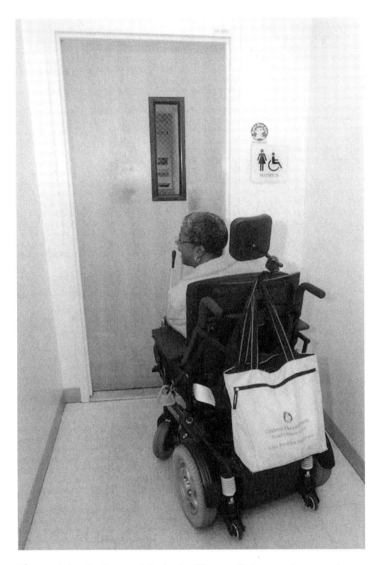

Figure 5.1. Bathroom blockade. Eleanor Peters again cannot
open a door in her clinic because it has no automatic opener. The
restroom, though, is hidden from public view, so staff members
have difficulty knowing when Eleanor requires assistance. There
is no intercom or way to signal the need for help. Fortunately, the
door does have a panel of textured glass, allowing persons inside
the bathroom to detect Eleanor sitting outside—presumably preventing them from pushing the door open and hitting her. The
raised threshold, even though slight, makes it harder for Eleanor
to roll into the restroom once someone opens the door.

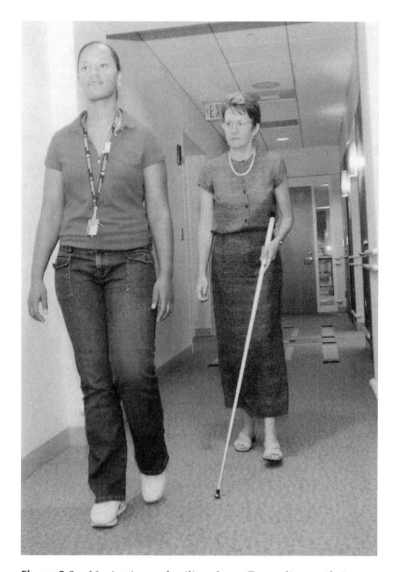

Figure 5.2.   Navigating unfamiliar places. Depending on their preferences and the situation, persons who are blind or have low vision use different strategies for navigating unfamiliar places, such as a clinic. They can walk a few steps behind a sighted guide, using a white cane or their limited vision.

ures 5.2, 5.3, and 5.4)—each demanding that staff ask patients' preferences and then respond accordingly. Service animals of various species now fulfill diverse needs, including assisting persons who are deaf or hard of hearing, persons with limited mobility, and individuals with specific health conditions, such as epilepsy (Allen and Blascovich, 1996). ADA regulations

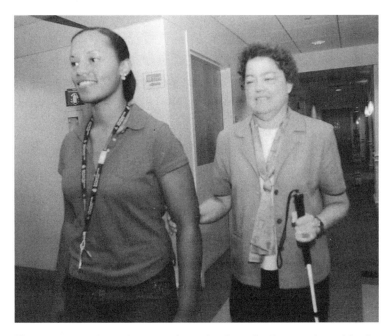

Figure 5.3. Taking the arm of a sighted guide. Doris, who is blind, walks one step behind a sighted guide, whose arm she holds lightly near the elbow.

stipulate that "generally, a public accommodation shall modify policies, practices, or procedures to permit the use of a service animal by an individual with a disability" [28 CFR Part 36, Sec. 36.302(c)(1)]. Instituting such policies does not guarantee that individual staff members will react appropriately to service animals. Although the few blind interviewees who use guide dogs reported minimal problems bringing their animals into medical facilities, some concerns did arise. While hospitalized, one blind woman missed her evening meal: upon seeing the woman's guide dog at her bedside, the food service worker delivering her tray refused to enter the room and left the tray outside without informing the supervisor. The worker, an immigrant from a culture that does not view dogs as house pets or as belonging indoors, had not received training about how to handle situations involving service animals. Nona Tidewell had one unfortunate incident:

> Most of the time I didn't have any trouble when I had a dog, but there was one doctor who flat out would not come in the room with my dog. He was just scared to death of the dog. There was nothing I could say to convince him that the dog wasn't going to jump right up and tear his throat out. I finally had to leave the dog out. The doctor wasn't letting that dog anywhere near him.

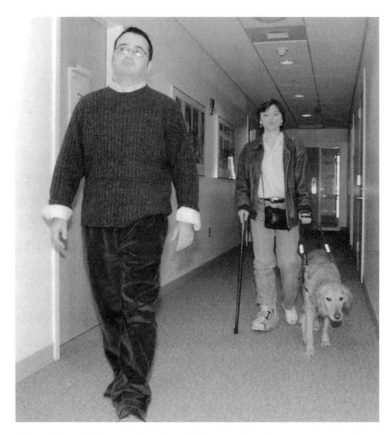

Figure 5.4. Using a guide dog. When Annie gives the command "follow," her guide dog follows a few paces behind a sighted guide. Here, Annie uses a cane to assist her ambulation: she fractured her foot while exercising at the gym and must wear a walking cast.

The physician's behavior violated the ADA, but Nona recognized that he had his own disability—uncontrollable terror of her dog.[2] Such occurrences are "so rare," said Nona.

Getting onto and off Examining Tables

Getting onto and off examining tables poses a challenge that some persons with physical impairments insist on facing independently and with aplomb. Louisa, born with spina bifida, has perfected her technique through years of frequent physician visits. Like a gymnast sizing up her approach to the vault, she positions her canes and twists her body just so, ending up seated atop the examining table in a few quick steps. However, for Louisa, as shown in figure 5.5, there's a catch. She is twenty-two weeks pregnant with her first child. Soon her pregnancy will make walking for long distances with her crutches slow and exhausting, and she anticipates moving to a manual wheelchair for the duration. Louisa certainly won't be able to spring onto fixed-height examining tables. Fortunately, her obstetrician has an examining table that lowers automatically—acquired to accommodate physical access for all women late in pregnancy, regardless of disability, but certainly a must for Louisa. (Late update: Louisa gave birth to a healthy, seven-pound boy—mom and baby are doing well!)

Many people do not have Louisa's physical strength or control. For them instead of accessible tables, clinicians often provide metal step stools or pull out small platforms from the foot of fixed-height examining tables (figure 5.5). Some interviewees find these step stools and platforms insufficient and even potentially dangerous: for example, persons with arthritis might experience considerable pain or their joints might suddenly collapse. Those with neurological conditions can have inadequate balance or strength to mount even one small step safely and twist their bodies to seated positions. Step stools or platforms may not effectively support the size or weight of obese persons.

Some persons accurately observe that they do not always need complete examinations. "If I go to my annual physical with my primary care physician," said Todd Paulson, "he's going to get me up on the table and do an appropriate physical exam. If I go in with symptoms of an upper respiratory infection, he can listen to my lungs through a stethoscope while I sit in my wheelchair." Todd, who has a college degree and professional job, feels patients should understand their needs and advocate for themselves. Some persons, however, may not have the knowledge to make such decisions or an aptitude for self-advocacy. Furthermore, making explicit requests, as did John Lonberg, does not always work.

Mounting examining tables is essential for some screening services that maximize long-term health and well-being. Persons with major mobility difficulties are less likely than others to receive certain screening services recommended by the U.S. Preventive Services Task Force, especially those requiring physical access to examining tables (table 5.1).[3] Among women eighteen to seventy-five who had not undergone hysterectomy, 81 percent without mobility difficulties received Pap smears compared with 63 percent of women with major problems (Iezzoni et al., 2000a).[4] Although multiple factors likely explain this finding, the absence of automatically adjustable examining tables poses one significant barrier (Andriacchi, 1997; Welner, 1998, 1999; Welner et al., 1999; Welner and Temple, 2004).

Pap smears need not be done in office settings. In one program specializing in women with disabilities, a trained nurse visits women in their homes and performs Pap smears as they lie in bed. Receiving Pap smears at home also spares women from traveling to physicians' offices, but it is costly. The program is struggling to find funding to continue providing services.

We also heard from the other side of the examining table—from a small, admittedly nonrepresentative group of clinicians, including practitioners *with* adjustable examining tables.[5] One physician proudly displayed his adjustable table—an ancient specimen that nonetheless still serves his patients well. This physician sees many elderly persons and individuals with long histories of diabetes who have amputations and other mobility problems. Despite its boxy appearance and faded orange plastic upholstery, his patients like the adjustable table, which allows them easier access and more independence and control.

Other physicians who practice in settings with automatically adjustable examining tables admit being uncertain how to use the equipment. Furthermore, in busy practices with multiple clinicians, scheduling specific patients for a particular room (e.g., the one room with an accessible examining table) is often logistically complicated. One physician admitted that, even when assigned a room with an accessible table, she never uses the automatic lift feature. She keeps the table fixed at a height convenient for her. "I'm busy," said the physician. "I've only got fifteen minutes per patient, and it

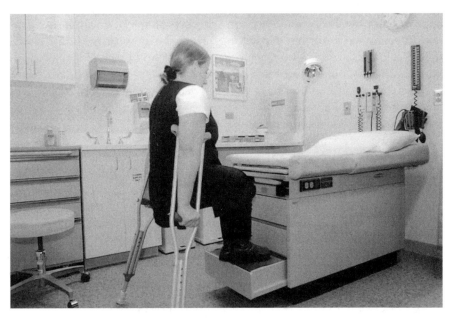

Figure 5.5.   Springing aboard. Louisa proudly demonstrates her technique for mounting fixed-height examining tables, wielding her canes and swiveling her body with athletic precision. Since she is pregnant, Louisa will soon find this complex maneuver unsafe.

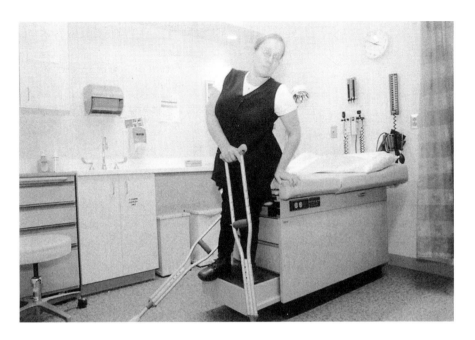

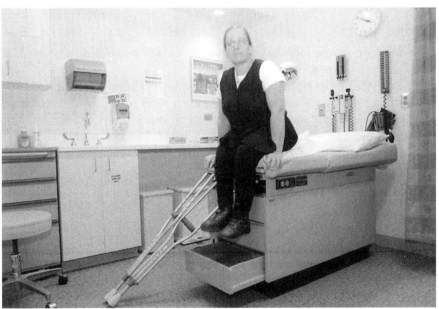

Figure 5.5. (*continued*)

Table 5.1.   Rates of Screening and Preventive Services That Require
Physical Accessibility

Service	Extent of Lower Extremity Mobility Difficulty (Percent)			
	None	Minor	Moderate	Major
"During this last check-up, did you have:				
Your height checked?	79.3	72.6	75.9	69.3
Your weight checked?	92.8	93.5	92.8	88.7
A vision test to check how well you see?"[a]	23.2	25.6	26.9	21.6
Had a Pap smear within past three years[b]	81.4	79.4	79.6	63.3
Had a mammogram within past two years[c]	63.5	58.3	51.5	45.3
Had a breast exam within past two years[d]	75.7	71.7	65.4	63.9

Adapted from: Iezzoni et al. (2000a, table 3).

[a]Asked only of persons age sixty-five and older.

[b]Asked only of women age eighteen to seventy-five years; figures only for women who did not report having had a hysterectomy.

[c]Figures for women age fifty and older.

[d]Asked only of women age thirty and older.

takes too long for the table to go up and down. My patients don't complain. They just get up on the table using a stool."

The physicians' comments highlight the importance of office practices, scheduling systems, practitioner training, and other structural factors for ensuring that accessible tables are both used and used properly. Simply having an automatically adjustable examining table does not guarantee easy or safe access for patients, as suggested by one physician's rueful story:

When I set up my practice in the community, I wanted to do things right. So I spent the extra money to buy an adjustable examining table, and I put it in a big room so that people in wheelchairs could get in and around the table. One day, a quadriplegic woman came in for a routine physical examination. I had my practice assistant help the woman get undressed and transfer onto the examining table—it all worked perfectly. The practice assistant held the patient's legs while I did her Pap smear, and as I left the room, I told the practice assistant to help the patient get off the table and dressed again. The practice assistant mustn't have heard what I said and left the room. The patient lay on that table for half an hour until someone came by the room and found her there.

Clearly, office staff must remember that persons who require help getting onto examining tables likely need help getting off.

Getting Tests and Procedures

"Every time I have a mammogram, there's a different technician," observed Suellen Mitchell, who is deaf, "and I have to go through the same spiel. When the technician leaves the room," or goes behind an opaque radiation shield, "how do I know when to hold my breath? I can't hear her tell me to hold my breath!" Halting respirations during mammography imaging limits chest wall motion that could blur the picture. "There should be a sign or some kind of visual information, like a red light for a deaf person to know when to hold her breath and for how long."

Persons with sensory and physical impairments face countless barriers to various medical tests and procedures. For individuals with physical impairments, these barriers range from difficulties getting into ophthalmologists' chairs for slit lamp examinations and glaucoma screening to mounting tables for radiological studies and magnetic resonance imaging. In addition, some tests, such as mammograms and certain X-rays, generally require patients to stand. Again, no one knows how often medical technologies and equipment are inaccessible or how frequently alternative strategies are needed to perform tests.[6] As for adjustable examining tables, accessible equipment often does exist.

As Suellen Mitchell indicates, hearing limitations demand specific communication accommodations when patients must obey instructions typically conveyed by spoken word. Particular problems arise during radiology and imaging tests when technicians disappear behind opaque protective screens or monitors without adequately instructing patients and providing accessible information, such as visual cues to communicate commands.

For some persons, accessibility concerns persist after the test, as patients are given additional instructions. "After a mammogram, they stick you in front of a video that tells you how to do breast self-exams," recounted one woman who is hard of hearing. "But the video's not captioned. So it's an absolute waste of time for me." Captions—texts of the spoken words simultaneously inset into the image on the television screen[7]—would allow persons with limited hearing to understand these instructional videos. Blind and low-vision persons also need this information in accessible formats, like large print or braille handouts, audiotapes detailing self-examination procedures, or voice-overs on videotapes describing visual images of self-examinations.

Inpatient Challenges

Jenny Hartwell uses a wheelchair because of multiple sclerosis (MS). She was hospitalized for an "exacerbation of MS—I was falling down. The bathrooms in the patient rooms are not accessible for wheelchairs; they're not big enough. So I had to go down the hall to the visitor's bathroom to wash up, to change clothes, to use the toilet." Her physician prescribed a new medication to control her muscle spasms, but Jenny thought the drug made her weak. "The next day, I went down to the visitor's bathroom and fell."

Jenny might have fallen even with a bathroom in her room, but needing to use a visitor's bathroom for all toileting activities clearly compromised her privacy and heightened the physical and psychic discomfort of being hospitalized. Jenny's situation is not unique. Patients' rooms in older hospitals, in particular, are sometimes too small for the many medical devices required by today's inpatients, such as pumps to administer intravenous medications and monitoring equipment. Having bathrooms large enough for fully accessible toilets, let alone wheelchair access and showering facilities, is seldom possible.

Nowadays, many acute care inpatients are so severely ill that they would be unable to safely shower or leave their beds or bedsides to urinate or defecate. Sponge baths, urinary catheters, bed pans, and bedside commodes substitute for independent bathing and toileting activities. Conflicts can arise when patients are capable of using a bedside commode or bathroom but need physical assistance to leave their bed and the nursing staff are either untrained, too busy, or unwilling to provide the help. Restrictive policies about who can assist patients, driven by liability concerns, exacerbate these tensions. "I used to work in a detox unit," one woman told me. "The detox program was twenty-eight days long, but there was no accessible bathroom or shower. People with disabilities weren't allowed to bring their PCAs [personal care assistants] along with them. Without their PCA's help, people wouldn't bathe for twenty-eight days."

Sometimes, persons with disabilities must enter hospitals for care that other persons ordinarily receive at home or as outpatients. Failures to listen and accommodate physical access exacerbate the anxiety of already stressful situations. Connie Wilder, in her late thirties, uses a power wheelchair because of muscular dystrophy. Connie needed a colonoscopy to determine whether she had colon cancer or worrisome polyps in her large intestine. On the day before colonoscopies, patients must swallow powerful liquids, like magnesium citrate, to "clean out" the colon (i.e., eliminate all feces) so that the colonoscope, a fiberoptic instrument inserted through the rectum, can visualize the bowel wall. Most people without mobility limitations perform bowel cleansing at home, but persons with disabilities that impede quick movement to the toilet are often hospitalized. Connie knew exactly what she required.

> I called the hospital in advance. I told them specifically what I needed: an egg-crate mattress and padded commode seat. They said there was no problem, but when I came in, they had none of it. I had to make a special trip back home to get what I needed. I brought back my PCA to train the nightshift how to transfer me. I had to bring in my own mattress and commode. I did all the work.

Help That Is Unhelpful

Sometimes efforts to make facilities physically accessible don't meet the needs of people with disabilities. "The bars in the bathroom are in the wrong place for a disabled person to transfer to the toilet," said Joe Alto, describing restroom facilities at his post-ADA clinic. "The bathroom door has a button to open going in but no button so you can get out." Buttons for automatic door openers are placed in positions such that doors swing open before the person who pushed the button can move out of the way. Signs indicating accessible routes are hung from high ceilings or in obscure locations, not easily visible to persons with mobility problems. Accessible entryways are inconveniently positioned in out-of-the-way locations or at the backs of buildings.

Steffie Giacommo, who is in her late forties and has a spinal cord injury, has watched changes in health care over the past decade. Modifications to improve accessibility have occasionally produced unexpected consequences. At her mammography center, "you would change and then go into another waiting room where you'd watch a video about breast self-exams." Recently, the facility bought an accessible mammography machine and installed it in a spacious room. "Now when I have my mammograms, they send me right to that room. I have to change in there and don't go into the big waiting room anymore. I miss out on the educational opportunities with the videotapes, and I don't get to sit with the other women and chit chat." From Steffie's perspective, much improved physical accessibility came with unwanted costs.

Are Accommodations Acceptable?

A physiatrist recently told me about her patient Maria, who had long used a wheelchair and recently developed breast cancer. The physiatrist referred Maria to a superb cancer center in their large midwestern city, but the center did not have adjustable examining tables. For Maria to receive complete physical examinations from her oncologist, nurses first helped her change into a flimsy hospital gown flapping open in the back. The nurses then summoned security guards who, holsters on hips, lifted Maria from her wheelchair onto the examining table. Embarrassed and humiliated after several such episodes, Maria refused to return to the cancer center. She could no longer bear to be lifted almost naked from her wheelchair by armed security guards.

The ADA does not stipulate precisely how patients should get onto examining tables; it only requires that patients receive equal services as other patients. By making assistance available, physicians' offices and clinics might technically meet ADA standards of accommodating persons with disabilities. In other words, having *only* high, unadjustable examining tables may not breach ADA requirements if trained office staff routinely and appropriately transfer patients onto the tables for essential clinical services.

Without trained personnel performing these transfers, patients can risk serious injury. At her women's health center, efforts to lift Samantha onto the standard-height examining table almost ended in calamity. "They didn't know how to lift me. I told them how to do it before they started, but things just fell apart. They tried to grab my arms to hold onto me, then somebody grabbed my legs. The nurse got scared and let go, then somebody else came and grabbed something. It was just a disaster!"

In contrast, Maria's transfer appeared safe, but did the cancer center breach ADA requirements by humiliating her? After all, she received the essential service—complete examinations by a skilled oncologist. Should how patients feel about their experiences determine the acceptability of alternative accommodations? It is hard to imagine health care providers explicitly sanctioning practices that outright humiliate patients. Nonetheless, anecdotal evidence suggests that these situations do occur, such as hospitalized patients with severely impaired mobility being forced to sit for hours in their feces because nurses are too busy or unsure how to transfer them to bedside commodes (Chan, 2003; Pérez-Peña and Glickson, 2003).

Sometimes, an alternative accommodation is clearly unacceptable. A geriatrician asked my advice about his office. He runs a private practice in an elegant old townhouse; many neighboring buildings, dating from the late nineteenth or early twentieth centuries, also house medical and dental practices. Patients must enter the geriatrician's charming, bow-fronted building by climbing its steep granite stairs: the building has no accessible entrance from street level. "I know my patients very well," the geriatrician explained, "and my back is good. When someone is scheduled who has trouble walking, I go outside and carry them up the stairs."

This solution—albeit well-meaning—suffers several major flaws. First, carrying patients up stairs likely endangers their safety; second, some people may view this transport as demeaning and disrespectful, crossing an immutable boundary of physical privacy; and third, the geriatrician risks his own well-being (i.e., his back may not be "good" for much longer). Carrying patients up stairs is not an acceptable alternative, and the geriatrician should seek an accessible office. Unfortunately, though, he has a five-year lease at a good price. Since his practice faces financial strains, with Medicare reimbursements failing to cover his costs, he does not have the resources to break his lease and find new, presumably more expensive, accessible quarters.

Some inappropriate accommodations could potentially compromise care. At one inner-city mammography center, which does not have wheelchair-accessible equipment, technicians routinely lift patients who cannot rise and hold them in place during their mammograms. This solution to inaccessible equipment has flaws, as does the geriatrician's strategy. Being held against a mammography machine is likely uncomfortable, as well as potentially unsafe and demeaning. Ensuring the technical quality of mammograms—and thus the ability of radiologists to make accurate readings—might sometimes prove difficult. Without adequate shielding, technicians holding patients might risk unnecessary X-ray exposure.

Two points deserve comment. First, accessible mammography equipment does exist; machines can lower to wheelchair height. The best solution is for mammography facilities to purchase accessible technologies. Second, women with disabilities are substantially less likely than other women to have mammograms as recommended. Many factors likely explain this finding including the competing demands of other complicated health problems; failure by physicians to recommend mammograms; "magical thinking" by women who believe that, with one disability, nothing else could go wrong; and patients' refusal to comply with recommendations (Welner, 1998). Women who find prior inaccessible mammograms distressing or uncomfortable are unlikely to return.

Accommodating Obesity

One woman who had a spinal cord injury almost thirty years ago jokes darkly that she weighs now what she weighed then—she hasn't been weighed since her injury, so of course she retains her youthful weight! Her clinicians do not have wheelchair-accessible scales, and none have suggested alternative approaches, like the hospital laundry room scale used by another paraplegic woman during her pregnancy.[8] Nationwide, persons with major mobility difficulties are only slightly less likely to be weighed than other persons (table 5.1). However, certain individuals with sensory and physical impairments are much more likely than others to be overweight, obese, and extremely obese (table 5.2).

Being unable to exercise for whatever reason, including disability, certainly contributes to obesity.[9] However, obesity itself is profoundly disabling, especially when persons weigh three hundred or more pounds. Extreme obesity can cause problems accessing and getting around health care settings—and even leaving home. Elsie Friar, in her early fifties, participated in our focus group by telephone because she cannot leave her home without substantial effort:

> I weigh about six hundred pounds, and my accessibility is not great.
> I have trouble getting through doors that are made for normal
> weight people. For the last few years, I've been pretty much stuck in
> my room. Not that I don't love my little room, but I know it would
> be much better for me health wise if I could get out more. I'd like to
> exercise. My mind is atrophying, and I'd like to go back to school.
> But doing things like that are only a dream right now.

Table 5.2. Overweight and Obese

	Weight Categories[a] (Percent[b])			
Impairment	Normal	Overweight	Obese	Extremely Obese
No impairment	40.5	35.4	19.4	2.5
Vision impairments				
Some	36.2	37.3	20.1	4.7
Blind or major	41.9	26.0	27.3	4.1
Hearing impairments				
Some	35.7	30.7	28.0	4.6
Deaf or major	31.9	38.4	22.8	2.1[c]
Lower extremity mobility difficulty				
Minor	27.2	36.5	26.7	6.6
Moderate	25.8	29.6	31.9	11.4
Major	29.7	30.3	28.2	9.6
Upper extremity mobility difficulty				
Some	26.4	39.1	25.2	7.6
Major	43.8	23.3	23.1	8.4
Difficulties using hands				
Some	30.3	30.4	27.1	9.7
Major	31.9	34.0	24.6	6.7
Any impairment	33.0	33.9	25.1	6.1
Any major impairment	32.4	30.6	27.3	6.9

Data source: 2001 Medical Expenditure Panel Survey.

[a]Normal weight = 18.5–24.9 kg/m^2; overweight = 25.0–29.9 kg/m^2; obese = 30.0–39.9 kg/m^2; extremely obese = 40+ kg/m^2.

[b]Percentages do not total to 100 because underweight individuals are excluded; figures account for age category and sex.

[c]Because of the small number of respondents, this estimate may be unreliable.

Elsie is currently battling her health insurer to obtain a hospital bed that automatically raises and lowers: otherwise, she has trouble getting in and out of bed. Not surprisingly, inaccessible medical equipment also poses enormous problems, but first she needs to get to medical facilities.

> Both my mother and grandmother on my maternal side had breast cancer. Up until this year, I've managed to get to this place where you can sit and get mammograms. This year, I just can't do it any more. I can't physically deal with the whole process; all the doors are way too small. Slowly, a lot of things I've clung onto every year have gone by the board. I didn't get a Pap smear this year, and I

have gum disease now but I can't get to the dentist. It's disheartening how I can't take care of my body because of difficulties getting access.

Elsie Friar's many dilemmas seem heartbreaking and extreme, but her situation is increasingly common. As rates of obesity skyrocket, health care facilities must care for growing numbers of persons who simply do not fit into standard bathrooms, operating room beds, gurneys, X-ray machines, ambulances, wheelchairs, blood pressure cuffs, waiting room chairs, and countless other devices and physical structures. Even facilities designed specifically for extremely obese persons, like centers performing bariatric or gastric bypass surgery, sometimes fail to provide safe and comfortable access. At one busy center, a toilet broke from the wall when a patient sat upon it. This accident undoubtedly humiliated the patient and generated considerable costs for the facility, which now needed to repair and substantially reinforce its plumbing fixtures.

Specialized equipment can accommodate extremely obese patients, but the costs are high. One hospital's obesity program bought a bed that contains a scale and can tip patients to standing positions; the price ($18,500) was five times that of standard motorized hospital beds (Pérez-Peña and Glickson, 2003, p. A13). The hospital purchased an oversize wheelchair for almost $2,500, eight times more than standard wheelchairs, and an operating room table for $30,414, almost twice the usual cost. Having the right equipment, though important, is only one step toward accommodating physical access. As in other contexts, staff must know how to use it.

Henry Ashley, who weighs 441 pounds but used to be much bigger, said that in one of his many hospital stays, he fell while trying to use a commode that was too small, broke his tailbone, and herniated a spinal disk. He described spending 14 hours on the floor while hospital workers tried to figure out how to lift him back into his bed. The hospital had a motorized device called a Hoyer lift that uses a sling to raise patients—prices start around $4,000—but, he said, no one there knew how to use it (Pérez-Peña and Glickson, 2003, p. A13).

Patients as Access Advocates

A recurrent refrain throughout our interviews was disbelief, consternation, and frustration that health care facilities—of all public accommodations—would not recognize, anticipate, and meet the needs of patients with disabilities. With ADA regulations on the books for more than a decade, why do so many physical barriers to care persist? "There's no enforcement," concluded one woman. "There's not enough advocacy." Nonetheless, demanding accommodations often does not work. Joe Alto decided to learn about the ADA so he could speak with greater authority: "If you tell doctors you want reasonable accommodations, they'll think you know what you're talking about, and they'll help you undress and do what has to be done."

Joe's strategy can carry risks. I asked one focus group if any participants mention the ADA when they encounter barriers. When she raises the ADA, Samantha finds that people "get very standoffish and almost offended, like, 'How dare you mention something like that?' It's like you are threatening them."

"People tend to get defensive," Caroline agreed. "They presume that you must be a bitter old bag."

"Well phrased!" laughed Marcia. "They really do get their backs up."

Interviewees recognize that it doesn't need to be this way—strategies do exist to make health care accessible. Over time, as older buildings are abandoned or renovated and new facilities built, presumably access will gradually improve. Interviewees find this slow pace unacceptable: they need access to health care now. They worry that competing priorities for constrained health care resources will stymie progress toward improving disability access. "There's technology for almost everything out there," said one man. "But unfortunately, the cost—how it looks on the ledger sheets—is one big problem."

Connie Wilder, though, won't accept that argument. "They should build hospitals and offices right in the first place," she says. "Being accessible is just the cost of business in health care." With the aging population and growing numbers of persons with functional limitations, Connie is right. Accessible facilities and equipment make getting health care easier for patients, as well as assist clinical staff to provide essential services, such as complete physical examinations. In the long run, health care quality can only improve, perhaps even with decreasing costs.

Challenges to Interpersonal Communication

For me, quality care is knowing that the doctor is really good technically but also is willing to take the time to communicate with me and explain what's happening every step of the way. Sometimes you get one and not the other. If you get both together, that's perfect.

—Marta Redding

Virtually all aspects of health care quality—from the safety of technical interventions to a sense of trust—build upon patient-clinician communication. At its most basic level, we define communication as "the transmission of information, thoughts, and feelings so that they are satisfactorily received or understood" (Daley, 1993, p. 73). However, this simple definition belies the sometimes torturous complexities of communication between human beings. Even when one conversational partner is a health care professional, trained explicitly to elicit, evaluate, and efficiently process information from another person, countless factors can disrupt communication. Mismatches of age, gender, culture, language, education, income, belief, social standing, and expectations can cause seemingly straightforward words to become barriers to complete and open communication. Adding complex medical terminology to this mix further heightens communication barriers.

Donabedian (1980) recognized two broad dimensions of health care quality: technical and interpersonal. Technical quality represents the application of medical science and technologies in ways that maximize the benefits to health while not simultaneously raising the risks. Interpersonal quality encompasses a range of attributes, including fulfilling patients' expectations, values, and aspirations and meeting professional ethical standards. Empathy and understanding—of clinicians for patients—foster interpersonal communication quality.

Generally called the *science* and *art* of clinical practice, respectively, technical and interpersonal dimensions of care frequently interact. "It is easy to see how the interpersonal relationship can influence the nature and success of technical management. One could also plausibly suggest that the nature of the technical procedures used and the degree of their success will influence the interpersonal relationship" (Donabedian, 1980, p. 4). Communication bridges these technical and interpersonal dimensions. Making accurate diagnoses and safely administering treatments require open and complete communication, as does ensuring that therapeutic goals match patients' desires. Good communication is essential to patient centeredness—respect for and responsiveness to individual patients' preferences, needs, and values (Institute of Medicine, Committee on Quality, 2001).

Disability can complicate communication. On a purely mechanistic level, sensory impairments, such as limited vision and hearing and cognitive and physical difficulties with choosing words and speaking, can affect the pace, nature, and content of discourse. As Marta Redding, who is hard of hearing, said, "Because you can't hear everything, you're sort of in a no-man's land of not knowing exactly what's happening." But many other factors also impede patient-clinician communication. For persons with hearing loss like Marta, two broad sets of barriers hamper effective communication—personal and environmental (figure 6.1). Personal factors include the attributes and attitudes of persons with hearing deficits and health care professionals; environmental factors encompass inhospitable physical environments, inadequate communication accommodations, and health care system problems. All aspects of these complex interactions occur within a broader societal context in which oral communication dominates explicit person-to-person interactions. Similar sets of barriers impair communication between clinicians and persons with other sensory and physical disabilities.

Such barriers can affect not only interpersonal relationships but also can compromise technical quality of care. Although clinicians are unlikely to consciously communicate dangerous health-related information to patients with disabilities, clinicians' complex attitudes or misperceptions about disability may result in the transmittal of incomplete or biased information or advice. According to Marta, "Doctors tell me that I don't have to worry about whether antibiotics are ototoxic." Marta thinks that her physicians feel that, since her hearing is already impaired, it doesn't matter if she takes medications that can potentially cause additional hearing loss. She now investigates every medication her physicians prescribe to learn about potential side effects.

This chapter and the following two address different aspects of communication. These chapters draw heavily upon what interviewees told us, so we make a disclaimer up front. Our interviewees may be more outspoken than average patients—more likely to perceive or comment upon communications lapses. Many persons with comparable disabilities in similar situations may hesitate to raise such concerns or may be satisfied with their experiences. In particular, persons from other cultures and traditions may have very different perceptions. As in other aspects of clinical care, some patients proactively self-advocate while others do not. However, ensuring patient-

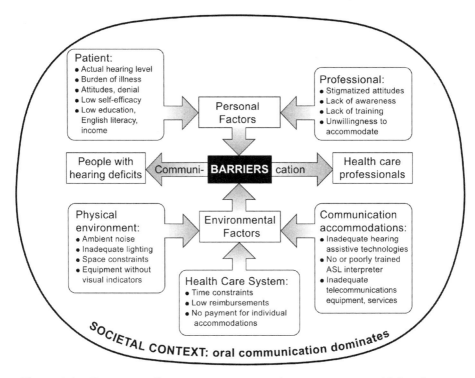

Figure 6.1. Barriers to effective communication between persons with hearing loss and health care professionals.

centered care requires that clinicians seek to understand the values and preferences of all patients, even those who are more reticent. This requires diligent, comprehensive, and sensitive patient-clinician communication. The interviewees' observations offer useful cautions about how disability can sometimes influence this communication.

The rest of this chapter concentrates on interpersonal aspects of communication and examines interactions about sexuality, mental health, and substance use—topics carrying sensitivities perhaps exacerbated by the overlay of disability. Chapter 7 explores communication etiquette during physical examinations, interactions with office staff, and telecommunications concerns, while chapter 8 focuses on technical communication about clinical topics. We start here by reviewing briefly general research findings about patient-clinician communication.

Communication Matters

Ensuring good communication between clinicians and patients goes well beyond a cosmetic or "warm and fuzzy" concern. More than fifty years of research show that good communication enhances clinical outcomes, such as improving blood pressure control and reducing medication side effects, as well as patients' comfort with their treatments and health care experiences. Some patients value interchanges that build patient-clinician relationships, confidence, and trust more highly than clinicians' technical competence (Mechanic and Meyer, 2000).

Good communication is not easy, requiring "not only a great deal of time but also very hard effort and skill on the part of physicians" (Thomas, 1974, p. 32). Entire textbooks offer instruction on these skills, training clinicians how to become careful and empathetic listeners and to understand how illness experiences fit into and shape patients' lives (Cassell, 1985a, 1985b; Stewart and Roter, 1989; Rollnick, Mason, and Butler, 1999). Most studies of patient-clinician communication have examined specialists or primary care physicians, demonstrating that physicians' characteristics and beliefs can influence communication. For instance, compared with male physicians, female physicians are more likely to inquire about patients' feelings and emotions, address psychological and social aspects of patients' conditions, use positive and supportive conversational styles, and actively seek patients' input (Roter, Hall, and Aoki, 2002). However, patients of female physicians are not necessarily happier with their care than those visiting male doctors (Schmittdiel et al., 2000).[1]

Physicians typically control the topics addressed during office visits. In one study, 32 percent of outpatient primary care visits focused narrowly on biomedical topics, while 33 percent included very limited discussions of psychological or social issues (Roter et al., 1997, p. 352).[2] Primary care physicians with more positive attitudes toward psychosocial issues make more statements conveying emotion, such as empathy and concern, and develop more collaborative relationships with their patients (Levinson and Roter, 1995).

Both patients and clinicians can influence how much the other communicates. By asking questions and expressing concerns, patients can elicit more information from clinicians than they otherwise might provide (Street et al., 2003). However, physicians report more difficulties communicating with patients whom they perceive as untrustworthy, manipulative, or noncompliant (Levinson et al., 1993). The value individual patients place on communication varies based on their sense of control, coping styles, desire for information, and expectations about the future. Compared with younger persons, elderly individuals generally ask fewer questions, interrupt their physicians less often, and express fewer opinions (Stewart et al., 2000). Elderly persons also are more likely to give socially desirable responses, exhibit gratitude, and avoid complaints. Persons who are middle-aged, female, and better educated are typically more assertive and expressive during medical encounters than elderly, male, and less educated individuals (Street et al., 2003). Persons who rate their overall health as fair or poor participate less during their health care visits than those reporting excellent or very good health (Kaplan et al., 1995).[3]

Race and ethnicity of both patients and clinicians can influence communication. Some, albeit not all, studies suggest that "racial concordance" (i.e., where patients and clinicians share the same race or ethnicity) can generate higher patient satisfaction, involvement during office visits, and use of routine preventive services (Cooper-Patrick et al., 1999; Saha et al., 1999). Health-related expectations and perceptions can differ systematically by race or ethnicity. When asked whether "recovery from illness requires good medical care more than anything else," 60 percent of whites agree with this assertion, as do 78 percent of black and Latino respondents and 87 percent of Asians (Murray-García et al., 2000, p. 305).[4] According to some studies, racial and ethnic minorities say their physicians invite them to participate in decision-making about their care less often than do white patients (Cooper-Patrick et al., 1999; Johnson et al., 2004).

Approximately one fourth of adult Americans are not functionally literate, and this group experiences communication difficulties on multiple levels, especially with medical vocabulary (Williams et al., 2002, p. 384). Roughly half of adult Americans have deficient reading and computational skills, such as those required to read a bus schedule or enter background information on a Social Security application (Parker, Ratzan, and Lurie, 2003, p. 148). "Health literacy may also be more reliant on domains of literacy such as oral (speaking) ability and aural (listening) comprehension that are not measured . . . [by] the tools currently used to measure health literacy" (Institute of Medicine, Committee on Health Literacy, 2004, p. 66). Compared with others, persons with low health literacy are less likely to obtain routine preventive and screening services, such as mammograms, Pap smears, and influenza or *pneumococcal* pneumonia immunizations (Berkman et al., 2004, p. 6). Inadequate health literacy is associated with worse glycemic control and higher rates of retinopathy among persons with type 2 diabetes (Schillinger et al., 2002). Poor health literacy also compromises patients' abilities to participate actively in their care and become effective self-managers (see chapter 11).

Few studies have explicitly examined communication between clinicians and patients with specific functional impairments. We examined satisfaction among Medicare beneficiaries with aspects of care relating to communication (Iezzoni et al., 2002, 2003), and the vast majority, regardless of disability, are happy with interpersonal aspects of their care (table 6.1). Nevertheless, persons with sensory and physical impairments report problems roughly twice as often as do persons without disabilities. In particular, more persons with disabilities express concerns that physicians seem hurried and do not explain medical problems. Such communication lapses can seriously compromise patient-clinician relationships. Patients who report that their physicians "do not always take enough time to answer questions" or "do

Table 6.1. Medicare Beneficiaries' Concerns about Interpersonal Aspects of Care (Percent[a])

Aspect of Care	No DA[b]	Very Low Vision	Deaf/HOH[b]	Major Difficulties		
				Walking	Reaching	Grasping
"Concern of doctors for overall health rather than just for an isolated symptom of disease"[c]	3.6	9.9	8.5	8.7	8.7	11.0
"Doctor often seems to be in a hurry"	11.6	18.3	18.7	17.9	17.9	15.8
"Doctor often does not explain medical problems"	7.1	14.2	12.9	14.7	15.3	16.7
"Doctor often acts as though doing you a favor by talking to you"	4.7	9.8	9.3	8.5	9.2	8.8
"Doctor tells all you want to know about your condition and treatment"[c]	5.4	10.2	9.6	11.0	11.1	11.6
"Doctor answers all your questions"[c]	2.5	6.4	4.8	6.1	6.3	5.9

Adapted from: Iezzoni et al. (2002, 2003).

[a]Figures account for age category and sex.

[b]DA = disability; HOH = hard of hearing; grasping = grasping and writing.

[c]Percentage dissatisfied with doctor's concern or communication.

not provide sufficient information" are likely to consider changing doctors (Keating et al., 2002).

Aspects of twenty-first century medicine heighten the urgency of open and clear communication between clinicians and patients with disabilities. Technological advances have fundamentally altered the anticipated end-points of many conditions. Largely because of antibiotics, for example, persons with spinal cord injuries now can live for decades. With improved treatments, illnesses that once rapidly caused death, such as certain cancers, cardiovascular diseases, and human immunodeficiency virus infections, can last for years. According to physician educator Eric J. Cassell,

> The basic struggle in chronic disease *is not against death; it is against disability.* . . . Of course, people die from chronic disease, but disability—the loss of function and independence—has always come first and marked their lives. Keep in mind multiple sclerosis, severe strokes, Tay Sachs disease, many cancers, and Alzheimer's disease. In considering these diseases personally and professionally, it is not the deaths of these patients that we find so awful but their lives. . . . There has been a natural presumption since antiquity that death is the worst fate. In the modern era we know more awful futures than death, and they are all related to disability. (1997, pp. 22–23)

Such perceptions are troubling and carry huge implications for patient-clinician communication. Certainly, severe physical and cognitive impairments can profoundly compromise quality of life, but who makes the ultimate judgments: persons living those lives or clinicians? Disagreements between clinicians and patients about the basic value and quality of patients' lives could irrevocably erode patients' trust in their clinicians, destroying the bedrock foundation of communication. Ruth Moore, whose "crumbling" spine posed risks of complete paralysis, worried about her physician's views:

> The neurosurgeon told me that he was only interested in quality of life and that in no way would he be looking to prolong my life if he didn't feel the quality would be acceptable. However, neither he nor anyone else has asked me what criteria *I* would use in judging what was an acceptable quality of life. I am very worried that if I get admitted unconscious or without the power of speech, he will take a decision based on *his* judgment and *his* criteria about what is an acceptable quality of life. (Morris, 1996, p. 62)

Anticipating such situations, everyone nowadays should communicate clearly and effectively their preferences for care under extreme scenarios (e.g., through a designated health care proxy or living will[5]). But as suggested by Ruth Moore, the stakes are especially high for persons with disabilities who fear that clinicians may not seek their views, respect their preferences, or value their lives.[6] Life-and-death decisions can, quite literally, rest upon the spoken and unspoken nuances of patient-clinician communication and all the myriad judgments underlying those interactions.

Communicating with Clinicians

Rick Abernathy, who is in his early fifties and has low vision, recently lost his primary care doctor when she left Distant Dunes for the city. Mr. Abernathy knows exactly why he had liked her so much—she treated him like a complete human being:

> What made our relationship positive was that she never looked at me as a patient. She looked at me as a human being. Whenever she talked about me, she never said, "My patient needs such and such." She always said, "Mr. Abernathy needs this or that." She made you feel like she really cares. She wants to know not just your mental or physical condition but how your life is. She wanted to know *me,* and she worked with *me.* That's what made it so special.

Mr. Abernathy fears she'll be hard to replace.

Virtually everyone, with and without disabilities, likely hopes for such caring and respectful interactions. But during clinical encounters, as elsewhere in daily life, disability is often "the elephant in the room"—even if not spoken of, its presence dominates and drives the discourse, in overt to subtle ways. "Attitudes toward disability and persons with disabilities by those who are able-bodied are a significant factor in the lives of persons with disabilities," wrote the clinical psychologist Rhonda Olkin (1999, p. 72). "Overall, such attitudes still are quite negative. . . . Attitudes toward disability are difficult to change. There are hundreds of studies on this issue and overall the results are not encouraging."

Growing up within a society that has historically marginalized persons with disabilities, clinicians may, consciously or unconsciously, share these views. As one primary care doctor told me, "My upbringing was like everybody else's—not to talk about it."

> As clinicians, we are subject to all the same factors that influence others, and are not immune to prejudice. Worse, we believe ourselves to be above all that, to be universally empathetic by training and skill. But our beliefs about disability, our responses to the fact of disability, to attractiveness, to loss of health, and so on, affect how we view the client, the role we think the disability plays in the client's character and presenting problems . . . and ultimately the treatment. (Olkin, 1999, p. 74)

Different sensory and physical impairments shape specific communication experiences. This diversity reflects obvious practical concerns, such as accommodating particular functional requirements. However, such differences also likely relate to an implicit hierarchy of disability in which persons with mental disabilities generally face the greatest difficulties, followed by those with impaired hearing (Charlton, 1998, p. 97). Persons who are blind or who have mobility impairments usually have easier times. Not surprisingly, interpersonal communication concerns dominated comments by interviewees who are deaf or hard of hearing.

An unswerving and exclusive reliance upon the medical model (see chapter 2)—perceptions that individuals with disabilities must adjust, adapt, or change their behaviors and expectations, presumably with professional help—poses a major impediment to communication between clinicians and persons with disabilities. Each can hold widely divergent views of the effects and implications of patients' functional impairments. Requiring patients to modify their behaviors and expectations simply may not comport with reality. For example, no amount of wishful thinking or individual adaptations will remove the barriers posed by inaccessible medical office buildings and equipment.

In clinical settings, however, completely rejecting the medical model also does not reflect certain realities. After all, clinical encounters specifically aim to address medical concerns of individual patients. Thus, clinicians face the challenge of transcending the medical model in their perceptions of patients with disabilities while simultaneously meeting patients' specific clinical needs. Mr. Abernathy's physician leapt this hurdle by caring about his multifaceted life—his overall wellness—while simultaneously treating his diabetes and heart condition to prevent the disease progression that could impede his larger life goals.

As did Mr. Abernathy, some interviewees reported excellent interpersonal communication with their clinicians. However, others raised important concerns, grouped into broad themes in the following sections. We highlight communication missteps where disability was the likely "elephant in the room"—the unspoken or sometimes obvious cause of the problem.

Basic Respect

Mr. Abernathy viewed his former physician as an anomaly. "A lot of people—even doctors—look at people with disabilities as being more or less a nobody," said Mr. Abernathy. "They figure, 'he's a cripple' or 'he's blind.' People with disabilities are not treated fair at all." Mr. Abernathy believes they don't get basic respect.

Lack of respect has different manifestations. Interviewees view clinicians' failures to involve them in decision-making or give them basic information about their conditions as devaluing their intelligence, motivation, and desire to understand and participate in their own health care. Jeb McCarthy's experiences exemplify this concern. In his late thirties, university-educated, and a teacher of deaf children, Jeb "was born deaf. My family is Deaf. I'm third generation Deaf." A few years ago, Jeb developed Guillain-Barré syndrome: paralysis starting in his lower extremities and ascending up his body. At the hospital, Jeb, who knew nothing about Guillain-Barré, "was freaking out without an [American Sign Language (ASL)] interpreter." He describes his experience in the intensive care unit:

> Four or five doctors would circle around my bed and talk about me.
> I didn't know what anybody was saying. They were touching me,
> they were checking me, they were talking about me, and I was lying
> there. Hearing people could at least hear what is going on and
> maybe have something to say about it. But not me. They come in,
> treat me like some object in a zoo, and leave.

Three days elapsed before an ASL interpreter arrived to interpret as Jeb's physician explained Guillain-Barré syndrome to him. (Jeb eventually regained full physical functioning.)

According to the interviewees, failure to take time and listen to them connotes lack of respect. Not only does the patient-clinician relationship suffer, but also clinicians may miss critical clinical information, putting technical quality at risk. As one woman who is hard of hearing said, "Unless doctors really listen to you, they can never find out what's wrong. Today, so many of them just spend five minutes with you—treat one little specific thing and not the whole person." When clinicians do take the time and listen, patients feel respected and valued. "My doctor tries to understand my day-to-day lifestyle, what I'm going through by being visually impaired, whether I'm dealing with some stress situation," said one woman. She feels that her physician attempts to fit her health concerns into the totality of her life experiences.

Interviewees perceive common courtesies—greeting people, introducing oneself, and looking people in the eye—as conveying respect. One blind man says he can tell the quality of nurses the moment they enter his hospital room. "You can't see her, but you know if you have a good nurse. Does she come in and announce herself, 'I'm going to be your nurse'? She's only doing her job, but it's her tone of voice, that she's got compassion."

For some persons with congenital or early childhood sensory or physical impairments, perceptions of disrespect and feeling devalued extend back to their earliest memories of clinical encounters. Vivid recollections of being excluded from decision-making as children—never being asked what they wanted as they sometimes endured multiple surgeries or lengthy hospitalizations—can leave people as adults feeling disrespected, marginalized, angry, or afraid (Saxton, 1987). Memories of such long-ago upsets are hard to erase and color adult expectations, with people anticipating the worst from every clinical interaction.

Brad Pepperill, in his late forties and born deaf to hearing parents, never knew why his tonsils were removed or what was happening during his hospitalization. He was terrified. "Hearing parents will explain to hearing children what is going on, but my parents couldn't sign." Even copious quantities of ice cream did not assuage his "suffering. I say, get an [ASL] interpreter in that situation to make the deaf child feel safe." Brad's daughter is now a teenager and is deaf like her father. He makes sure she has a sign language interpreter during her medical visits. Brad doesn't want his daughter to experience the fears and sense of isolation that he did.

Finally, some persons believe that the disrespect they confront springs from multiple sources—disability is only one factor. Being of minority race or ethnicity, poor, low social standing, or having other socially stigmatized personal attributes compounds negative perceptions of disability. Several black interviewees with mobility difficulties recounted falling or being assaulted without people rushing to their aid. Their stories contrast starkly with those of white interviewees, who sometimes complained about crowds gathering, anxious to help (Iezzoni, 2003). Even without conclusive evidence of racism, these discrepancies are hard to dismiss. "One time I was on the train, and when I was getting off, for some reason I just fell," said Jackie Ford, a human services counselor with multiple sclerosis (MS) who is black. "Do you know that people just walked right over me? Literally just walked right over me! If it wasn't for one old white man who helped me up, I would still be on that ground." Ms. Ford had a message for her physicians:

> A neurologist told me that because of my gait being off, I should walk with my head down. I said, "Never." He said, "What?" I said, "Never. I will not walk with my head down." He said, "But your MS puts you in a situation where you have to watch where your feet are going." I said, "No. I do it my way." Walking with my head down makes me feel less of a person.

For Ms. Ford, holding her head erect conveys her self-respect.

The Third Person

Interviewees repeatedly recounted being referred to in the third person: Instead of addressing patients directly, clinicians speak to someone else in the room, such as the patient's companion, an interpreter, or another professional. Akysha Nanuet, who is deaf, described typical experiences:

> When I'm there with [a sign language] interpreter, the nurse always looks at the interpreter. It's hard for me to get eye contact. But I'm the patient. I don't want them speaking to me in third person. I want them to speak directly to me. Don't refer to me as "she." I feel ignored when they do that.

Perhaps their clinicians are unaware of standard procedures for communication with patients using sign language interpreters. The same principles apply as for oral foreign language interpreters: keep eye contact with and speak directly to patients, not to interpreters. Some clinicians rationalize that speaking directly to interpreters and invoking patients in the third person is quick and efficient (San Augustin, Atchison, and Gracer, 2004). Feeling rushed, with the office clock ticking, these clinicians neglect basic interpreter etiquette.

Circumventing patients and communicating with companions can pose problems. Patients may not understand fully what they need to know to manage their health care or make informed decisions. "Sometimes doctors want to tell other people in our families and not us about a given medical problem," said one blind man. In such situations, he feels marginalized and inadequately informed. "In order for me to understand what's going on, doctors need to explain it to *me*"—not his family member. Unless clinicians talk directly to patients, clinicians might not appreciate patients' knowledge of their conditions or treatment regimens. Technical quality of care, such as adherence with care plans, may suffer.

Ineffective Communication Causes Inequities

As noted in chapter 1, the Institute of Medicine (Committee on Quality, 2001, p. 42) lists equity—equal quality regardless of patients' personal characteristics—among its six essential features of a health care delivery system. Absent communication virtually ensures that some persons with disabilities will receive lower quality care. Interviewees who are deaf or hard of hearing repeatedly raised concerns about simply not having essential information communicated to them. Especially when physicians communicate through writing notes, people feel they get abbreviated input, the bare minimum required: "Even when the doctor does write to me, I don't get all the details that I would otherwise." According to Jeb McCarthy, the man who had Guillain-Barré syndrome:

> If a doctor gives options to a hearing person, then they have choices. But a deaf person doesn't get the explanation about our options. We are not aware of our options, so our choices have always been limited. We may pick up information incidentally. But why aren't we getting that information from the people that are supposed to be advising us?

Some deaf interviewees admitted not knowing even such basic health information as risk factors for HIV infection until mid-adulthood.[7] Jeb McCarthy did not learn about routine dental hygiene until he attended Gallaudet University[8] and visited a deaf dentist. "For years, every time I brushed my teeth, my gums would bleed," he recalled. No hearing dentist had ever talked to him about this problem. On Jeb's first visit to a deaf dentist, "the dentist told me all kinds of things. I didn't know that flossing helps gum disease! I keep wondering why I didn't have that information a long time ago."

Although note writing and lip reading sometimes provide effective communication with deaf and hard of hearing individuals, often they do not (Barnett, 2002a, 2002b; Iezzoni et al., 2004). Miscommunication can ensue, with mismatches between clinicians' perceptions and patients' realities: clinicians erroneously assume that patients accurately "hear" (or know) what they are saying. This problem compromises both technical and interpersonal communication. According to Denise Harding, in her mid-thirties:

> Hard of hearing people often think we hear things that are very different from what was actually said, and we have no way of checking that information. . . . You're really concentrating to hear what you think the doctor's going to say, but if you don't hear the questions right, then you can't answer them right. Doctors could come up with a whole different diagnosis if you answer the questions wrong. . . . That happens to us all day long. We're constantly negotiating what we're going to make an issue about hearing and what we're going to ignore.

These concerns stoke Denise's anxieties from the moment she enters the clinic. After all, "most of the time you're not going to the doctor because everything's peachy keen." Being worried about accurately understanding what clinicians say magnifies the usual stresses of health care encounters.

Numerous factors contribute to ineffective communication. Deaf and hard of hearing persons report difficulties understanding words when lip reading, especially when physicians speak quickly, turn away, bow heads, have foreign accents, or wear beards or masks. Even in the best circumstances, lip reading is generally inadequate: Only 30 to 45 percent of English sounds are unambiguously visible on lips (Barnett, 2002a, 2002b). Multiethnic populations pose additional challenges. "I have one doctor from India, one is Hispanic, and another is Danish," recounted a man who is hard of hearing. "They speak in a variety of accents which took me some time to understand." He feels it is his responsibility to ask physicians to repeat statements that he cannot understand. But one woman finally gave up on "a marvelous, marvelous doctor, renowned in his field. I really wanted to stay with him, but he had a beard and talked very fast. I couldn't understand a word he said."

Some interviewees would rather write notes than read lips "because you don't want to miss anything." However, older persons who are hard of hearing can find note writing difficult because of low vision, arthritis, or fatigue. In one study, less than 20 percent of deaf individuals reported fluency in written English, and more than half reported slight or no understanding of written English (MacKinney et al., 1995, p. 134). When English is learned as a second language (e.g., as for persons educated using ASL in some Deaf schools), deaf persons may have difficulty understanding written English, especially complicated medical terminology. Certain aspects of sign language and English grammar and syntax differ importantly, occasionally producing basic misunderstandings. As one deaf man who spent several years at college said:

> The doctor will write some big hundred-dollar word on a piece of paper. I write, "Please, just regular English." Doctors don't know what to do, so they call the nurse. I feel stupid. When I leave the office, I understand maybe only half of what the doctor said. After two or three days, I have to find an interpreter to call the doctor because I'm not satisfied. I don't want to take the wrong drugs. I don't want to do the wrong thing.

In addition, multitasking clinicians often fail to provide familiar visual cues typically used to verify comprehension. Without these reassuring affirmations, some patients feel lost. "When you communicate verbally, you want feedback," asserted one man who is hard of hearing; "some kind of check to know that you're registering with people." He rarely gets such cues from his physician, whose "head is buried in the chart."

Inadequate communication can sometimes embarrass patients. "You write notes back and forth," recalled Brad Pepperill, "and the doctor wrote 'C-O-K-E.' I said, 'Yes, a lot.' Suddenly, there were three people trailing me to the bathroom for a urine test. I thought they were trying to keep me from running away! I didn't understand where that was coming from. I thought he meant do I drink Coca-Cola. Why didn't he write the whole word 'cocaine'?" With hearing patients, such miscommunication is likely quickly identified.[9]

Not Getting It

Sometimes, interviewees worry that clinicians "just don't get it"—they fail to make basic connections between sensory or physical impairments and what patients need. One deaf woman visited an emergency room for an injury, but hours passed while she waited on the gurney to see the physician, and the promised sign language interpreter never arrived. She needed to use the restroom, but the nurses did not understand as she gesticulated with her hands. "They kept telling me, 'Just calm down,' to be patient for the interpreter to arrive, to wait until tomorrow. But I needed the restroom right away!"

Failure to think through the implications of patients' functional impairments can compromise clinicians' ability to give patients useful advice. It erects invisible walls between patients and clinicians, as patients realize that clinicians are unlikely to suggest practical, reality-based solutions to their daily concerns. According to one woman who uses a manual wheelchair:

> I love my physician dearly, but she doesn't know a lot about spinal cord injury. One time my shoulders were really hurting. So she told

me, "Don't use your arms so much." I'm a paraplegic, and all I have is my arms! I do everything with them, even talk with them. I told her she was absurd to say something like that to me.

Some interviewees sense skepticism among clinicians about conditions that can elude technologically driven assessments or quantification. "Chronic fatigue syndrome, immune dysfunction syndrome, environmental allergies, or fibromyalgia all still raise this attitude in the medical community," observed one woman. "They think it's all psychological. Even with doctors who were fairly good about it, the attitude's very subtle, but it's still there."

Hope

Finally, according to a survey of Medicare beneficiaries, about 80 to 85 percent of people, regardless of disability, depend on physicians to help them feel better physically and emotionally (Iezzoni et al., 2003). For some interviewees, this translates into seeking hope from their clinicians—wanting them to communicate positive or upbeat messages, the possibility of restoring or improving sensory or physical functioning. Some clinicians might worry about conveying false hopes or raising unrealistic expectations.[10] Indeed, the concept of hope is complicated for persons with chronic impairments, as people "are impelled at once to defy limitations in order to realize greater life possibilities, and to accept limitations in order to avoid enervating struggles with immutable constraints" (Barnard, 1995, p. 39).

Experts have studied how people "adjust" to impairments, identifying the "stages" they pass through to reconcile themselves to new limitations. Theoretically, these stages follow a tidy sequence, progressing forward to ultimate "acceptance." However, people do not generally proceed, lock step, through such neat stages (Rohe, 2005). While the word "adjustment" suggests attainment of an ultimate, reconciled state, living with impairments often requires continuous adaptation and accommodation. About three to five years after disability begins, people typically stop talking about how it happened—"it's a moot point" (Olkin, 1999, p. 60). As one wheelchair user told me, "If a cure comes, fine. But in the meantime, you've got to live."

People vary widely in their perceptions of their functional impairments. Persons with significant impairments may prize even limited abilities "since they have adjusted their life styles and expectations to take account of their condition. This may be particularly true of young disabled men and women" (Dolan, 1996, p. 559). People with disabilities also diverge in their hopes and aspirations and their thoughts about the role of clinical interventions, spiritual forces, and personal willpower in achieving their individual goals. Sanford Peck, in his late fifties, credits his faith for getting him through the aftermath of a stroke. "You've got to have hope. People see me all the time, moving and on the go. They stop me in the street and say, 'How you doing?' I just get into my spirit life, have hope and faith, and I don't give up. I think I can do anything I want to do. I just take my time to do it."

Hopelessness and despair can prove infectious, insinuating themselves into the patient-clinician relationship. "Chronically ill or disabled people being cared for by action-oriented professionals who thrive on dramatic results may be at special risk for this reaction" (Barnard, 1995, p. 54). In other words, if clinicians cannot work medical magic and restore patients' lost functioning, they too can withdraw that all-important empathy and emotional support. Patients perceive this and become angry, frustrated, and demoralized. Vic Domenico, in his late twenties, had a low thoracic-level spinal cord injury more than three years ago and has worked tenaciously to avoid a wheelchair. Vic walks painfully at a snail's pace, feeling that his physicians' attitudes threaten his recovery.

"Initially, they said I would never walk again," said Vic, "but I was able to walk. Now the doctors say I can't improve any more. Other people tell me that I can improve through physical therapy." Vic finds these contradictions "really frustrating. My doctor says she doesn't expect me to improve, but she's the one who told me I would never walk again when I got injured. She doesn't give me any hope. A doctor that doesn't give you hope is not a good doctor. I'm thinking about changing doctors."

In Vic's situation, the continuum between real and false hopes stretches wide. He and his physician seem at loggerheads as they navigate this treacherous divide. Given Vic's injury and the time elapsed, using a wheelchair would likely offer quicker, safer, and more comfortable mobility than constantly struggling with canes. He could still walk with canes whenever he wishes, using the wheelchair only to travel long distances. Vic needs to discover this himself, perhaps guided by understanding and empathetic clinicians.[11] Hope for a better life differs importantly from hope for a cure or to walk again.

Balancing reality-based expectations against hope is inevitably an imperfect game. "When I had my stroke, my [physical] therapist was fitting me for a brace and getting me in a wheelchair," Sanford Peck recalled. "I said, 'What's going on? I can't run around the beach in Hawaii in a wheelchair!' She said, 'But Mr. Peck, you had a pretty bad stroke. You might never walk again.' I just wouldn't hear it. Four days later, I started walking with a cane. If I'd listened to her, I would have gave up."

Discussing Potentially Sensitive Topics

As discussed earlier, disability is often a culturally sensitive and value-laden topic. Expanding conversations to cover other socially delicate or difficult subjects can prove challenging, even during discussions with health care professionals. In the following sections, we touch briefly on sexuality and reproductive health, substance abuse, and mental health.

Sexuality and Reproductive Health

"My doctor said, 'Miss Tidewell, you don't want no birth control. You're visually impaired,'" recalled Nona. " 'What's that got to do with it?' I said. 'Everybody got a life. Blind people do just as much as sighted people!' I don't stay at home and sit in no corner."

Today, sexuality is viewed as a central aspect of health and human behavior, not simply as a matter of reproduction. However, physicians often do not raise sexuality with patients, regardless of disability. Some clinicians feel uneasy discussing sexuality, a discomfort communicated to patients (Sipski, Alexander, and Sherman, 2005). As one woman observed, "They don't ask able-bodied people about sex either. Sex is a topic that no one likes to talk about except over coffee."

Only 39.8 percent of all women under age fifty, regardless of disability, report that physicians ask them about contraception, compared with 19.2 percent of men (table 6.2).[12] Similarly, regardless of disability, only 24.8 percent and 27.3 percent of women and men, respectively, report that their physicians inquire about sexually transmitted diseases.[13] Just 14.7 percent of women with major lower extremity mobility difficulties report their doctors asking about contraception, compared with 33.1 percent of men with similar impairments.

In considering sensuality and sexuality, "a woman's self-concept and body image . . . can influence how a woman with a disability or chronic illness may interact with others" (Whipple and Welner, 2004, p. 347). Significant mobility problems represent perhaps the most visible functional impairment. Some clinicians might view women with impaired walking as asexual or uninterested in sexual activity (Beckmann et al., 1989; Becker, Stuifbergen, and Tinkle, 1997; Quint, 2004; Kirschner et al., 2005).[14] In the public's mind, these women do not have the "physical grace or ease" central to "male notions of attractiveness" (Asch and Fine, 1988, p. 16).

> In short, attractiveness is linked to virtue, to all that is desired, especially by men of women. In the cultural imagination, beauty is linked to goodness and nurturance, the traits most sought after in women both as lovers and as workers. . . . Unfortunately for the disabled woman, only a few attributes count toward attractiveness in the United States, and a woman's bodily integrity is one such requirement. . . . The woman with a disability, whether apparent or invisible, may display less than the norm or the fantasized ideal of bodily integrity, grace, and ease. The very devices she values for enhancing free movement and communication (braces, crutches, hearing aids, or canes) may repel men seeking the fantasized flawlessness.

Table 6.2. Queries about Contraception and Sexually Transmitted Diseases

| | "During Your Last Check-Up, Were You Asked about . . . ?"[a] (Percent[b]) | | | | | |
| | Contraception | | | Sexually Transmitted Diseases | | |
Impairment	All	Men	Women	All	Men	Women
All persons	31.6	19.2	39.8	25.8	27.3	24.8
Blind or very low vision	34.5	25.3	40.5	28.5	23.0	32.2
Deaf or hard of hearing	31.1	22.2	36.9	26.4	28.9	24.8
Lower extremity mobility difficulty						
Some	30.2	24.3	34.1	24.9	24.8	25.0
Major	21.9	33.1	14.7	25.1	32.6	20.2
Upper extremity mobility difficulty						
Some	21.4	11.0	28.3	22.8	16.3	27.2
Major	34.2	30.6	36.2	26.6	13.7	34.1
Difficulty using hands						
Some	13.0	8.6	15.8	16.8	18.4	17.1
Major	21.2	19.5	22.4	21.4	16.3	23.4

Data source: 1994 National Health Interview Survey Disability and Healthy People 2000 supplements.

[a]Respondents reporting routine check-up within the last three years were asked whether their physician inquired about contraception ("the use of contraceptives"; asked only of persons younger than fifty years of age) and sexually transmitted diseases (asked only of persons younger than sixty-five years of age).

[b]Findings for all persons account for age category and sex; analyses by sex account only for age category.

Given these societal attitudes, clinicians may believe that addressing reproductive issues with women who use mobility aids is moot. As one woman commented about her doctor, "They think you're sitting in a wheelchair. What makes you think you can have sex with somebody? That's a no-no." Disability arriving with older age can compound matters. "People look at me as someone who's aging and single," said a woman in her mid-sixties. "'You're old. You don't need sex.' But I don't feel that old." Some women report physicians encouraging them to be sterilized or use long-lasting forms of birth control to avoid pregnancy at all costs, under the assumption that they could not adequately care for a child.

In contrast, men with mobility impairments present clinicians with dueling images and concerns. On the one hand, society often sees men with limited mobility as damaged, just as they do women (Asch and Fine, 1988; Morris, 1996). Nonclinicians find questions about erectile function titillating, especially when the subjects are famous men with spinal cord injuries. The reporter John Hockenberry (1995, p. 97), who is married with children, recounted a conversation with an airline flight attendant. Having seen Hockenberry transfer effortlessly from his wheelchair into his seat, the flight attendant expressed admiration and then asked, "Can you, I mean, can your body, I mean are you able to do it with a woman?" Hockenberry was understandably stumped by how to respond.

On the other hand, especially in the era of Viagra and other drugs for managing erectile dysfunction, as well as penile prostheses and other mechanical options, clinicians should address erectile functioning with men with physical impairments and diseases (e.g., diabetes) that can affect it. Even among our interviewees, the men reported that clinicians raised sexuality more often than the women. Joe Alto's neurologist and MS nurse asked him, "Do you still feel it down there?" His MS and certain medications could cause impotence, and Joe's clinicians want to guard against that. But they give him other messages, too. "They say, 'Don't you be promiscuous because we don't want you to have multiple sclerosis and AIDS. Don't catch any other diseases. Be very careful and know what you're doing.'"

Some male interviewees reported clinicians also talking to their spouses—conversations that could be very helpful to both patient and partner. One man with diabetes described discussions with his physician while hospitalized following leg amputation:

> My doctor did ask about sex. I'm fifty-nine years old, and he says to me, "How's everything going in that department?" I said, "No problem, I don't think." He wondered how it would be for me with just one leg. We don't have sex like we did when we were thirty, but that's the way it goes. Then he took my wife aside and asked how she felt with the disability part. He said, "It might change your sex life looking at your husband without his leg. Can you deal with that?" She told him she could deal with that very well.

Even with clinicians, conversations about erectile functioning can sometimes seem awkward. "I go to a urologist for [intracavernosal] injection therapy," said one wheelchair user in his early forties.[15] "It's funny how physicians are uncomfortable talking about some things. This urologist, he's absolutely wonderful, but just looking at him, I could tell he wasn't promiscuous in his younger days. So when I asked about using injection therapy, I could see he was much more uncomfortable than I was."

Other sexual stereotypes can sometimes affect discourse. Akysha Nanuet, who is deaf, black, and lesbian, feels that this combination discombobulates some clinicians, as well as sign language interpreters.

> People make a lot of assumptions, cultural assumptions, just by looking at me. They see that my skin color is dark, that I'm black.

They assume which part of town I live in. They ask me about drug use all the time—excuse me! They assume I'm extremely promiscuous. Hello—that's not me! The [sign language] interpreter comes in, and the doctor asks about intercourse, penetration. I say, "I don't do that. I'm a lesbian." I can see the shift in attitude on their faces. I can see there's some discomfort. Maybe they don't even know how to think about lesbian sex—I don't know. The interpreters are embarrassed. They don't want to ask the questions.

Failure to address sexuality and reproductive health issues represents not only a lapse in interpersonal communication but also an important potential quality problem. Some physical impairments carry consequences for sexual functioning that deserve discussion with clinicians. Health care professionals "should possess enough knowledge about sexuality and the specific disability/illness to impart limited information. Moreover, they should . . . know their limits" and refer patients to specialists, as appropriate (Sipski, Alexander, and Sherman, 2005, p. 1595). For many women with physical or manual dexterity limitations, contraception presents significant challenges. They may not be able to handle over-the-counter barrier contraceptives, and they could face greater health risks from oral contraceptives, such as deep venous thrombosis (blood clots), than other women (Drey and Darney, 2004; Quint, 2004). Unintended pregnancies could pose huge emotional dilemmas for women with certain physical disabilities, especially if they face heightened health risks (e.g., from urinary tract infections, autonomic dysreflexia) during pregnancy, labor, and delivery.

Low rates of screening for sexually transmitted diseases across men and women represent another troubling quality shortfall, particularly for people with certain conditions. Spinal cord injury, MS, spina bifida, and other conditions can impair pelvic sensations, decreasing awareness of symptoms and prompting misdiagnoses (e.g., of urinary tract infections). Untreated sexually transmitted diseases, especially in women, can have serious consequences, such as pelvic inflammatory disease and compromised reproductive health.

The bottom line is that neglecting reproductive health issues with patients with disabilities represents not only substandard care but also contributes to patients' perceptions of stigmatization. "People think we have no feelings, no flesh," said Eleanor Peters, who is a grandmother. "We're told we shouldn't have sex or shouldn't have kids. We may not be able to run around the track, but we do have brains and desires and feelings."

Mental Health

For many people, mental health represents another sensitive topic. Failures to diagnose and treat depression are widespread, across virtually all demographic groups. Given the power and effectiveness of today's psychotropic medications for many patients, these lapses needlessly perpetuate emotional pain and suffering among millions nationwide. Dissemination of practice guidelines for detecting depression may have recently improved diagnoses among ethnic and racial minorities, but African Americans and Latinos remain less likely than whites to receive antidepressant medications and specialty mental health care (Miranda and Cooper, 2004).

Identifying mental health problems, especially depression, requires careful attention among persons with sensory and physical impairments.[16] Compared with others, they report much higher rates of feeling frequently depressed or anxious; having serious difficulties coping with day-to-day stresses; and experiencing phobias or strong fears in situations where other people generally would not (table 6.3). Persons with major lower extremity mobility difficulties commonly describe emotional problems, with 33.6 percent reporting often feeling depressed or anxious. Among these persons, 20.4 percent report that feeling depressed or anxious seriously interferes with their abilities to work, attend school, or manage their daily activities over the preceding year.[17]

Table 6.3.   Reports of Mental Health Problems

Impairment	Responded "Yes" to Mental Health Questions[a] (Percent[b])		
	Depressed	Stressed	Strong Fears
No disability	3.4	1.3	2.5
Blind or very low vision	24.8	14.2	13.2
Deaf or hard of hearing	16.8	8.9	10.5
Lower extremity mobility difficulty			
Some	23.6	13.2	13.9
Major	33.6	20.3	17.4
Upper extremity mobility difficulty			
Some	26.4	15.1	15.5
Major	35.7	21.5	19.4
Difficulty using hands			
Some	24.7	14.1	16.0
Major	34.1	20.9	21.6

Data source: 1994–1995 National Health Interview Survey Disability supplement.

[a]Depressed = "Are [you] FREQUENTLY depressed or anxious?"

Stressed = "Do [you] have SERIOUS difficulty coping with day-to-day stresses?"

Strong fears = "Do [you] have phobias or UNREASONABLY strong fears, that is, a fear of something or some situation where most people would not be afraid?"

[b]Findings account for age category and sex.

Despite these important findings, flipping these percentages on their heads gives a different perspective: Even with major walking difficulties, 66.4 percent of persons do *not* report feeling frequently depressed or anxious. Olkin (1999, p. 206) warns that therapists can misdiagnose patients with disabilities "when they harbor mistaken beliefs about what and how strongly people with disabilities should and shouldn't feel." In addition, by expecting persons with disabilities to fixate on sensory or physical losses, clinicians might miss treatable depression. "If the clinician has the 'expectation of mourning' . . . , the disability will be expected to produce depression, the depression may not be diagnosed as a separate disorder, and hence a treatable condition will be overlooked" (Olkin, 1999, p. 207). Depression may, however, be easier to treat in some disabilities than others (Olkin, 2004).

Beyond depression, clinicians may also misdiagnose other types of mental health problems. For example, clinicians may diagnose a patient's justifiable anger at oppression or injustice as a personality disorder. Clinicians may erroneously interpret strong self-advocacy as narcissism, entitlement, or grandiosity. Much of the language ordinarily used by others to describe persons with disabilities carries implicit connotations of mental or emotional states:

> Disabled people are frequently described as *suffering from* or *afflicted with* certain conditions. . . . Although some people may experience their disability this way, these terms are not used as descriptors of a verified experience but are projected onto disability. Rather than assume suffering in the description of the situation, it is more accurate and less histrionic to say simply that a person *has a disability*. . . . [Similarly] the ascription of passivity can be seen in language used to describe the relationship between disabled people and their wheelchairs. The phrases *wheelchair bound* or *confined to a wheelchair* . . . imply that a wheelchair restricts the individual, holds a person prisoner. Disabled people are more likely to say someone *uses a wheelchair*. (Linton, 1998, pp. 26–27)

Social and economic vulnerabilities among many persons with disabilities further complicate mental health assessments. "I'm on a $600 income with $400 rent," said Sylvie Park, in her mid-thirties with post-polio syndrome. Daily, she must concentrate on financial survival—clearly a struggle: "I can't even get my medications." Sylvie feels that her physician thinks her pain and physical weakness represent emotional problems. "The doctor automatically assumes it's some mental disability. But I know my body's inner pains. When I can't move my leg, he always thinks it's depression." Sylvie lives in rural Distant Dunes and has few health care options.

Despite the complexities, clinicians must address mental health concerns among all patients, including those with disabilities. Oftentimes, patients themselves recognize their own risks. "I've read about mental health," said a woman in her fifties. "People with hearing loss are at much higher risk for depression. When you think about it, you're not hearing everything that's said. It's not always easy to assert yourself, especially if you don't have an understanding audience. So, what's the most common thing many people do? Withdraw. Hearing loss is actually much more than just a medical problem. It also has a major impact on you socially and on your self-esteem. . . . To me hearing loss and mental health are twin issues that go hand in hand."

Substance Abuse

Substance abuse, as well as tobacco use, poses another set of sensitive issues. Some clinicians may feel that persons with disabilities "suffer" enough and therefore ignore behaviors they view as giving solace to "damaged lives" (Schaschl and Straw, 1993). However, "people with disabilities use alcohol and illicit drugs as much as, if not more than, the general population" (Ford et al., 2004, p. 315). Substance use threatens patients' health and even lives. In addition, it can affect patient-clinician relationships, as in Vic Domenico's case.

"When I first got injured and I couldn't walk, I slipped into a deep depression and turned to drugs," Vic said. "I was on Baclofen, Valium, Neurontin, and some other medications, but I was so distraught. My mind couldn't think straight. A bag of dope would take away all the pain." Vic felt that he was addicted not only to dope but also to the prescription medications. The difference was that the prescriptions did not relieve his pain.

Vic and his physician reached an impasse. Vic felt she didn't want to "give me strong medication because I may get addicted. But I'm already addicted to her prescriptions! When you have a spinal cord injury like mine, the doctors can't comprehend or don't know how to help you with that pain. If you hurt twenty-four hours a day, and your doctor can't do anything for you, you're going to turn to other drugs."

Vic stopped using dope. "I'm clean now. I'm not on any illicit drugs, but I hurt. I'm not going to turn back to dope because it only makes my rehabilitation much harder." But Vic's perception that his physician fails to appreciate his need for better pain control is "one of the reasons why I want to change doctors. Maybe then I can get prescribed some medication that'll help with my pain."

People with disabilities face substantial health risks from tobacco, alcohol consumption, and illicit drugs, including heightened likelihood of dangerous secondary conditions, such as falls, decubitus ulcers, and depression. Despite this, screening for chemical dependency among persons with disabilities often falls short (Rohe, 2005). Sometimes behaviors attributed to disability can mask symptoms of substance abuse, leading to delays in identifying the problem (Ford et al., 2004). Regardless of disability, physicians ask patients about illicit drug use relatively infrequently and query roughly half of patients about tobacco and alcohol use (table 6.4). However, persons with disabilities generally use tobacco at higher rates than do others.[18] Physicians ask people with major lower extremity mobility difficulties about tobacco use 30 percent less often, although 47.3 percent of these individuals report using tobacco.[19]

However, figures such as those presented in table 6.4 represent broad population-based statistics, which may mask important differences within selected subgroups. For instance, the 1990 and 1991 National Health Interview Surveys asked detailed questions about hearing, allowing researchers to separate prelingually from postlingually deafened individuals and to determine more precisely the extent of hearing loss. Using those data, Barnett and Franks (1999) found that prelingually deafened persons (see preface) were roughly half as likely to smoke as hearing persons; smoking rates among postlingually deafened individuals were similar to those of hearing persons. Rates of alcohol use did not differ between persons with and with-

Table 6.4. Queries about Tobacco, Alcohol, and Illicit Drugs (Percent[a])

Impairment	Tobacco Use[b]	"During Your Last Check-Up, Were You Asked About . . . ?"[c]		
		Tobacco	Alcohol	Illicit Drugs
All persons	26.3	53.2	43.7	25.3
Blind or very low vision	33.3	57.3	50.8	27.2
Deaf or hard of hearing	34.8	53.5	44.6	28.0
Lower extremity mobility difficulty				
Some	38.6	55.8	46.2	26.2
Major	47.3	44.2	34.3	24.9
Upper extremity mobility difficulty				
Some	41.2	60.3	56.5	33.5
Major	39.1	56.4	48.5	23.7
Difficulty using hands				
Some	44.5	50.3	46.5	24.5
Major	29.3	46.3	39.0	22.8

Data source: 1994 National Health Interview Survey Disability and Healthy People 2000 supplements.

[a]Findings account for age category and sex.

[b]Currently smokes or uses other tobacco products.

[c]Respondents reporting routine check-up within the last three years were asked whether their physician inquired about:
   Tobacco = "Whether you smoke cigarettes or use other forms of tobacco?"
   Alcohol = "How much and how often you drink alcohol?"
   Illicit drugs = "Whether you use marijuana, cocaine, or other drugs?"

out deafness, regardless of age of deafness onset. Barnett and Franks speculate that cultural factors may contribute to lower smoking rates among prelingually deafened persons, may of whom identify with the Deaf community. Marketing images promulgated by tobacco advertisers may appeal less to culturally Deaf persons, who in any case are often less exposed to tobacco marketing (both aurally because of deafness and visually if persons have low English literacy).

Cultural factors—notably societal biases relating to race and ethnicity—can affect clinical care around substance abuse. Akysha Nanuet believes that her black skin explains why physicians always ask pointedly if she uses illicit drugs, seemingly assuming she does. Jenny Hartwell, also black, described "a friend who is disabled and black. She has a movement disorder that makes her look like she's drunk." When Jenny's friend "goes to the hospital, the first thing they see is she is black and looks homeless. 'You must be on drugs. What kind of drugs are you taking? Are you on liquor?'" Her friend feels stigmatized—on many levels—the minute she rolls through the hospital door.

7

Etiquette during Physical Examinations and Interactions with Office Staff

Interpersonal interactions during physical examinations and medical procedures convey volumes about respect, empathy, and understanding. Many people, regardless of disability, find physical examinations stressful and uncomfortable (Gabbard and Nadelson, 1995). Sometimes, these anxieties generate abnormal physical findings, such as "white coat hypertension"—when persons with normal blood pressures have elevated readings only in their physician's office. However, specific sensory and functional impairments, compounded by complex attitudes and expectations among both patients and clinicians, can make physical examinations and other office encounters especially unnerving for some persons with disabilities.

This chapter examines interpersonal interactions from the moment patients enter health care settings through the process of physical examinations and procedures. As discussed in chapter 5, persons with disabilities can confront numerous physical barriers during this journey; here, we focus on human-to-human communication that either helps or poses additional hurdles. We also consider issues raised when patients try to contact clinicians or office staff by telephone. Given the dearth of publications on these topics, we rely largely on interviewees' reports to describe these experiences and their perceptions of them.

First Contacts

Often, when patients have long-term relationships with particular clinicians, the office staff recognizes and welcomes them, knowing how to accommodate their needs. Familiarity can breed comfort. Furthermore, working well with one patient with disabilities may help staff think about how best to assist others. As a blind woman said, "If you've gone there for a while, they become more sensitive and educated to your needs. The more they interact with a certain disability, the more comfortable they become with other disabilities, from the doctors to the nurses to the technicians."

At the Receptionist's Desk

First contacts often set the tone for patients' subsequent experiences during a health care visit. Anxieties frequently start at the receptionist's desk. Desks above wheelchair height and sliding glass windows, for example, erect immediate communication barriers, both in a metaphorical and an actual sense. "You're talking to a secretary through a glass that nobody can hear through," a deaf woman observed. "You can't really lip read through glass either. So I don't know what they're saying to me."

When people already feel sick or worried, confronting difficulties at the front desk can exacerbate their anxiety. A man described receptionists waving their hands before his eyes to satisfy themselves of his visual deficit. "Then they talk to you all loud, like you're deaf. Wait a minute! I'm not deaf, I'm just blind!" Harry Spicer, who is deaf, feels unwelcome the moment he enters the office:

> They have a stereotype of a deaf person with all these negative connotations. . . . When they see you are deaf, you can see them backing off. There is no system set up for communication. They should have some protocol ready for communicating with deaf people so that they know how to deal with us.

Although Harry confronts such responses multiple times daily in the hearing world, he believes that clinicians' offices should be more sensitive, anticipating patients' diverse needs. Optimally, trained staff should follow established procedures for recognizing and addressing these needs as patients arrive (see chapter 13).

At the receptionist's desk, office staff generally focus on two primary tasks: determining whether the individual belongs there (e.g., has an appointment); and collecting information about insurance coverage, health histories, and other topics, as well as any payments. They therefore solicit and exchange information with newly arrived patients on sensitive subjects. Privacy often becomes an early casualty. People who are blind, have low vision, or have manual dexterity problems frequently need assistance filling out routine paperwork, typically attached to clipboards, handed over by front desk staff. Optimally, staff should take patients to private spaces to help them fill out these forms, but often this does not happen. Office personnel are too busy to leave their positions, or there are no private areas available. Interviewees report waiting rooms full of people overhearing entire conversations as receptionists help them complete required forms.

Provisions of the Health Insurance Portability and Accountability Act of 1996 (HIPAA, P.L. 104-191) aim to prevent such breaches in privacy and confidentiality (U.S. Department of Health and Human Services, 2003).[1] However, despite these HIPAA regulations, busy offices, cramped spaces, and poorly trained staff mean that failures to protect patients' privacy will still likely occur, especially for persons with sensory and physical disabilities. "We don't walk around with a sign that says, 'I have a hearing loss; shout at me,'" one man observed. He thinks his "in-the-ear hearing aids" provide obvious clues about his hearing loss. "But I'm still surprised at the number of times I go up to the receptionist and they don't look up. So the hearing aids aren't a cue. I finally have to say, 'Excuse me, I have a hearing loss. Would you mind repeating that, please?' I have to announce it to the whole waiting room."

Denise Harding, who is hard of hearing, trades off privacy against the chance for improved communication. "In a couple of doctors' offices, I've taken a Magic Marker and written 'HARD OF HEARING' on the front of the chart." Denise hopes that "receptionists will see that before they see me. At least it sometimes starts them thinking about things."

Waiting and Waiting Rooms

Most patients view waiting rooms with trepidation, anticipating lengthy sojourns. But waiting rooms present special challenges to persons with physical and sensory impairments. Privacy and comfort can vanish. Inadequate space sometimes forces persons who use wheelchairs to sit in public hallways, where they risk notice by passersby and must endure such irritations as busy foot traffic, poor lighting, and uncomfortable temperatures. Then, patients waiting in hallways must trust office staff to remember to fetch them once their appointment time comes.

Persons who are deaf or hard of hearing worry about not knowing when they are called for their appointments. While waiting, some people do nothing except watch to be called. "I can't relax in the waiting room," admitted a deaf woman. "I jump every time the door opens. I can't just read a magazine. I have to be hypersensitive and alert." People report missing appointments scheduled months before. One woman described a common experience:

> I told them I was there and that I was deaf. I had them make notes
> everywhere that I was deaf. And then I sat down. I waited a whole
> hour and nothing happened. I checked with them and they said,
> "We called you a long time ago." I said, "Oh, really? You knew I
> was deaf." I'd had to leave work to make that doctor's appointment,
> and then I missed it!

Lengthy waits frustrate many people, and no one knows whether certain patients routinely wait longer than others. In 2001, 52.5 percent of persons without any impairments waited fifteen or fewer minutes in clinicians' offices, as did 44.5 percent of persons with any major impairment.[2] At the other extreme, 16.3 percent of persons without any impairment waited more than thirty minutes (6.1 percent, more than an hour), as did 22.0 percent of persons with major impairment (8.6 percent longer than an hour). Thus, persons with disabilities spend longer times in waiting rooms at slightly higher rates than other individuals.

For some persons with disabilities, prolonged waiting dominates their daily life. They wait constantly—for accessible transportation (chapter 9), for assistance in stores, and even to meet basic needs. "I have to wait for long stretches before I can go to the bathroom," admitted one woman wheelchair user. "I have to wait for the PCA [personal care assistant] to come. I get very jealous when I see other women going to the bathroom and I can't go." So when people perceive they're waiting longer than other patients, this rubs a raw nerve: "They think disabled people don't have anything better to do than just wait around."

Some waits are not only inconvenient but also counterproductive. Despite her early appointment, Carmen Valdez's physician decided to see her last, anticipating that interacting through a sign language interpreter would consume considerable time (chapter 4). By the time the physician finally called Carmen, the interpreter had left, costing the physician money and Carmen time and aggravation. Lengthy waits can exacerbate certain impairments, as for one woman with severe back pain:

> I was in so much pain all the time. When I got to the doctor's office, he would arrange a room that I could lie down in because I just couldn't sit up for very long. I'd seen him over a long time, and he realized that was an access need for me. If I didn't have somewhere to lie down, I would just lie on the floor in his waiting room. I don't think he liked that.

Getting Settled in Examining Rooms

Once patients are called for their appointments, they must get to the examining room—sometimes with detours to be weighed, have blood pressure checks, or receive other routine assessments—and prepare for the visit. These steps introduce new stresses. Denise Harding, who is hard of hearing, described common anxieties:

> You can't hear the receptionist. You hope you'll know when they call your name. Then you go into another room, and they tell you to take off some of your clothes, all of your clothes, or none of your clothes. If you get that wrong, you're in trouble. I can't tell you the number of times I've opened the johnny [hospital gown] in the back when it was supposed to be the front and opened it in the front when it was supposed to be the back! . . . Then you don't hear the doctor at the door. They come in, and you don't know whether you've taken the right clothes off. Each thing seems little in itself. But when it all happens one after the other, you feel very anxious.

Getting to examining rooms presents challenges to some persons who are blind or have low vision, especially if routes are not clearly marked by braille or raised letter signage. Some interviewees described good experiences, where office staff simply asked what assistance they wanted and complied with their wishes. But other interviewees reported medical office staff providing help in unwelcome forms. According to Nona Tidewell, who is blind, "Instead of coming up and saying, 'Miss Tidewell, I'm So-and-so. I'm going to take you in the room now,' they grab you, they snatch you, they push you." Nona believes, "You always have to educate: 'Let me show you how to be a good sighted guide.' They always appreciate me doing that."

Wheelchair users can find themselves involuntarily pushed. "The staff at doctors' offices and hospitals sometimes tries to push your chair without telling you," reported Libby Cooper. She wonders whether staff does this for their own convenience (i.e., to move Libby where they'd like her to go) rather than hers. In any case, asking Libby first not only demonstrates respect but also lessens risks to staff. "My chair has automatic locking brakes so you can't move it," said Libby. "Sometimes people come up to push the chair and almost go over top of me. I tell people, 'If you want me to go somewhere, just ask me.'"

As described in chapter 5, some people with mobility problems need assistance getting undressed and onto examining tables. Sometimes patients arrange their own help, by bringing a family member, friend, or paid personal assistant. But others must ask office staff, generally a nurse or practice assistant, for help getting undressed and later dressed. Nowadays, most office staff willingly assists patients who need help with their clothing. "They do what they have to do," said one woman wheelchair user matter-of-factly.

Patients then await the clinician's arrival. Persons who are deaf or hard of hearing may not hear a knock at the door. If patients are not quite ready, they therefore do not have the opportunity to request more time. Clinicians can catch people undressing or inadequately draped, an embarrassing and distressing experience for some patients (Gabbard and Nadelson, 1995). If interior curtains to shield patients from open doorways are not drawn, patients can risk additional uncomfortable exposure. Then again, having clinicians pop out from behind such curtains can startle deaf or hard of hearing patients who are unaware that the clinician has entered the room.

Persons who are blind or have low vision must determine who has entered the room—easily accomplished if clinicians introduce themselves. This doesn't always happen. "This doctor never spoke to me," recalled Judi Pitt, who is blind. "He just came in, opened the chart, and started to do things. He never said hello. It was like I was invisible." Judi, though, spoke up, telling the physician to greet her and introduce himself whenever he comes into the room. "If you walk into this room right now, say, 'Hi, I'm So-and-so.' Say who you are."

Physical Examination and Procedure Etiquette

Examining patients with certain physical impairments requires clinical skill and knowledge. Clinicians must consider such factors as risks for autonomic dysreflexia (especially for persons with high spinal cord injuries, see note 12, chapter 4); appropriate handling of catheters, stoma, ventilatory support equipment, braces, orthotics, and other devices; management of spasticity and other movement disorders; and safe positioning on examining tables (Peters, 1982; Welner et al., 1999; Welner and Temple, 2004). For various reasons, some patients may be unable to perform the actions clinicians typically request during standard examinations.

> Severe motor, cognitive, and communication impairments make it difficult or impossible for some patients to follow through with directions from the physician, and they limit certain traditional physical examination maneuvers. Creativity is often required to accomplish the examination. Expert examination skills are particularly necessary in such situations. (Ganter et al., 2005, p. 8)

Some people with disabilities avoid medical encounters whenever possible precisely because of these challenges, so they approach clinic visits with heightened anxiety and even distrust (Welner et al., 1999; Kirschner et al., 2005).

Effective communication and proper etiquette during physical examinations are therefore essential, not only to ensure high-quality exams but also to make patients as comfortable as possible and thus likely to return for future care. Even something as simple as carefully draping patients can provide invaluable reassurance (Peters, 1982; Gabbard and Nadelson, 1995). Patients and clinicians should ideally function as partners during physical examinations. Most people with disabilities know what works best for them—for effective communication and physical movements—and clinicians would likely benefit from asking their advice (Ferreyra and Hughes, 1984; Welner et al., 1999).

Some interviewees told graphic stories about physical examination and procedure etiquette gone awry. Despite diverse details, the message of most stories boils down to one point: failure by clinicians to communicate effectively that something unpleasant is about to happen. Warning blind persons about imminent needle sticks exemplifies this concern. "When I'm going to have blood drawn, I always ask them to let me know when they're going to do the actual pricking," said a blind man. Being warned helps him "psychologically prepare for it."

Unpleasant Surprises

During physical examinations or procedures, patients often find themselves positioned so they cannot see what is about to happen, regardless of their visual acuity. The quintessential example of such a situation involves women undergoing pelvic exams and Pap tests. For Pap smears, women typically lie on their backs, legs spread apart, with feet positioned in stirrups; clinicians, seated between the woman's legs, insert a speculum to spread the vagina and reveal the cervix. Women cannot see when the clinician is about to insert the speculum, so this step can come as a surprise. Even when clinicians warm the speculum under hot water, many women find its insertion uncomfortable (Welner et al., 1999).[3] Good clinicians talk women through the procedure, describing each step just before it happens.

Because of risks of cervical cancer especially among sexually active women, Pap testing should begin in early adulthood. Often, this represents the initial foray beyond the pediatrician's office, and their first Pap test experience can affect young women's perceptions of clinical encounters for years to come. Bridget Becker was fortunate in her initial Pap test, but it taught her what to request in future encounters. Bridget, deafened in early childhood, reads lips and speaks sign language.

> For my first Pap smear, I went to an RN [registered nurse] who was a family friend. I didn't have a sign interpreter. There I was in the stirrups, and the nurse disappeared. I said, "I can't see you." So she would stand up and tell me what she was about to do and then disappear between my legs to do it. She was this little jack-in-the-box, jumping up and down. It was very funny, but it helped me to understand the process. Looking back, I thought, "Oh lord, bring in an interpreter! Don't do this jack-in-the-box thing between my legs." The positive thing was we had communication. The negative was the way she had to do it. It took a lot longer because she kept popping up and down. I just wanted to go home.

Unfortunately for Kate Cather, who is also deaf, her first Pap smear was "awful." Her clinician told her virtually nothing. "They didn't tell me what they were going to do. There I was in the stirrups—I couldn't see what was going on. The doctor didn't say to me, 'This might be uncomfortable,' or tell me how much pain to expect. I never went again." Kate, in her late twenties, needs periodic Pap screening to detect cervical cancer, which is treatable at early stages but can kill when found late. However, citing this trauma caused by faulty communication, Kate refuses to get another Pap smear. Not surprisingly, deaf women with access to sign language interpreters appear much more likely than those without interpreter services to receive Pap testing (MacKinney et al., 1995).

Even when patients can see what clinicians are doing, fears can arise when patients do not understand specific actions. Harry Spicer recalled his first testicular examination—screening to detect testicular cancer, which generally responds well to treatment. "I was scared," Harry admitted. "I didn't know if I was being molested or raped, or if this was a sexual advance."

Harry believes that hearing doctors talk hearing patients through "the entire exam. But when the patient is deaf, they just do it. We don't know what's coming, what's going on, or how long it's going to last. Some doctors keep on talking and forget I'm deaf.'" To reassure Harry, "All doctors have to say is, 'I need to check this. I'm going to touch you here.'"

Several interviewees described acute care situations that left them traumatized. The common thread was complete communication breakdowns: clinicians simply failed to explain what they were about to do. Teddy Grady, in his late fifties and blind, was rushed to the emergency room after an accident. "The first thing they slapped on me was a neck brace. They put it all around my mouth, all around my nose." No one told Teddy why he needed the neck brace, which also covered much of his face. "I didn't know what they're doing to me. I couldn't even breathe." Technicians wheeled Teddy downstairs for X-rays and left him in a room for four or five hours. Being unaware of his surroundings and what was happening compounded Teddy's terror about his injuries.

Brad Pepperill's experience humiliated him and caused considerable pain. Brad, who is deaf, had "a cyst between the cheeks of my buttocks. They did not warn me that they were going to slice it open." Brad lay prone on the procedure table, erroneously thinking that the injection he had just had had drained the cyst. Instead, the injection only provided local anesthesia preparatory to lancing and draining the cyst. "They patted me on the shoulder and gave me the thumbs up. I don't know if they thought it was funny. Why couldn't they show me the knife and say, 'I'm about to cut'? They did two cuts. I wanted to scream. Oh my God, I didn't know what that was for!"

The location of his cyst certainly left Brad vulnerable. In identical circumstances, a hearing person would also likely feel embarrassed. But as Brad said, "If I was hearing, they would have talked me through it. I would at least have known. But being deaf, there I was on my stomach looking at the view until I felt the knife." Brad thought the physician could have shown him anatomic pictures and described what was about to happen. "It was rude the way they communicated with me. It wasn't comfortable for me at all. I felt like an idiot."

Making Accommodations

Sometimes the only accommodations required to facilitate communication involve simple courtesy. Melvin Schwartz, who is in his mid-seventies, hears better in his right ear than he does his left. His physician always makes sure she comes around to Melvin's right side when she wants to speak with him. During his recent hospitalization, Melvin's doctors and nurses also remembered his preference. "They would talk to each other, and I couldn't hear what they were saying. When they wanted to talk to me, they would talk directly to my right ear."

Simple accommodations occasionally require bending rules. For example, many institutions limit the access of family and friends to surgical suites. Granting selected exceptions to this rule makes sense. George Corrigan and his wife are both hard of hearing. "When my wife had a baby, she had a C-section [Caesarean section delivery]. I was in the operating room with her. They were telling us all this stuff to do, even though she wasn't having a vaginal birth. But everyone was wearing masks." The masks prevented George from reading the clinicians' lips. The delivery team allowed George's mother-in-law into the surgical suite; she heard the instructions and spoke them to George, who read her lips.

Some facilities require people to relinquish their hearing aids during major operative procedures. These rules may have excellent rationales, but they can cause problems for patients. "They made me leave my hearing aids with my mother," Denise Harding recounted. "Afterwards, they told me, 'You took a long time to come out of anesthesia. We kept talking to you.' But I couldn't hear them! There was no way for me to understand what was going on and get pulled out of the anesthesia. It's very scary." Later, in her hospital room, Denise had trouble hearing when the nurses spoke to her through an intercom. "I had them put signs at the nurses' station that I was hard of hearing. But no one read the signs. They'd talk to me over this loud-speaker, but I couldn't hear them." Because of this, Denise thought the nurses never responded when she rang her call button.

Sometimes, requests to change rules require balancing competing interests, as with Carmen Valdez's plea about her screening mammogram. "My favorite [sign language] interpreter happens to be male," Carmen said. "I told them that I want the interpreter in there with me during the mammogram. It was okay with me if he saw me in that condition. But the office person said this man could not come in with me." Likely the mammogram center's policies prohibited men from passing beyond their outer door to avoid surprising, embarrassing, or distressing their virtually exclusively female clientele. But for Carmen, the interpreter's absence meant she could not communicate effectively with the mammography technicians. Carmen blamed bruising on her breast from the mammogram on inadequate communication.

Finally, clinicians should not assume that someone who assists persons with daily activities is necessarily welcome during clinical encounters.[4] Men and women with disabilities are vulnerable not only to physical but also emotional abuse, especially when they have substantial sensory or physical impairments and must depend on others to assist with basic needs. From 10 to 13 percent of women with physical disabilities report physical, sexual, or emotional abuse within the prior year (Young et al., 1997; McFarlane et al., 2001). Over time, 31 to 83 percent of women with disabilities experience abuse, double to quadruple the rates among nondisabled women (Nosek et al., 2004, p. 335). Although domestic partners are the primary perpetrators, disabled women also report abuse by mothers, brothers, paid personal assistants, and health care providers.[5] Elder abuse is increasingly recognized, with approximately 1 million cases annually nationwide, and it is most often committed at home by spouses, children, other relatives, or paid caregivers (Marshall, Benton, and Brazier, 2000, p. 42). Allowing abusers to remain in the room during clinical visits can have serious consequences. Patients obviously could not freely reveal the abuse to clinicians, and patients may suffer further trauma, psychic and physical, when they return home.

Connie Wilder pays a personal assistant to help with activities she can no longer manage independently because of muscular dystrophy. Connie's personal care assistant (PCA) drove her to a gynecology appointment and helped Connie get undressed and onto the examining table. Connie felt "taken aback" at what happened next.

> During the exam, the gynecologist asked my PCA, who I didn't know that well, to stay in the room to hold my legs in the stirrups. Then the doctor started asking me all these questions, like if I was sexually active. I didn't want to answer in front of the PCA, but I didn't feel comfortable telling the PCA to leave—I didn't want to hurt that relationship. It was very uncomfortable. I did not go back to that doctor.

In deciding not to ask her PCA to leave, Connie weighed her own sense of exposure—both physical and emotional—against the risk of losing the PCA. Personal assistants are hard to find and retain (see chapter 9). The gynecologist erred in putting Connie in this difficult position. A better approach would have been for the *gynecologist* to request that the PCA leave the room during all aspects of the clinical interview. For holding Connie's legs during the Pap smear, the gynecologists should have involved the nurse or clinical assistant or asked Connie's preferences about whether she wanted the PCA's help.

Telephone Communication

Telephones provide an essential conduit for patient-clinician communication, as well as the vehicle for such routine tasks as scheduling appointments, obtaining insurance referrals, and refilling prescriptions at pharmacies. In addition, growing numbers of health care providers aim to improve patient care via the telephone, such as by using interactive, computer-controlled programs to routinely solicit information from patients (e.g., about their blood pressure levels, medication use, diets, physical activities) and then provide advice and instructions (Friedman et al., 1997). Despite its impersonal aura, some patients form positive personal relationships with telephone-linked care (Kaplan, Farzanfar, and Friedman, 2003), and telephone-based programs can improve clinical outcomes as well as satisfaction with care (Waterman et al., 2001).

Nowadays, roughly 25 percent of contacts between internists and their patients occur via telephone. At one academic primary care practice, telephone callers were younger than the average patient (41 compared with 49 years old) and more likely to be female (71 versus 59 percent; Delichatsios, Callahan, and Charlson, 1998, p. 581). Seventeen percent of calls about symptoms involved the upper respiratory tract, with 16 percent pertaining to orthopedic, 15 percent to dermatologic, and 14 percent to gastrointestinal problems. Thirty-eight percent of patients who called viewed telephones as an acceptable conduit for obtaining medical care, while 17 percent did not: "Can't discuss things over the phone . . . have to point to where it hurts" (p. 583).

Thus, telephones are now integral to clinical care, despite remaining questions about their appropriate roles. Certainly, clinicians should optimally impart sensitive clinical information, such as test results suggesting new diagnoses, in person, where they can appreciate fully patients' reactions and patients have more opportunities to ask questions. The trade-off is time. Busy clinicians generally find it easier to schedule telephone calls than face-to-face appointments. Some patients prefer to know bad news sooner rather than later, regardless of how it arrives.

Telephones can prove a double-edged sword for persons with disabilities. On the one hand, telephones enhance the convenience of communication for persons who face considerable challenges in getting to clinicians' offices or other settings (e.g., to drop off prescriptions at pharmacies). Patients might willingly trade off the convenience of speaking to clinicians by telephone, even on sensitive topics, against the effort of journeying to clinics or offices. On the other hand, some persons with vision, hearing, and manual dexterity difficulties can find operating and accessing telecommunications technologies challenging.

Persons with sensory and physical disabilities, especially younger persons, report dissatisfaction with their telephone access to clinicians more often than others. Among Medicare beneficiaries younger than age sixty-five, 12.8 percent of persons reporting major sensory or physical disabilities are dissatisfied with the "ease of obtaining answers to questions over the telephone about treatment or prescriptions," compared with 5.9 percent of persons without these disabilities (Iezzoni et al., 2002, p. 375). Among Medicare beneficiaries older than sixty-four, the numbers dissatisfied with telephone access are 7.8 percent and 4.4 percent, respectively, for persons with and without major disabilities. Medicare beneficiaries who are blind, deaf, and very hard of hearing report the highest levels of dissatisfaction with telephone communication.[6]

The Americans with Disabilities Act and Section 255 of the Telecommunications Act of 1996 require that telecommunications services be accessible to persons with disabilities (see chapter 13). Teletypewriters or telecommunications devices for the deaf (TTY or TDD, often used synonymously), telephone relay services, and video relay services provide accessible telephone services to persons who are deaf or hard of hearing. Today, the major barrier to telephone communication involves clinicians' willingness to acquire and learn how to use accessible equipment and services.

Rick Abernathy never has trouble with his physician returning his calls. When his low vision suddenly blurred further, Rick called his doctor. "They called me right back and asked if I had a headache along with it. I said 'yeah,' and they told me what medicine to take. The blurring went away. I've had no problem communicating with the receptionists or the doctors."

Rick Abernathy's brief story suggests that his physician's quick response was critical. Blurring vision accompanied by headache could portend a life-threatening emergency. Perhaps his physician's telephoned instructions spared Rick from calamity. However, this story highlights an important challenge posed by telephones—winnowing out urgent calls that require immediate attention from numerous mundane contacts. Although this imperative applies to all callers, individuals with complex medical conditions develop complications more often than do others. For instance, when Sylvie Park, who has post-polio syndrome, switched her antiseizure medication, strange symptoms appeared.

> Two weeks ago I called the doctor's office because I was having a reaction to medication—that's what it turned out to be. I was taking this one seizure drug, and I was fine. When I switched drugs, my muscles started jumping. So I called, and the nurse was going to get back to me that day. I waited overnight and waited the next morning. I waited for four days. I kept calling and leaving messages. The nurse never did call me back. I finally went to the emergency room.

Sylvie, like many other discouraged telephone callers, resorted to visiting an emergency room. One study found that 33 percent of callers would go to emergency departments if they cannot reach their physicians by telephone (Delichatsios, Callahan, and Charlson, 1998, p. 583). A telephone call from her nurse or doctor could perhaps have resolved Sylvie's medication side effect and prevented a costly visit to the emergency room.[7]

Thankfully, most calls are not emergencies. Nonetheless, even something as simple as making an appointment can prove challenging, especially for persons who are deaf or hard of hearing. Interviewees describe being unable to understand when office staff mumbles, speaks with heavy accents, or talks rapidly. Automated telephone menu systems (e.g., for scheduling appointments, ordering prescription refills, obtaining test results, or leaving messages) often frustrate callers and consume considerable time. Offices frequently do not have TTYs or staff does not know how to use the equipment. Some office staff refuses to take telephone or video relay calls, claiming "we're too busy right now." The comments of one woman, in her mid-sixties and hard of hearing, typify these complaints:

> I get extremely stressed out on the telephone. Just making phone calls is bad enough, but making them to a doctor's office is horrible. You tell them that you have a hearing loss: "Would you please speak slower and speak up?" But even if they do slow down, if they have a heavy accent, I can't understand them. They have trouble speaking up.
>
> What gets me the most in the doctor's office is that you have to push all these buttons for this or that. I had to go through seven or eight buttons to get a test result! You have to hear all the instructions to push the right buttons. It takes double time for me because I have to keep going back to the previous menu to know what the hell they said. I find the telephone extremely scary.

Marta Redding, who is also hard of hearing, tries using the telephone relay service (see box 13.3) to deal with lengthy automated menus. That doesn't work either: "Very often the relay can't keep up with them because the menu's too fast." The communication assistant in the relay cannot type instructions to Marta quickly enough to respond to the automated telephone commands. "So by the time they get the first two or three items on the menu typed to you, the thing is finished. They have to keep calling back and going over it again and again and again."

Nonetheless, Marta and other interviewees like using the relay with their TTY because the TTY prints out what the relay communications assistant says. That gives Marta a written record of her conversation, reassuring her about accurately understanding what transpired over the telephone. In particular, Marta wants to hear her test results correctly. "With a relay, you can read accurate numbers, assuming that the relay operator does it right. . . . But doctors don't want to mess with it. They don't know how to do it, and they don't want to learn. As far as they're concerned, it takes too long."

Clinical Competence and
Technical Communication

"The first thing I expect from my doctors is that they be well informed and professional," George Corrigan replied when asked to define good quality health care. "I expect to ask a lot of questions and either get answers or referrals to appropriate people to get the answers. I want them to give me an unbiased opinion free from any pressures from health insurers or drug companies. . . . I want to know that my physician is working for me and not for anybody else."

Mr. Corrigan's emphasis on competence and objectivity reflects his personal priorities. "Look," he said to his fellow hard of hearing interviewees, "we're men, and men use doctors differently than women. Women have a more holistic approach to their bodies and their health. Men, we tend to wait till there's a crisis to go to the doctor." His concentration on competence may also relate to what happened several years ago. "I was working very hard, putting in ten- or twelve-hour days," Mr. Corrigan recalled. "I developed what I thought was an ulcer. My primary care physician put me on a prescription acid blocker. That didn't help. Two months later, he suggested I change my diet. . . . Four months later, I'd been to the emergency room three times, doubled over in pain. I was admitted for emergency gallbladder surgery. It's normally a forty-five minute procedure, but it took two and a half hours, the gallbladder was so swelled up."

Mr. Corrigan thinks his primary care physician's diagnostic failure flowed inevitably from today's health care system. Financial and time pressures made his physician go "for the easiest, least expensive thing to treat." But he wonders whether his being hard of hearing contributed to incomplete or inaccurate communication with his physician, prolonging the misdiagnosis. "Sometimes when you're talking to doctors, you don't feel like you're connecting. Because we're hard of hearing, the first thing we do is to slow things down. But doctors tend to go through a checklist real fast." Mr. Corrigan accepts some blame for his diagnostic delay. "It's my responsibility to be aware of what's going on with my body . . . and to make my needs known."

Nonetheless, he feels the ultimate responsibility rests with his physician. After all, evaluating symptoms and making diagnoses is his doctor's job.

Complete, open, and accurate communication between patients and clinicians is essential to ensuring the technical quality of care—making accurate diagnoses, evaluating therapeutic alternatives, and managing disease over time.[1] Even in this technical context, communication is a two-way street. Just as clinicians ask patients questions to elicit essential information, so too do patients question clinicians to learn more about their conditions and to understand prognoses and treatment options. As described in part III, fully appreciating these clinical concerns enhances patients' abilities to manage their health conditions effectively.

Drawing on the conventional metaphor, this chapter addresses communication about the science rather than the art of clinical care—the search for "objective" facts and evidence, the touchstones of technically competent care. However, communication—even about narrow technical or clinical matters—is rooted in larger meanings. As medical educator Eric Cassell wrote, patients do not simply provide facts but instead convey "facts along with explanations, interpretations, and understandings." For their part, clinicians hear those facts within their own frameworks of meanings and interpretations. "It is not the patients' fault that doctors often provide interpretations or understandings that are different from the patients'" (Cassell, 1985b, p. 22).

This gap between the interpretations of patients and their physicians—even around the meaning of signs, symptoms, side effects, and other clinical observations—can loom especially large for some persons with disabilities. Numerous interviewees worry that their clinicians do not know enough about patients' specific functional impairments to render safe and effective care. Patients' suspicions that clinicians do not understand medical features of their disabilities can complicate communication from the outset.

Some interviewees—especially those with relatively rare conditions—may have unrealistic expectations about what primary care or even some specialists can reasonably know about their specific disorders. However, most interviewees do not expect all clinicians to know absolutely everything about their conditions. They do want clinicians to remain open to new ideas and to be concerned enough to concede knowledge gaps. When clinicians admit they must seek expert advice or refer patients elsewhere, many interviewees feel reassured that clinicians are taking their concerns seriously. In some instances, patients themselves are experts about certain aspects of their disabling conditions and can help their clinicians decide what additional input is needed (chapter 11). This chapter considers such communication about technical aspects of care, examining both in-person interactions as well as written information.

Communication and Competence in Technical Care

During my second year at Harvard Medical School, when we first moved from classrooms into clinics, each student received a small, rust-brown volume embossed with gold letters: *The Art of Medical Care and Caring.* We were poised to learn about eliciting patients' histories and performing physical examinations, and two "loyal alumni" wanted to remind us that "compassion and care for the patient is equal in importance to the full understanding of molecular biology and pathophysiology."[2] The little book contained several works from famous physicians from the early twentieth century—a time when most technical clinical information came from questioning and examining patients, not diagnostic tests. One essay, an address by Frederick Cheever Shattuck to 1907 medical graduates of Yale University, identified seven essentials for success in clinical practice.[3] First came knowing medical science, then "thoroughness":

> Form the habit of it from the start and deal with each case which comes to you as if it were the only case in the world. Never forget that mistakes come far more from not looking than from not knowing, from taking things for granted. Collect all your facts. For failure to do this there is no excuse. . . .
>
> In history taking there is a chance for the exercise of much art. The way in which a person tells his story in itself teaches you much about his case. . . . Just remember that people generally care little how you collect your facts. They want to help you to help them, and are ready to accept your methods, especially if tactfully applied. (Shattuck, 1907)

Zipping forward almost a century, clinical educators have developed entire curricula around the clinical interview. Exhortations continue about gathering complete and accurate information, placing primacy on patients' stories.[4] "The patient's history of the illness or report of symptoms, behaviors, and feelings . . . is usually the most essential element in making diagnoses and decisions" (Cassell, 1997, pp. 96–97). Tact alone is no longer sufficient to ensure complete and accurate communication about technical clinical topics. Clinicians' interview styles, interest, and involvement relate directly to the quantity and quality of information elicited from patients (Frankel and Beckman, 1989, p. 87). An empathic communication style during the clinical interview can improve the effectiveness of care. "The feeling of being understood by another person is intrinsically therapeutic: it bridges the isolation of illness and helps to restore the sense of connectedness that patients need to feel whole" (Suchman et al., 1997, p. 678).

During clinical interviews, patients judge their clinicians along various dimensions, ranging from assessing their clinical competence to their compassion. "Patients are trying to discover whether physicians are taking them seriously, are on the right track, or are empathetic" (Cassell, 1997, p. 148). Some patients rarely articulate their feelings directly or explicitly, instead giving clues about their emotional concerns and offering clinicians opportunities to respond with empathy (Suchman et al., 1997). Most people seek substantive knowledge from their clinical encounters about their specific conditions and treatments. In addition, some persons desire general health information, including advice about modifying lifestyles and health behaviors, addressing social isolation and stress, and wellness and preventive care.

Many people want clinicians to understand how their conditions affect their daily lives and physical and emotional well-being. Increasing reliance on sophisticated biomedical knowledge is widening the gulf between "illness" experiences of patients and "disease" as construed by practitioners. According to physician and anthropologist Arthur Kleinman:

> By invoking the term illness, I mean to conjure up the innately human experience of symptoms and suffering. Illness refers to how the sick person and the members of the family or wider social network perceive, live with, and respond to symptoms and disability. . . . [Illness includes] the patient's judgments about how best to cope with the distress and with the practical problems in daily living it creates. . . . Disease, however, is what the practitioner creates in the recasting of illness in terms of theories of disorder. . . . The practitioner reconfigures the patient's and family's illness problems as narrow technical issues, disease problems. . . . For the practitioner, the patient's complaints (symptoms of illness) must be translated into the *signs* of disease. . . . Clinicians sleuth for pathognomonic signs—the observable, telltale clues to secret pathology—that establish a specific disease. This interpretative bias to clinical diagnosis means that the patient-physician interaction is organized as an interrogation . . . (1988, pp. 3–4, 5, 16)

Questioning alone often will not elicit the information clinicians need to make their diagnostic judgments. By careful listening, clinicians must also follow where patients lead as they tell their stories.

Given the diverse and weighty goals attached to the clinical interview, evidence about what actually happens during these encounters is troubling. One seminal study of physicians' behavior during office visits examined audiotapes of 74 encounters (Beckman and Frankel, 1984). Physicians allowed just 17 (23 percent) patients to complete their opening statements about their clinical concerns. In 51 (69 percent) visits, physicians not only interrupted patients' opening statements—after an average of 18 seconds—but also steered the ensuing discussion toward one specific topic. In only one of these 51 visits did the physician allow patients to return to their opening statements. Although physicians typically worry that allowing patients to continue uninterrupted would take too much time, no completed opening statement by patients lasted longer than 150 seconds (Beckman and Frankel, 1984, p. 694).

Another study analyzed audiotapes of 537 primary care visits and found that 32 percent focused narrowly on biomedical topics, while another 33 percent primarily addressed biomedical issues but added some psychosocial topics as well (Roter et al., 1997, p. 352). During both types of visits, 17 to 19 percent of physician talk involved interrogation (asking questions), while 22 to 27 percent represented providing information to patients. For both visit types, physicians spoke 40 percent more than patients, with physicians controlling interview topics and direction. Although biomedical topics dominated 65 percent of visits, both patients and physicians expressed less satisfaction with biomedically focused visits than with those that included psychosocial concerns.

Few studies have looked explicitly at the link between patient-clinician communication and safe, effective care. One study of adverse drug events in primary care found that 63 percent of ameliorable events occurred because physicians failed to respond to patients' reports of problems, while 37 percent stemmed from patients not telling their physicians about drug-related symptoms (Gandhi et al., 2003, p. 1560). Often patients had symptoms for months without visiting or calling their physicians or changing their medications. This situation highlights an irony of today's medicine: "The complexities and discomforts of modern therapeutics have made it even more important for us to understand the patient's experience" (McWhinney, 1989, p. 28). Ensuring safe and effective care requires knowing patients' subjective perceptions—information sometimes discredited as unreliable by scientifically oriented professionals.

According to depositions in malpractice lawsuits, plaintiffs often blame fundamental breakdowns in interpersonal relationships with their clinicians for whatever went wrong. A review of forty-five plaintiff depositions from settled lawsuits found that 32 (71 percent) cited "relationship issues." Problems fell into four broad themes: "desertion" or not being available to patients (31.6 percent); devaluing patients' and/or families' views by not listening or by discounting their opinions (28.9 percent); dysfunctional delivery of information, including failures to provide explanations and timely updates, insensitive provision of bad news, and blaming patients and/or families for bad outcomes (26.4 percent); and not understanding the perspective of patients and/or families (13.1 percent) (Beckman et al., 1994, p. 1368).

In general, people who report fair or poor health are less satisfied with their medical care than those who report better health (Gerteis et al., 1993). This makes sense. Persons with greater clinical needs have more interactions with the health care system and therefore more opportunities for disappointment and mismatches in expectations between patients and clinicians. They are more likely to need timely care and information about their conditions, prognoses, and therapeutic options. Because of lower physiologic reserves, persons in poor health recover less quickly and fully when medical mishaps do occur.

Few studies have examined how persons with sensory and physical impairments assess the technical quality of their care. Primary care physicians often fail to recognize fully patients' functional deficits (Nelson et al., 1983; Wartman et al., 1983; Calkins et al., 1991, 1994) and are uncertain about when to refer patients to rehabilitation specialists (Hoenig, 1993). Nurses' and physicians' assessments of patients' functioning sometimes disagree with patients' perceptions, and these discrepancies can compromise patients' understanding of treatment plans following hospital discharge (Reiley et al., 1996; Calkins et al., 1997).

Nonetheless, almost all Medicare beneficiaries, with and without disabilities, believe their physicians are competent and well-trained (table 8.1). Persons with impairments, however, report higher rates of dissatisfaction with other technical aspects of care. In particular, more than 13 percent report having health problems that they would like to discuss with their physicians but do not.

Clinicians' Training about Disabling Conditions

Most Americans identify a physician as their usual source of health care, with roughly two thirds seeing family physicians or general practitioners (table 8.2). The specialty of physician "usual sources" varies little between persons with and without disabilities, although persons with disabilities are slightly more likely to visit internists and other medical and surgical specialists. Health insurance presumably drives many decisions about who people designate as their usual source of care, with insurers restricting persons to professionals considered primary care physicians—the "PCP." However, for individuals with rare or complex sensory or physical impairments, this may mean their designated PCP has little specific clinical knowledge about their condition (Oshimi et al., 1998). PCPs still need to coordinate care among appropriate specialists, an essential primary care function regardless of patients' disability status. However, as some interviewees observed, when specialists direct the vast majority of care, the role of PCPs becomes less clear.

The overall structure of basic medical education has changed relatively little in nearly a century, despite the growing prevalence of chronic disabling conditions. Traditionally, medical schools have emphasized the diagnosis and treatment of acute problems, as well as the search for scientific knowledge leading to cures (Institute of Medicine, Committee on a National Agenda, 1991; Cassell, 1997). Schools do not ignore functional impairments and lifelong progressive conditions, but students learn primarily about their acute manifestations and technical therapeutic interventions, such as surgeries and treatments for acute exacerbations. Because most clinical educa-

Table 8.1. Medicare Beneficiaries' Concerns about Technical Aspects of Care (Percent[a])

Aspect of Care	No DA[b]	Very Low Vision	Deaf/ HOH[b]	Major Difficulties		
				Walking	Reaching	Grasping
"Doctor is competent and well-trained"	0.7	2.1	1.5	1.5	1.5	1.7
"Doctor is very careful to check everything when examining you"	4.1	10.4	9.0	8.6	9.1	9.3
"Doctor has a good understanding of your medical history"	2.5	5.2	4.6	5.4	6.5	6.8
"Doctor has a complete understanding of the things that are wrong with you"	3.5	8.9	7.0	8.6	9.5	9.6
"Often has health problems that should be discussed but are not"	6.0	14.2	13.5	14.2	13.3	15.0
"Availability of care by specialists when needs it"	2.2	7.8	8.4	6.2	7.2	8.2
"Follow-up care received after an initial treatment or operation"	2.3	7.0	7.5	5.7	7.6	8.2
"Has great confidence in doctor"	3.5	7.8	7.7	7.9	8.4	9.1
"Overall quality of the medical services received in the last year"	2.7	8.1	8.0	7.2	7.9	8.2

Adapted from: Iezzoni et al. (2002, 2003).

[a]Percentage dissatisfied with aspect of care; figures account for age category and sex.

[b]DA = disability; HOH = hard of hearing; grasping = grasping and writing.

Table 8.2 Specialty of Usual Source of Care

Impairment	Practitioner Specialty[a] (Percent[b])					
	FP/GP	Internal Medicine	Pediatrics	OB/GYN	Other MD	Non-MD
Nonimpairment	68.7	18.4	6.1	2.4	3.6	0.8
Vision impairments	64.7	21.6	3.9	3.2	6.0	0.6[c]
Hearing impairments	66.7	20.4	4.5	1.5[c]	5.8	1.1[c]
Lower extremity mobility difficulty	64.4	20.7	3.3[c]	0.7[c]	8.1	2.7[c]
Upper extremity mobility difficulty	63.7	22.8	1.4[c]	0.5[c]	8.6[c]	3.0[c]
Difficulty using hands	68.1	19.0	4.7[c]	0.3[c]	7.2[c]	0.7[c]
Any impairment	66.1	20.7	4.1	1.8	6.0	1.3
Any major impairment	70.0	20.3	2.9[c]	0.5[c]	4.5	1.8[c]

Data source: 2001 Medical Expenditure Panel Survey.

[a]FP/GP = family or general practitioner; OB/GYN = obstetrician and gynecologist; other MD = surgery and other medical specialties; non-MD = nurse, physician assistant, and other non-physician.

[b]Figures account for age category and sex.

[c]Because of small number of respondents, this estimate may be unreliable.

tion still happens in hospitals, students gain little insight into how patients function at home or rebound from short-term exacerbations. By primarily seeing acutely "sick" patients, trainees can undervalue patients' functional abilities and usual quality of life, absorbing "the impression that the chronically ill are problem patients for their failure to improve and for their frequent need of physicians' services" (Kleinman, 1988, p. 257).

Medical schools generally do not offer formal didactic training in assessing patients' physical, sensory, cognitive, and emotional abilities to function in daily life (Cassell, 1997; Institute of Medicine, Committee on Assessing, 1997; Iezzoni, 2003). They rarely require clinical rotations in rehabilitation medicine or training with interdisciplinary clinical teams about functional impairments (Institute of Medicine, Committee on a National Agenda, 1991, p. 231). "Rehabilitation has been one of the major advances in American medicine since World War II, yet it remains peripheral in the educational process" (Cassell, 1997, p. 166).

General medical postgraduate training programs (internships followed by residencies) also offer little formal teaching about functional evaluations. Beyond such specific assessments as vision testing and neurological exams, "primary care providers are not typically trained to recognize the general health care needs of people with disabling conditions" (Institute of Medicine, Committee on Assessing, 1997, p. 181). By practicing in outpatient clinics, most residents do have opportunities to observe how functional impairments affect people's daily lives. Many learn to refer patients with functional concerns to physical or occupational therapists, although primary care physicians may not know exactly what these professionals do (Hoenig, 1993; Iezzoni, 2003). Some primary care residencies, including family medicine, as well as osteopathic programs, offer more training in functional topics.

After completing formal training, physicians continue to learn, often reporting that each patient brings new insight. Many primary care physicians do eventually acquire skills in assessing sensory and physical impairments. After all, 20 to 40 percent of their adult patients likely have one or more disabling condition. Some physicians find special mentors or role models who teach them, while others learn with experience. But as one physician said about caring for persons with disabilities, "There's a sort of haphazard, random interaction between me, my nurse practitioner, and home care nurses—my eyes and ears on the ground at home. It's not a satisfying process. I don't have a strategy with defined goals." He regrets that he has no one to teach him about evaluating and improving functioning and quality of life. "I'm not growing in this area" (Iezzoni, 2003, p. 146).

Views of Clinicians' Technical Competence

Some interviewees worry that their physicians—primary care doctors and sometimes even specialists—have little scientific or practical knowledge about their conditions. These perceptions lead directly to uneasiness about how far patients should trust or rely on their physicians' clinical judgment. Jena Foster articulated these concerns. With a condition similar to spina bifida, Jena requires expert urological care. Deciding that "as an adult I need a little bit different care than when I was a child," Jena changed her doctors.

> I was born with my disabilities. I'm twenty-five years old. I've been going to the hospital for children my whole life, and I was nervous to switch over. A couple of appointments with adult doctors didn't go so well, so I'm thinking, "Why did I do this?"
> . . . I felt the doctors had very little knowledge. I needed to do a lot of explaining, but I didn't think it was necessary to explain things to *the doctor!* That in itself made me uneasy. I've had excellent care my whole life. Now I'm throwing all my trust into people whom I don't know that I do trust. Now I go to each doctor thinking, "Do I have to educate them from day one about everything?"

For some interviewees, diagnostic delays precipitated concerns about physicians' clinical knowledge. Some persons spent years searching for a diagnosis once disabling symptoms began and were especially troubled when physicians seemed unwilling to admit ignorance. As one man said, "A doctor doesn't like to tell a person he doesn't know what's wrong with you."

After diagnosis, delays in devising treatment frustrate some persons. For instance, Marta Redding calls her dual conditions—hardness of hearing and tinnitus (ringing or buzzing in the ear)—the "double whammy. Tinnitus can be debilitating—people have committed suicide." Marta found that "most doctors don't know what to do about it. You get the run around for a long time before you get put in the right direction. It's not curable, but it's manageable." As Marta said, patients spend time, energy, and money finding clinicians who can help. Interviewees sense that some physicians are simply stymied, uncertain how to adapt interventions for persons with functional impairments. Sometimes, patients step in, filling the knowledge gap. "Nine times out of ten, I'm educating the doctor," observed one woman with a spinal cord injury. "If the doctor is at all egotistical . . . it's very frustrating to educate."

Referrals to specialists offer an obvious solution to specialized needs. Some persons require sequential referrals up a hierarchy of technological sophistication. Involving specialists can risk splintering care, as different physicians address their area of expertise but neglect other clinical concerns. Coordination then becomes key to ensuring good technical care, such as preventing dangerous interactions among medications. Some interviewees view specialists as their primary clinicians. That strategy can backfire if specialists are not trained to coordinate all aspects of care, including screening and preventive services and overseeing medications for common, coexisting medical conditions. Some specialists are also ill equipped to handle inevitable acute episodic conditions, such as colds and sinusitis.

For some people, finding the right specialist is difficult, exacerbated by restrictive health insurance policies and limited physician referral networks. Some interviewees report independently combing through lists of potential specialists, unsure whom to choose; others rely on their primary care physicians to suggest appropriate specialists. Then, all clinicians caring for a patient must communicate with each other. "When I was hospitalized, all my doctors came, and they didn't just look at the disability," reported one woman. "The primary care doctor came and my neurologist and psychiatrist, and they all agreed that my medications were at odds with each other. I was taken off four prescriptions, and the fifth one was cut in half. I don't know that you could ask for more, with them all working together."

Inevitably, people with disabilities will develop new medical conditions, especially as they age. Diagnosing new conditions is sometimes straightforward, uncomplicated by coexisting disability. Dwight Eaton, in his mid-fifties, developed prostate cancer four years previously:

> I was very fortunate. The doctor I had was the head of the urology department, a prostate cancer expert. He never deprecated me because I was blind. He noted that I was a young man to have the disease and said we should take an aggressive course. He kept repeating, over and over again, "You're a young guy. You deserve a shot."

Presumably, Dwight's clinicians immediately evaluated his prostate when he first reported urological symptoms. Confusing urological symptoms with blindness is unlikely! But delays in diagnosing new medical conditions can occur when clinicians assume that all symptoms relate to someone's underlying impairment. This happened to Penny Hanks, in her early fifties with a C-6 spinal cord injury from a car crash.

"I was injured thirty years ago, and I was healthy for many years," Penny observed. "The past few years I've felt as though I were falling apart in so many ways, so I've started to see doctors. For five years or so, I had a really hard time finding someone that I could relate to. I'd go in, explain the problem, and they would say, 'It's probably nothing, but I'll order this test for you.' In some cases, they were very expensive tests." None of the tests found anything wrong.

Physician after physician dismissed Penny's symptoms, attributing them to decades of living with spinal cord injury. Finally, "I found this doctor who is a woman. She's new, so she had all the time in the world to spend with me. She found the problem. I had symptoms that I'd always looked at in isolation. But when you brought them all together, it ended up being a pituitary problem." Penny likes her "young doctor. She thinks very broadly." Unlike her older peers, the young doctor recognized that spinal cord injury alone did not explain all Penny's symptoms.

Pain

Patients' and clinicians' perspectives can collide over the frequently vexing topic of pain. Pain is the sentinel symptom of the most common reason for adult disability—arthritis. Depending on the nature of their disability, roughly one third to one half of older women living in the community cite musculoskeletal pain as the main cause (Leveille, Fried, and Guralnik, 2002, p. 768).[5] Women reporting widespread musculoskeletal pain are 2.5 to 3.5 times more likely than other women to experience difficulties with walking, lifting, or activities of daily living (Leveille et al., 2001, p. 1038).[6]

Controlling pain is much in the news. Addictions of high-profile personalities to prescription painkillers and the media blitz from pharmaceutical companies marketing pain medications keep this topic constantly in the public eye. Despite new therapies, many persons remain unresponsive to mainstream medical interventions. The dark side of pain control involves complex societal and personal fears of addiction, illicit drug use, and its myriad destructive consequences, stoked by questions about whether patients' pain is "real."

> If there is a single experience shared by virtually all chronic pain patients it is that at some point those around them—chiefly practitioners, but also at times family members—come to question the authenticity of the patient's experience of pain. This response contributes powerfully to patients' dissatisfaction with the professional treatment system and to their search for alternatives. . . . Reciprocally, chronic pain patients are the bête noire of many health professionals, who come to find them excessively demanding, hostile, and undermining of care. A duet of escalating antagonism ensues, much to the detriment of the protagonists. (Kleinman, 1988, p. 57)

Vic Domenico and his physician are at loggerheads over how to control Vic's pain from a spinal cord injury (chapter 6). In the past, Vic found that "a bag of dope would take away all the pain." But now that he is clean, Vic wants his physician to respect and respond to his need for pain control. He believes that he is already addicted to the medications she prescribes (e.g., for his spasticity), but Vic remains in pain. "Give me some drugs that are going to help me."

Primary care physicians see many persons with such conditions as arthritis and back pain and likely feel confident addressing pain in those clinical contexts. But they often have little knowledge about pain in other physical impairments and can make erroneous assumptions. The experiences of Steffie Giacommo, paraplegic from a spinal cord injury, typify this concern. "I was having unrelenting abdominal pain," Steffie recalled, "and I don't get ill very often. So, when I complained to my physician, she told me to go to the emergency room. I'm a nurse, and I thought I was having appendicitis.

"By the time I got to the emergency room, the pain was really unbearable. The first thing out of the physician's mouth was, 'You feel pain? But you're paralyzed!' He couldn't get the concept that I could still feel pain." Steffie's trust in the physician's clinical competence eroded. "It made me really nervous to see a physician that doesn't understand the pain process."

By midnight, eight hours after Steffie's arrival at the emergency room, "nothing much had been done. They put me in this room by myself, never put the call bell near me, and kept telling me that I shouldn't be in pain because I'm a paraplegic. They never gave me any medication, nothing to ease the pain. They didn't even help me get to the bathroom." Steffie left, and, "The next day at 6 p.m. the pain just subsided. The abdominal X-rays had showed a gas pocket that wasn't moving. I thought that must be the cause. But the physician wouldn't listen to me."

Other interviewees with spinal cord injuries described clinicians performing small procedures on their lower bodies or limbs without local pain control, incorrectly presuming that they would not feel pain. Clinicians withheld pain medications that they would routinely administer to other patients. Caroline Patrick, who is tetraplegic from a spinal cord injury, described her experiences with a "not very glamorous procedure, a hemorrhoidectomy." Afterwards, "my fanny was sore. I told the nurse, 'I need Tylenol.' She says, 'Why? You can't feel.' I said, 'Just because I'm a C-5 quad, doesn't mean I still can't feel pain.[7] Some people do, some people don't. You have to ask.'" The physician was also skeptical, but he finally prescribed something to control Caroline's pain.

The sensory and physical manifestations of spinal cord injuries *do* vary widely across patients. Some persons might feel pain while others, with ostensibly similar injuries, do not. After tracking persons for five years following spinal cord injury, one study found that 81 percent reported some pain; among those, 53 percent described their pain as severe and 5 percent as excruciating (Siddall et al., 2003, p. 251). People with incomplete spinal cord injuries (perhaps Vic Domenico) can become hypersensitive to pain, experiencing intense discomfort from minor stimuli. Therefore, clinicians must ask and listen to patients who are, after all, experts in their perceptions of pain. Fortunately, no interviewees sustained serious injuries or complications (such as autonomic dysreflexia, see note 7, this chapter, and note 12, chapter 4) from invasive interventions without pain medication.

Explaining Technical Topics

George Corrigan's complaints about technical explanations likely echo those of many other persons, regardless of disability. "The biggest communication difficulty that I have with physicians is the complexity of the information. I couldn't even pronounce 'laparoscopy,'" the surgical technique used to remove his gallbladder. "There's lots of questions I want to ask. I read a lot, and I want surgeons to feel like I'm an intelligent patient. I want to know what the procedures entail, what the risks are going to be. But if there's a lot of complex, Latin-based, multisyllabic words, then forget it! I'm not going to get it."

George Corrigan and other interviewees feel that physicians sometimes avoid providing detailed technical information to them, assuming that because of their disability they are either unable to understand or uninterested in knowing about their conditions (see chapter 6). Nonetheless, Mr. Corrigan and his counterparts do want this information, even if technical language momentarily escapes them (e.g., if they cannot infer these unfamiliar terms while lip reading). They believe that clinicians bear the responsibility of providing clear and understandable explanations of technical topics in accessible formats.

Communicating effectively with persons with visual impairments perplexes some clinicians. Since their work depends heavily on visual input (e.g., seeing anatomical structures), these physicians have trouble conveying information in another format. One blind man described his physician's bafflement at trying to explain technical issues to him without drawing or showing him pictures:

> One of my doctors who's a specialist for a long time couldn't explain anything to me. To him everything's so visual. He couldn't understand how I could conceive what he was trying to tell me. When I talked to him, he'd say, "Well, that's complicated." And I'd say, "You know, I'm a pretty smart guy. You could try to explain it to me." After I convince him, he finally explains things to me, and it's fine.

Some interviewees report not having adequate technical knowledge to ensure the safety and effectiveness of their care—medication side effects, symptoms to watch for, activities to avoid or pursue, or other aspects of care. They have thus faced heightened risks of the medical errors and adverse events endemic to the U.S. health care delivery system (Institute of Medicine, Committee on Quality, 1999). George Corrigan worries about what might happen "if the doctor gives some verbal instruction, I misunderstand, and I carry out what I thought he said." One deaf man believes that his physician, who insists on writing notes, gives him only the "barest information about medications." One time his physician prescribed a medication without warning him to avoid alcohol—apparently a known dangerous interaction. "I took the medicine, and then I drank alcohol and started throwing up. I didn't have the information that I needed."

Blind interviewees report not having comprehensive information about medications in accessible formats. As one man said, this leaves him vulnerable: "If I'm a sighted person and my doctor doesn't give clear directions on how to take the medicine, at least I can read the print instructions. This is much harder for me to do as a blind person. I have to get somebody else to read the thing to me."

In certain situations, clinicians do not consider fully how their proposed treatments might interact with patients' sensory or physical impairments. This leaves people uncertain what to do. Steffie Giacommo confronted this situation when her physician recommended shoulder surgery: "They don't understand that, if you're a paraplegic and have shoulder surgery, you're in bed for three months." Without her arms, Steffie cannot transfer out of bed or onto the toilet or operate her manual wheelchair. "Who's going to come in and take care of you physically, personally, as well as house-wise? Doctors don't go that step beyond the surgery."

"Or think about whether you're going to be able to follow their instructions," added Connie, who has muscular dystrophy. "The doctor says, 'Go home and put your feet up.' I can't put up my feet without help. They don't ask, 'Do you have someone at home to put your feet up?'"

Steffie thinks she knows the right questions to ask because she is a nurse. She worries that patients without that training do not know what to ask and could slip through the cracks when physicians don't understand disability-related issues. As one woman wheelchair user said, "They tell me what they want me to do, but they have no idea how I'm going to do it. And nobody comes up with any ideas for me."

Being responsible for the safety of another family member raises the stakes, as well as the anxiety level of persons with disabilities. George Corrigan's wife, Helen, is also hard of hearing. Helen thought she heard correctly when her son's pediatrician gave her instructions about his medication, but she became unsure when she filled the prescription. When she read the directions, "I'm thinking this doesn't sound right. Instead of putting down a 0.5 dose, they put 5." Could Helen trust her hearing and memory of the pediatrician's instructions? Helen followed her intuition and called the pediatrician, averting a medication error. "My son could have been seriously injured by this prescription mistake."

Making Written Information Accessible

Clinicians now dispense considerable personal health information on paper, such as written instructions for prescription medications, post-discharge activities, and self-management programs. However, for people to read information, clinicians must provide it in accessible formats. For persons who are blind or low vision, accessible formats include braille, large-print texts, audiotape recordings, videotapes or DVDs with oral descriptions, and computer diskettes (see chapter 13).

Braille, created in the early nineteenth century, is used worldwide to convey written information in a tactile format (box 8.1). Unlike sign language

Box 8.1. Braille

Louis Braille (1809–1852)

Louis Braille, who accidentally became blind at three years of age, invented braille as a teenager studying at the Royal Institute for Blind Youth in Paris. Most teachers only talked to the students, and few books were available with raised print letters. Charles Barbier, a former soldier, visited the school and told students about "night writing," a code based on twelve raised dots that let soldiers share secret information without speaking. Braille trimmed the raised dots to six, further honed his system, and published the first braille book in 1829.

What Is Braille?

Braille is not a separate language or vocabulary. Instead, braille uses patterns of one to six raised dots to represent letters, numbers, punctuation, and words. Braille therefore offers another way to write or read English or other written languages. Almost every country worldwide uses braille.

The Braille Code

Different arrangements of one to six raised dots represent every character in the braille code. Each dot has a numbered position (1–6) in the braille cell (see figure 8.1). Different patterns of dots indicate each letter in the alphabet. Numbers are formed using the first ten letters of the alphabet (a–j) and a special number sign (dots 3, 4, 5, and 6). Braille also has 189 special characters, called contractions, used as shorthand for certain words (such as five dots indicating "and" and four for "the") and groups of letters within words (such as three dots indicating "ing" and four dots for "ed").

Ease of Braille

Raised print letters, used since the early 1800s, are actually very difficult to read by touch and harder to write. In contrast, skilled braille readers can read one hundred to two hundred words per minute.

Adapted from: American Foundation for the Blind, What Is Braille? www.afb.org/braillebug/Braille.asp, accessed August 12, 2004 (see box 4.1), braille is not a separate language. Instead, braille uses patterns of one to six raised dots to represent letters, numbers, punctuation, and words (figure 8.1). The precise number of braille readers in the United States is unknown, although persons who were born blind or become blind by early adulthood use braille more often than those who lose vision in old age.[8] For persons who are both blind and deaf, braille is a primary means of communication. Many blind persons know enough braille to decipher signs or read braille labels, although they may not read entire books in braille.

With today's technologies, producing braille texts, signs, labels, and other physical formats is relatively cheap and easy. Creating other accessible formats should be fairly easy in many circumstances. For instance, producing large-print texts merely requires font sizes of fourteen points or higher, depending on the needs of individual readers. Since so much printed information originates from computer files, producing computer diskettes or CDs should also pose few technical problems.

Despite legal mandates to provide written information in accessible forms (see box 13.1), blind and low vision interviewees report rarely receiving in-

The Braille Cell

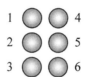

The Braille Alphabet

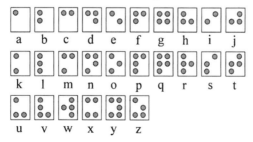

Braille Numbers

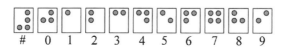

Figure 8.1.   The braille code.

formation they need in formats they can use. One woman complained about the tiny print on prescription package inserts. "The print is very small even for someone who can read 20/20. My sister and my mother try to read it to me, but they always have such a difficult time." To enlarge images of the texts, another woman reads package inserts "under my CCTV [closed-circuit television[9]]. But it's so cryptic, you can't even understand it anyhow. For $150 a bottle for some of these pills, you'd think they could afford a [audiotape] cassette with all that information."

For persons with visual disabilities, the inability to tell which bottle holds which medication poses a huge problem. Some interviewees ask their pharmacists to put large print or braille labels on their pill bottles, but not all drug stores will do this. Carrie uses a low-tech solution to distinguish among her many pill bottles. "I stick rubber bands over some bottles. Then there are different shaped bottles. I just remember what's what." What happens when Carrie's pharmacist refills her prescriptions choosing bottles with different shapes? Carrie lives alone and has no one who can, at a moment's notice, read her prescription labels. Because she does not have critical information in an accessible format, Carrie risks taking the wrong medication and potentially endangering her health.

9

Pushing against Boundaries
of the Health Care System

In the United States, clinicians, health insurers, and policy-makers generally compartmentalize issues related to disability, erecting walls around needs deemed inside and outside the health care system (see chapter 3). But the needs of many persons with disabilities defy tidy packaging, zigzagging across health care, welfare, housing, transportation, education, and other social sectors. Leaping these entrenched boundaries is challenging, at best. Meeting needs in only one sector, while helpful, leaves persons vulnerable on numerous other scores.

This final chapter of part II pushes against the conventional boundaries of the health care system, largely circumscribed by standard health insurance coverage policies. We briefly address assistive technology, personal assistance services, public transportation, and accessible housing. In addition, we touch upon dental services which, although critical to overall health, generally fall outside the perimeter of standard health insurance. These topics do not encompass all concerns of persons with disabilities. Our list notably excludes education, employment, and income support, as well as urban and community planning. Our areas hew closely to the boundaries encircling health care, occasionally crossing the border and gaining health insurance coverage—albeit sometimes only within Medicaid.

Special programs already exist that meet needs beyond traditional health care. For instance, PACE—Program of All-Inclusive Care for the Elderly—provides not only comprehensive health care but also meals, adult day care, transportation, assistive technologies, and other services to nursing home–eligible persons age fifty-five and older living in communities who qualify for both Medicare and Medicaid.[1] "The profile of a typical PACE participant is like that of the average nursing home resident: she is eighty years old, has about eight chronic medical conditions, and needs help with three activities of daily living" (Lynn, 2004, p. 75). Nonetheless, PACE participants generally require fewer expensive hospitalizations and report better quality of life than do equally frail older persons outside PACE. Despite its laudable twenty-year record, PACE remains small, with fewer than fifty PACE sites nationwide. Although PACE and similar programs set high standards for all-inclusive care, disseminating these models more widely presents considerable challenges.[2]

Assistive Technologies

According to the Technology-Related Assistance for Individuals with Disabilities Act of 1988 (P.L. 100-407, nicknamed the "Tech Act"), assistive technology is "any item, piece of equipment, or product system, whether acquired commercially off-the-shelf, modified, or customized, that is used to increase, maintain, or improve the functional capabilities of an individual with a disability." Assistive technologies can restore a person's ability to live his or her daily life independently and efficiently. These technologies span the gamut, with numerous products now available to address wide-ranging sensory and physical functional needs.

Assistive technologies reside at that fractious border between covered and uncovered benefits: sometimes health insurers reimburse assistive technology purchases, and sometimes they do not (chapter 3). Bright lines exclude certain assistive technologies from coverage, including eyeglasses and hearing aids, computers with synthetic speech systems, and accessible telecommunications devices.[3] In Medicare parlance, these technologies qualify as "convenience items," "self-help devices," or "not medically necessary" and therefore fall outside payment boundaries. Certain Medicaid and private health insurers cover some of these items.

Health insurers could not possibly cover every device—or associated needs, such as home renovations and wheelchair-accessible automobiles—without bankrupting costs. Unfortunately, however, for many persons these items do not represent simply enhanced convenience or luxuries but the opportunity to live independently, become employed, and have a safer and fuller life. So the rhetorical and unanswered question is: who will or should pay for assistive technologies if persons with disabilities cannot afford them?

Certain assistive technologies fall within payment boundaries but generally with explicit restrictions. For instance, Medicare covers mobility aids that people need to function within their homes but not devices used only for going outside. Established nearly forty years ago, these rules ignore three crucial facts: dramatic advances in the technological capabilities of wheelchairs; widespread societal recognition of the rights of persons with disabilities to participate fully in community life; and court rulings (notably *Olmstead;* see note 1, preface) requiring community accommodations for persons with disabilities to live as independently as possible outside institutions (Medicare Rights Center, 2004). Medicare rules governing power wheelchair purchases are especially restrictive, covering motorized equipment only if persons cannot operate any type of manual wheelchair in their homes.

After decades of building wheelchairs primarily for institutions, manufacturers finally recognized the diverse needs of customers living in communities. This consumer revolution began in the late 1970s, when Marilyn Hamilton crashed her hang glider into a California mountainside and became paraplegic. Unhappy with existing wheelchairs, she challenged two fellow glider pilots to build an ultralight wheelchair using aluminum tubing as found in their gliders. The resulting wheelchair weighed twenty-six pounds instead of the standard fifty and sold under the name "Quickie."[4]

> Hamilton's wheelchairs put people—users and those around them—
> at ease. Instead of chrome, Hamilton's chairs came in a rainbow of
> hot colors. The customer could personalize a chair in candy apple
> red, canary yellow, or electric green. . . . Quickie chair riders were
> neither sick nor objects of pity. They just got around in a different
> way. "If you can't stand up," Hamilton likes to say, "stand out."
> (Shapiro, 1994, p. 212)

Some observers credit Quickie designs with bolstering the disability rights movement of the 1980s by transforming images of wheelchair users from conventional institutional stereotypes to independence and freedom.

Quickie's market success and demands for new technologies—such as ultra-lightweight manual wheelchairs, motorized scooter wheelchairs, wheelchairs for sports and recreation, and power wheelchairs with specialized capabilities—attracted many competitors to the wheelchair market (Karp, 1998). Some companies sell directly to consumers through the Internet, magazines, and other venues. However, health insurers still typically limit reimbursement to the least expensive equipment, starting with low-end manual models. They generally do not cover wheelchairs that, albeit more expensive, provide greater safety, functionality, and independence to users. Without insurance coverage, many persons cannot afford wheelchairs. Insured people who cannot walk are 40 percent more likely than the uninsured to have wheelchairs (Iezzoni, 2003, pp. 225–226).

Persons with progressive chronic conditions face an additional problem. Insurers typically pay for only one piece of equipment every five years or per an enrollee's lifetime (or time with the insurer). Therefore, with increasing debility, people must think ahead and purchase equipment in anticipation of the worst. These situations pose financial and psychological difficulties, as people must acknowledge deficits they do not yet have—and likely hope never to have. "I had a [multiple sclerosis] MS patient who wasn't safe with her walker anymore," a physical therapist told me. "She wanted a scooter. But because of the progression of her disease, a scooter was not the answer. Medicaid is only going to pay for one mobility aid for the next five years, and she's going to need an electric four-wheeled wheelchair before that. It was really tough to get her to accept that electric wheelchair because that's looking down the road. We convinced her that she needed the wheelchair to be safe."

After equipment arrives, many people require mechanical adjustments to match their new technology—especially complex power wheelchairs—to their bodies and mobility needs. Insurers often do not pay for this fine tuning, although ill-fitting chairs can cause pressure ulcers and other complications. Sometimes people find their equipment does not work for them and they abandon it. Most equipment cannot be rented or borrowed before making purchases, so people have little sense of how the technology will work in their daily lives. People abandon mobility aids more than any other assistive device, especially in the first three months.

> Technology abandonment can have a series of repercussions. For individuals, non-use of a device may lead to decreases in functional abilities, loss of freedom and independence, increases in expenses, and risk of injury or disease. Device abandonment also represents ineffective use of limited funds by federal, state, and local government agencies, insurers, and other providers. . . . The single most significant factor associated with technology abandonment is a failure to consider the user's opinions and preferences in device selection—in other words, *the device is abandoned because it does not meet the person's needs or expectations.* (Scherer, 2000, p. 118)

Obtaining repairs presents another hurdle. The downside of sophisticated circuitry is its tendency to go awry: Fixing complicated power wheelchairs costs more than the nuts and bolts needed to restore standard manual wheelchairs that are malfunctioning. Although insurers theoretically cover necessary repairs, obtaining reimbursable repairs is frequently frustrating, pitting the wheelchair user's definition of "serviceable" equipment against that of the insurer's. Horror stories surface periodically about power wheelchair users, unable to cope at home because of broken equipment, being forced by their health insurers into nursing homes. In these instances, health insurers calculate that placing persons in institutions costs them less than the $20,000 to $30,000 required to replace sophisticated power wheelchairs.[5]

Thus, dollars inevitably shadow decisions about which wheelchair technology insurers will cover for individual consumers. Given their relatively higher costs, power wheelchairs attract the greatest scrutiny: Medicare spending on power wheelchairs grew 450 percent between 1999 and 2003 (Centers for Medicare and Medicaid Services, 2003b). In 2003, federal investigations unearthed unscrupulous vendors bilking Medicare for millions of dollars in fraudulent charges. In response, requests for Medicare power wheelchair purchases now face intensive review.[6] Denying power wheelchairs could force certain persons into institutions, not only compromising their quality of life but also adding to total health care costs (Janofsky, 2004).

The bottom line is that people who can no longer walk safely and independently need wheelchairs—just as persons with different impairments need other assistive technologies. Without essential equipment, their lives are needlessly restricted, even unsafe, and potentially less full and productive than they otherwise might be. In certain circumstances, more expensive equipment could save dollars down the road. Marcia McDonough's situation exemplifies this trade-off. Marcia has a rotator cuff injury: damage to the muscles around her shoulder joint caused by self-propelling her heavy manual wheelchair (see chapter 11). She wants an ultra-lightweight model, but it costs more, and her health insurer will not cover it:

> How can this understanding of better equipment get into the heads of the medical community and the insurance companies? They should understand that if you've got a heavy wheelchair that was giving you a repetitive stress injury in a shoulder or a wrist or an elbow, the cost to them for putting you in rehab and getting you back to 100 percent health is ten, fifteen, twenty times greater than paying the few extra bucks for the better wheelchair. They should just go ahead and buy the right chair.

Personal Assistance Services

Although he grew up in the 1950s and 1960s, Mark O'Brien's life probably differed little from that of severely disabled polio survivors from earlier generations. The late poet, who had polio at age six, spent virtually every moment between then and his early twenties lying supine on a cot, a gurney, or in his iron lung. During what would have been his high school years, O'Brien rarely left his home and saw few people outside his immediate family. His parents tended to all his physical needs, even holding the telephone to his ear when a relative called. Isolated and alone, O'Brien watched lots of television.

"One of the interesting shows was *Ironside,* on Thursday nights; the main character was the only disabled person on TV"—albeit played by the late Raymond Burr, a barrel-chested and able-bodied mountain of a man. "The premise was that a chief of police, paralyzed by a gunshot wound, worked as a consultant to the San Francisco police. He used a wheelchair, he had a live-in attendant, and he seemed energetic and strong. Still, the situation was ridiculous; among many other impossibilities, the attendant worked twenty-four hours a day" (O'Brien, 2003, p. 63).

O'Brien, however, also had round-the-clock attendants—his parents. His guilt at burdening them turned into " 'learned helplessness.' I didn't feel I could control anything . . . [My parents] had total control over my life. . . .

I wondered how I could get away from home, where I could go, who would take me, and what I would do" (2003, pp. 60, 63). O'Brien finally found that independence in the Disabled Students Program at the University of California (see chapter 10).

Personal assistance services (PAS, also sometimes called personal care assistants or PCAs) provided the services essential to O'Brien's independence. Disabled Students Program attendants—men and women in their twenties who generally treated him like a regular person—assisted O'Brien with physical functions from toileting to writing examination papers as he dictated responses. But he controlled their actions: he requested assistance, and they provided it under his direction. That control defined O'Brien's independence.

Ensuring PAS is a leading goal of today's disability rights movement. Obtaining assistance with essential daily tasks and activities can allow persons with even significant impairments to live safely and comfortably in their homes. Today, roughly 19 percent of persons with disabilities use personal assistance or help from someone in bathing, getting dressed, preparing meals, and other basic activities (Harris Interactive, 2004). Various disability rights organizations view the scope of PAS differently: some seek inclusive definitions while others narrowly circumscribe services to basic personal care, hygiene, and light household tasks. Most agree, though, that PAS offers cheaper alternatives to costly institutionalization in many circumstances.

Nonetheless, the problem with PAS is paying for it. Admittedly, 77 percent of persons with disabilities needing these services receive personal assistance from family members or friends—at unknown costs to those individuals—but 29 percent use home health aides or other paid providers (Harris Interactive, 2004). Traditional Medicare does not cover PAS (after all, PAS does not treat illness or injury), but some Medicare managed care, Medicaid, and certain private insurers do. Insurers generally dispense PAS benefits using one of three approaches: (a) cash payments directly to the disabled persons, who then hire and supervise their personal assistants; (b) payments to case managers, who organize, oversee, and reimburse the personal assistants; or (c) vouchers given to clients to exchange for authorized purchases (Mahoney et al., 2004). Methods for arranging and compensating PAS are generating considerable attention, especially anticipating increasing needs with aging "baby boomers." Giving cash payments directly to consumers is popular among many persons with disabilities who feel they best know their needs and are fully capable of managing their own PAS.[7] Others worry about personal assistants receiving adequate protections as employees and whether some persons with disabilities can, in fact, competently oversee their own care and cash disbursements.

State Medicaid budget cuts raise additional concerns. Even if states do not eliminate PAS, some persons with substantial disabilities fear being forced into nursing homes if states ratchet back their PAS coverage (Perry, Dulio, and Hanson, 2003). MiCASSA legislation—the Medicaid Community-

Based Attendant Services and Support Act—would allow Medicaid recipients of all ages who qualify for institutional care to substitute community attendant services and fund their transition from institutions to homes (covering essential items including rent, bedding, and basic kitchen equipment). Community attendants would assist with such activities as toileting, bathing, eating, transferring, meal planning and preparation, shopping, and household chores, permitting people with disabilities to live as independently as possible in the least restrictive settings. The MiCASSA legislation, which aims to redirect Medicaid dollars away from nursing homes and into community-based services without generating additional expenditures, had not yet passed Congress by mid-2005.

Apart from payment issues, recruiting, managing, and retaining good personal assistants can pose considerable difficulties, especially when salaries are low and benefits limited or absent. Although personal assistants give persons with disabilities "independence" through theoretical control over routine physical needs and activities, in actuality, complicated interpersonal dynamics can reinstate dependence. Immediately after his spinal cord injury, cartoonist John Callahan lived with a personal assistant who liked vodka and stock car racing and questioned why Callahan felt compelled to do his bowel program everyday (answer: because it was medically essential). The personal assistant, an elderly man, consumed three hours each morning getting Callahan out of bed and dressed and rarely took him outside the apartment. "Nearly every day for six months I sat by the breadboard [in the kitchen] with my cigarettes, which he had to light for me, until it was time to go back to bed. This is going to be my life, I thought" (Callahan, 1989, p. 90).[8]

As described in chapter 7, clinicians often do not understand the role of personal assistants. When offices are inaccessible, relying on patients' personal assistants to lift them onto examination tables can potentially breach important privacy boundaries. Connie Wilder's gynecologist kept her personal assistant in the room during a physical examination, asking questions Connie felt uncomfortable answering in front of the personal assistant. Furthermore, physicians may not understand the role personal assistants serve in essential daily activities. "The neurologist says, 'You've still got help at home?'" said one woman with MS, who fell and can no longer maneuver unaided to use the toilet. "'God! That's expensive and must make you crazy.' He didn't say another word. Now if I can't stand and pivot, how the hell can I go to the bathroom? Actually, he doesn't think, not about the practical things."

Dental Services

Dental problems are not simply a cosmetic concern. Tooth decay causes considerable pain and discomfort, and potentially life-threatening dental infections can extend deep into tissues of the head and neck. Infected teeth can seed the bloodstream with bacteria during routine brushing or flossing, risking infection of the heart valves and other cardiac complications. Periodontal disease and eroding gums contribute to these problems, sometimes leading to tooth loss. Approximately 18 million American adults have lost all their teeth, primarily because of dental caries and periodontal disease (Chow, 2002).

Little is known about whether rates of dental disorders differ for persons with and without disabilities. Certainly, persons with manual dexterity problems could find brushing and flossing their teeth difficult, leaving them at higher risk for tooth decay and gum disease. Personal assistants could perform these tasks but perhaps not with diligence and care—although persons without disabilities also fail at daily dental hygiene. Two factors bode poorly for many persons with disabilities: high costs of dental care alongside limited insurance coverage; and the inaccessibility of dental offices and chairs for people with significant physical impairments.

General health insurance rarely covers dental care, and the interviewees recounted numerous instances of being unable to afford services. Medicare reimburses dental procedures associated with cancerous tumors and jaw injuries but not the extraction of an impacted tooth, regardless of its complexity (American Medical Association, 2003, p. 214). States can cover routine and restorative dental care as optional services under Medicaid, but with budget shortfalls many states have reduced or eliminated this coverage. Some employers offer dental insurance on their menu of employee benefits, but private coverage often carries large deductibles, copayments, and strict limitations on total expenditures. Thus, high costs and lack of insurance coverage may place dental services beyond the reach of many persons with disabilities.

Inaccessible facilities pose another major barrier. One wheelchair user finally got dental insurance, "but I can't find a dentist that's handicapped accessible." Another woman goes to the dental clinic at a large medical center, but says "you can barely get into the office with a wheelchair—the dental chair takes up so much room. Some of the dental chairs don't move down, so you can't get onto them. Then, if you want to stay in your own [wheel]chair, the dentist can't stand next to you because the dental chair's in the way." In all focus groups, interviewees raised serious concerns about accessing dental care.

Public Transportation

Survey data find that more than 90 percent of persons with and without disabilities rely on private cars to visit their health care providers (see chapter 4). Presumably, many individuals with disabilities get rides from family members or friends. Without this option, other persons with disabilities have little choice and must use taxis or public transportation to see their doctors. Although Medicaid sometimes reimburses cab fares to and from health care appointments, few other insurers do. Therefore, many persons with disabilities depend on public transportation systems, with decidedly mixed results. Sometimes people miss medical appointments because of transportation difficulties, while others wait for hours for rides.

Accessible public transportation, with its promise of independence and easy movement, led the disability rights agenda in the 1980s.[9] Transportation issues varied by region, depending on whether goals involved retrofitting old systems (as in New York City and Boston) or building new networks (as in the San Francisco Bay Area and Washington, DC).[10] Title II, Subtitle B, of the Americans with Disabilities Act mandates that public transportation must be "readily accessible to and usable by individuals with disabilities, including individuals who use wheelchairs" [Section 222(a)]. However, transportation systems reflect regional terrains, decades-old policy decisions, and shifting population patterns, with some systems offering better access than others.

Depending on local factors, public transportation for people with disabilities generally gravitates toward either services separate from the main public systems (so-called "paratransit") or integrated systems accessible to all.

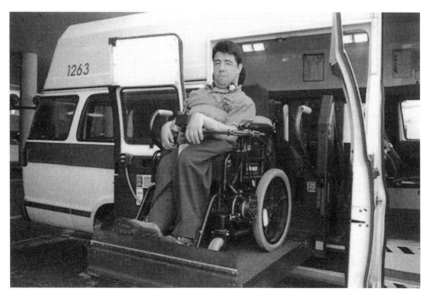

Figure 9.1.   Accessible transport. Stevie uses public paratransit vans to travel wherever he needs to go, including to and from work. When he goes someplace special, like to his doctor, Stevie must schedule his trip for hours before his appointment to ensure he arrives on time.

Paratransit programs, such as those used by Stevie (figure 9.1), vary some-what in the nature of vehicles, scope of services, costs, and passenger requirements from region to region. Most, though, require passengers to make appointments well in advance (unless clients have regularly scheduled trips, such as to and from work), and few have earned rave reviews from their riders. Concerns about poor reliability and availability of accessible transportation remain a prominent issue among disability rights advocates.

Metropolitan Boston melds fixed route and paratransit approaches through accessible public buses on all routes, accessible subways, and trains (to the relatively limited extent feasible given Boston's antiquated facilities), and a "demand response" system known as The RIDE. Intentions do not always match reality. Essential accessibility equipment, such as wheelchair lifts on public buses and elevators at subway stations, often malfunctions.

With fleets of large vans with automatic wheelchair lifts, The RIDE paratransit service carries people who cannot manage the fixed-route systems alone or who need to go someplace that accessible buses, subways, and trains do not reach. To qualify for The RIDE, persons must pass a medical determination, based on documentation from their physicians. For efficiency, RIDE vans often load multiple passengers simultaneously, meaning that riders sometimes take numerous detours before reaching their final destinations. RIDE users who have time for such delays tolerate the inconvenience, balanced against very low fares and good accessibility. But Eleanor Peters, who uses a power wheelchair, frequently finds herself frustrated with the system:

> There have been times when I have actually had to miss a doctor's appointment because of The RIDE. It may look bad on the patient, but it's definitely not our fault. . . . I have to use The RIDE every day, so I'm talking experience. I always tell them that I have to be places a half hour earlier than I really do, and they still sometimes either get me there late or they don't get me there at all. So The RIDE can be a real nightmare if you have to rely on it for medical appointments or school or work.

Routinely, RIDE passengers arrive hours early in our clinic just to ensure they make their appointments, then sit waiting to be taken home afterwards.[11] As one woman said, "Usually you end up there at 9:30 in the morning for an 11:30 appointment, and then you have to wait until 2:30 to go home."

Public transportation can break down entirely in rural regions. "I've sat down and cried before because I have to get somewhere and I've got no way to get there," a blind resident of Distant Dunes reported. Facing financial losses, their one accessible transportation service, "You Call, We Haul," had gone out of business. Now disabled persons in Distant Dunes have few transportation options. "Sometimes you can't get to the doctor."

Accessible Housing

Joe Alto's MS had progressed, but because his apartment did not have an accessible entrance, he didn't get a wheelchair: he couldn't have rolled it in or out, so, "I was stuck in my house for ten years." But Joe felt that things could have been worse. During his admissions for MS flares, hospital personnel could have learned about his inaccessible housing. "If you're crippled and can't go up and down the stairs, and you live in an apartment without an elevator," said Joe, "the hospital will send you to a nursing home. They're not supposed to send you home." Being forced into a nursing home was his greatest fear. Joe finally found an accessible apartment and got his wheelchair.

Most private homes and smaller apartment buildings pose inconveniences, outright impediments, and dangers—such as stairs, insubstantial railings, narrow doorways and halls, lack of grab bars, cramped bathrooms, doorbells and alarms without visual cues, and inadequate lighting—for people with sensory and physical disabilities. Thus, many persons like Joe Alto confront barriers daily within their own homes, limiting their independence and potentially compromising safety. Among persons with major walking problems, almost 19 percent report difficulties using their bathrooms, and 66 percent must climb stairs to enter their homes.[12] Just over 24 percent of injuries occur inside people's homes—the most common place injuries happen (Warner, Barnes, and Fingerhut, 2000, p. 23).[13]

In recent years, policy-makers have recognized links between home environments and health, both physical and emotional (see chapter 16). Risks to children's cognitive development posed by lead-based paint and exacerbations of asthma related to building disrepair and pest infestations are two prime examples. Views of this connection are expanding, with growing appreciation of mental stress and anxiety associated with dilapidated housing, as well as the need to foster independent community living. "For various population groups—the elderly, the handicapped, and vulnerable families with children—housing policy is increasingly emphasizing the goal of independence. . . . This goal can only be achieved if it is explicitly shared by the housing, health, and related sectors" (Newman, 1997, p. 190). Independence demands accessibility, but nationwide, relatively few private houses and small apartment buildings are truly accessible. A 1995 federal housing survey found that only 20 percent of 20.6 million privately owned, multi-family rental properties had at least one "handicapped accessible" unit, as did just 12 percent of 8.8 million privately owned, single-family rental properties (U.S. Census Bureau, 2002a, 2002b).

The Fair Housing Act Amendments of 1988 (FHAA) gave persons with disabilities important protections in housing, representing the first time antidiscrimination provisions relating to disability extended to the private sector.[14] Prior to 1988, owners, landlords, and housing management companies could reject applications from persons with disabilities to purchase or rent properties, basing decisions on subjective judgments. The FHAA prohibits owners from refusing to rent or sell housing to someone because of disability or to charge them higher rents, sales prices, or security deposits. In addition, the law mandates that new construction of multi-family dwellings with four or more units must be physically accessible, and it ensures that persons can adapt their residences to accommodate their disabilities. However, most existing private properties predate federal and state accessibility laws. In addition, it remains unclear whether laws mandating accessibility of new construction are vigorously enforced.

In some states, Medicaid pays for modest home modifications, such as installing grab bars in bathrooms and ramps at entryways, but Medicaid does not fund major structural renovations. Medicare and most private insurers will not pay even to install grab bars for persons at risk of falling. So, we circle back to situations like Joe Alto's. His ten-year forced isolation in an inaccessible home likely led to profound depression, a secondary disability that was possibly preventable. "If you tell a person they can't do nothing, that's like telling them to go home and die," Joe observed. "If you lose hope, you don't want to live no more." Thus, housing woes can carry significant clinical consequences.

Luckily, Joe's wheelchair and new accessible home restored his optimism and sense of mission. Joe now aims to educate everyone he possibly can about building accessible environments—changes that could benefit everyone. He recently chalked up one major victory, with his dentist: "I couldn't get into his office with my wheelchair, so I talked to him, and he built a ramp!" According to Joe, if people speak up, accessibility will improve.

III

IMPROVING HEALTH CARE FOR
PEOPLE WITH DISABILITIES

Using Universal Design to Accommodate All

Walter Masterson, in his late fifties, was a business executive who frequently flew abroad to negotiate corporate deals. One summer after a lengthy trip, he returned home with a limp, which persisted into the fall. Prodded by his wife, he finally consulted a physician: "I came in for a variety of torture tests, which were essentially measuring the nerves' response to being stabbed and jolted. The net result of all that was that an expert diagnosed me with ALS"—amyotrophic lateral sclerosis or Lou Gehrig's disease. Over the next two years, Mr. Masterson progressed through canes, leg braces, walkers, and manual wheelchairs. "Just recently, I got an electric wheelchair for outside. So, that's the state of things—increasing weakness in my legs that has taken me from limping to not being able to walk at all" (Iezzoni, 2003, p. 31).

Mr. Masterson adapted his environment to his changing physical realities—widening doors, installing stair lifts, renovating bathrooms, and building wheelchair-accessible paths in his backyard. "I've put a lot of money in my house and the various toys and tools that I need to get around. Most people don't have anything close to the kind of money I've spent on this," he ruefully admitted. Although his renovated home accommodated his needs, few other settings did. "They don't build bathrooms in the standard American house that can deal with a wheelchair. We can't visit friends for any length of time because I can't use their toilet." Instead, Mr. Masterson's friends visited him.

Mr. Masterson began looking at home and abroad for accessibility solutions. "I've done some international travel in a wheelchair, and despite its multiple shortcomings, the United States is *way* ahead of just about any place in Europe in some things," like building ramps and curb cuts. "In Europe, it's a normal occurrence to find yourself marooned on a sidewalk where the only way you can go is back." But in private spaces, "other countries are far, far ahead of us. Maybe they don't do the streets real well, but they do houses and bathrooms a lot better—any place in Scandinavia, Holland, Germany." He recalled a bathroom he had visited in a northern European airport:

These people had thought it through. Somebody had said, "Okay, we're going to build a toilet. Right. Here are all the people who have to use it." And so they built one that had a facility for all those people. They just did it. The toilet had a pulley system that could have lifted a car! There were five or six different ways you could use it depending upon what condition you were in when you encountered it. Its only purpose was to get whoever needed it onto the toilet. I've never seen a mechanism like that anywhere in the States.

Mr. Masterson was especially impressed that the accessible toilet "wasn't any place special. It was just in an ordinary municipal building," clearly reflecting a routinely inclusive attitude. He also admired private dwellings offering numerous built-in features—from lighting, to communication devices, to security systems, to physical spaces, to fixtures and appliances—to accommodate the full range of people who might eventually use them. "Inside the home, there are architectural splendors that a lot of folks in Europe have worked out" to welcome people like Mr. Masterson.

Although he didn't use the phrase, Mr. Masterson's description of the European airport toilet—and the thinking that produced it—exemplifies universal design: the notion of considering all potential users when designing places, information, communication, and other items, services, and policies to maximize their usefulness and appeal to everybody. "Universal design is human-centered design with everyone in mind. . . . If it works well for people across the spectrum of functional ability, it works better for everyone" (Adaptive Environments, 2004). In part III, we recommend building solutions to improve health care experiences of persons with disabilities around the principles of universal design. The chapters touch briefly on various universal design concepts and strategies, and appendix 1 lists selected Internet sites that offer details about the universal design approach.

Evolving Catalysts for Universal Design

The origins of universal design trace back to the 1940s, when several factors forced policy-makers to start recognizing and removing barriers within public and private spaces. Thousands of disabled veterans from World War II empowered by the "GI Bill" demanded and gained access to colleges and workplaces. New social policies moved persons with severe physical disabilities then residing in institutions out into communities. In its early stages, deinstitutionalization generally segregated persons with disabilities within specialized "barrier-free" environments.

Starting in the 1960s, the growing disability rights movement emphasized independent living in communities, shifting away from segregation toward inclusion—making entire communities and the tools of daily life accessible to persons with disabilities. The late Edward V. Roberts, sometimes called the father of the independent living movement, initiated this change as a student at the University of California at Berkeley in the early 1960s. Roberts, who was paralyzed from polio since age fourteen and required a respirator to breath, sued to gain admission to this prestigious university, which had initially rejected him. Once there, he formed a political action group, the Rolling Quads, which aimed to make Berkeley a barrier-free community.[1] Their ultimate goal was to maximize independence and self-reliance of persons with disabilities who previously had lived in isolation and dependence. Roberts later recalled:

> We secured the first curb cut in the country; it was at the corner of Bancroft and Telegraph Avenue. When we first talked to legislators about the issue, they told us, "Curb cuts, why do you need curb cuts? We never see people with disabilities out on the street. Who is going to use them?" They didn't understand that their reasoning was circular. When curb cuts were put in, they discovered that access for disabled people benefits many others as well. For instance, people pushing strollers use curb cuts, as do people on bikes and elderly people who can't lift their legs so high. So many people benefit from this accommodation. This is what the concept of universal design is all about. (Fleischer and Zames, 2001, p. 40)

Design, or sometimes "redesign," to eliminate barriers and ensure access thus became central to ensuring civil rights for persons with disabilities. "Lack of access to buildings, programs, and transportation was more than an oversight. It was discrimination pure and simple, another kind of segregation" (Potok, 2002, p. 50). Previous civil rights legislation barring discrimination based on race, ethnicity, and gender sought to ignore these characteristics, striving to judge people based on individual merit. But disability rights advocates recognized that they could not achieve their goal by an approach that more or less "ignored" disability. Instead, disability must first be acknowledged, then the path to civil rights cleared by tearing down barriers.

In the United States, laws began targeting specific obstacles, starting with the Architectural Barriers Act of 1968. Section 504 of the Rehabilitation Act of 1973, the Americans with Disabilities Act (ADA) in 1990, the Telecommunications Act of 1996, other federal statutes, and numerous state and local laws mandate additional actions to make public and private places, services, information, and communication accessible to persons with disabilities (see chapter 2).[2] However, despite the immense importance of these laws, their subsequent regulations and implementation produced unintended consequences. Designers seemingly pay attention more to meeting minimum requirements of regulatory codes than devising proactive and creative ways to include all persons. The resultant designs to facilitate access often appear separate and unequal, perpetuating the segregation the disability rights movement aimed to eliminate. For example, I routinely find wheelchair-accessible entrances tucked discreetly to the side or rear of buildings and elevators placed far from centrally positioned escalators, even in new construction.

By the 1980s, a powerful catalyst for universal design began attracting worldwide notice—rapidly aging populations, especially in developed nations. Interests of the disability rights and aging communities converge in their shared goals of maximizing independence and facilitating daily life within communities. This imperative applies to all persons at some point in their lives. As disability rights activist Ed Roberts observed:

> I look around, and I notice that a lot of us are getting gray. As we
> get older, we realize that disability is just a part of life. Anyone can
> join our group at any point in life. In this way, the disability rights
> movement doesn't discriminate. So those of us who are temporarily
> able-bodied and working for access and accommodations now get
> older, and the changes they make will benefit them as well. (Flei-
> scher and Zames, 2001, p. 40)

In 1987, the World Design Congress, including representatives of private industries and the public sector worldwide, passed a resolution urging designers everywhere and in all sectors to consider aging and disability in their work.

History offers numerous examples of products initially designed to benefit persons with disabilities that later attracted diverse users. Charles Thurber patented the first successful typewriter in 1843, initially developed to assist persons who are blind (Shapiro, 1994). The father of Kenneth Jacuzzi invented a pool with warm swirling waters to relieve the pain of his son, who had developed rheumatoid arthritis as a boy. The convergence of designs targeting persons with disabilities with mainstream marketplaces accelerated in the 1980s, with the growing purchasing power of aging consumers. For instance, OXO International introduced "Good Grips" kitchen utensils, designed initially for persons with arthritis in their hands (Story, Mueller, and Mace, 1998). With their oversized handles and aesthetic designs, these products enticed enthusiastic customers with and without arthritis. Television captioning, initially invented to accommodate hearing impairments, finds avid users among hearing patrons of pubs, sports bars, health clubs, and other noisy places tuned in to television.

Today, private industries are the vanguard of universal design. The worldwide marketplace, not regulatory imperatives, motivates them: few industries are legally required to design accessible products. Instead, diverse consumers and global competition provide strong catalysts for universal design, as private manufacturers strive to develop user-friendly products for as many potential customers as they can. Consumers' needs drive design.

Principles and Practice of Universal Design

The late North Carolina architect Ronald L. Mace coined the term "universal design" but recognized its limits.[3] Mace, who had polio as a child and used a wheelchair and ventilator, did not view universal design as a new concept. Furthermore, he acknowledged the impossibility of ever satisfying the needs of absolutely everyone. Mace viewed universal design as a mindset or orientation rather than an absolute. Designers should endeavor to create products, programs, places, and policies that have as universal an appeal as possible.

Adopting a universal design mindset first requires an appreciation of the full range of human abilities and how they vary within populations and across ages, environments, and personal circumstances. Mace and colleagues grouped human abilities within eight broad categories—cognition, vision, hearing, speech, body function, arm function, hand function, and mobility—and considered the implications for design within each area. Diversity in the sensory and physical functions we consider in this book carries important consequences for universal design, as described by Story, Mueller, and Mace (1998, pp. 19–33). Designs to accommodate variations in human abilities must consider differences in basic functions. Table 10.1 suggests factors that designers might think about to accommodate differences in various core functions.

Table 10.1. Design Considerations to Accommodate Variations in Human Function

Function	Designs Must Consider Differences in:
Vision	Perceiving visual detail; focusing on objects up close and far away; judging distances; seeing objects in the center and periphery of the visual field; perceiving contrasts in color and brightness; adapting to high and low lighting levels; tracking moving objects
Hearing, speech	Perceiving and recognizing high- and low-pitched sounds; separating auditory information from background noise; localizing sources of sounds; carrying on conversations
Arms	Range of motion; coordination; strength, including pushing, pulling, lifting, lowering, carrying; reaching up, down, forward, backward
Hands	Grasping; squeezing; rotating and twisting; pinching; pulling and pushing
Lower extremity	Walking; running; jumping; climbing; kneeling and rising; lowering to sit and rising from a seated position; standing upright; balancing on one foot; operating foot controls

Adapted from: Story, Mueller, and Mace (1998).

Principle 1: Equitable Use

The design is useful and marketable to persons of all abilities and does not stigmatize or disadvantage any group.

- Provide to all users the same means of use: identical when possible, but otherwise equivalent
- Avoid isolating or segregating any users
- Make any provisions for safety, privacy, and security equally available to all users
- Make the design appealing to all users

Principle 2: Flexibility in Use

The design accommodates persons with wide ranges of individual abilities and preferences.

- Provide choices in methods of use
- Accommodate right- and left-handed access and use
- Facilitate the user's accuracy and precision
- Provide adaptability to the pace of individual users

Principle 3: Simple and Intuitive Use

Use of the design is easy to understand, regardless of the user's experiences, knowledge, language skills, literacy, or current concentration level.

- Eliminate unnecessary complexity
- Make design consistent with expectations and intuition of users
- Accommodate wide range of literacy and language skills
- Array information consistent with its level of importance
- Provide effective prompting and feedback during and after use

Principle 4: Perceptible Information

The design communicates necessary information effectively to users, regardless of ambient conditions or sensory abilities of user.

- Present essential information in different and redundant formats (pictorial, verbal, tactile)
- Maximize "legibility" of essential information
- Design instructions or directions to be easy and easily described
- Make information compatible with various techniques or devices used by persons with sensory limitations

Box 10.1. (*continued*)

Principle 5: Tolerance for Error

The design minimizes hazards and adverse consequences from accidental or unintentional actions.

- Make the most used elements most accessible; eliminate, isolate, or shield hazardous elements; arrange elements to minimize hazards and errors
- Warn users about hazards and errors
- Provide fail-safe features to prevent injuries or misuse
- Discourage unconscious actions in tasks requiring vigilance

Principle 6: Low Physical Effort

Persons can use the design efficiently and comfortably, with minimum effort and fatigue.

- Allow user to maintain neutral body position
- Require reasonable operating forces for use
- Minimize repetitive actions
- Minimize sustained physical effort

Principle 7: Size and Space for Approach and Use

The design provides appropriate size and space for approach, reach, manipulation, and use regardless of user's body size, mobility, or posture.

- Provide clear lines of sight to important elements for any seated or standing users
- Make access to all components comfortable for any seated or standing users
- Accommodate variations in hand and grip size
- Provide adequate space for use of assistive devices or personal assistance

Adapted from: Story, Mueller, and Mace (1998).

After considering this spectrum of human abilities, designers must then determine how best to make products or environments comfortable and usable by the widest range of persons. Based on suggestions from architects, engineers, product designers, and environmental design researchers, Story, Mueller, and Mace (1998) specified seven principles to direct universal design projects and evaluations. Each principle includes several guidelines, indicating key required elements (box 10.1). Several examples suggest how these principles apply to actual designs. For instance, locating elevators adjacent to escalators avoids segregating or stigmatizing users with varying mobility abilities (Principle 1). Big-button telephone keys accommodate users with low vision, manual dexterity difficulties, and persons in a hurry (Principle 2). Easy-to-understand icons in signs and labels minimize the need for reading (Principle 3). Door levers that users can operate with closed fists or elbows or arms full of packages provide broader accessibility than conventional door knobs (Principle 6).

Applying these seven principles requires two things: an understanding of the goals and purposes of what is being designed; and an appreciation of the full range of relevant abilities of potential users. Although these principles obviously apply to physical products, equipment, and spaces, designers can easily adapt them to developing policies, procedures, and even interpersonal communication strategies for clinicians and patients. Again, universal and human-centered design represents a mindset.

Throughout the remainder of part III, we urge designers—in our instance, clinicians, health care managers, payers, and developers of medical products and equipment—to adopt universal design principles. Putting principles into practice requires consulting with persons with disabilities about their needs and preferred approaches for reconfiguring health care delivery. Designers cannot assume that even well-meaning and experienced clinicians appreciate fully the functional implications of various disabilities. Without asking and involving persons with disabilities in designing spaces, procedures, and policies, clinicians, managers, and other health care providers are unlikely to anticipate the breadth of function-related issues and concerns.

This caution applies to me, too. I could not get around outdoors without curb cuts in sidewalks, and I know—as Ed Roberts said—that many other people also benefit from them. But Bonnie tells me that some types of curb cuts are dangerous for her as she walks with her white cane. If the curb cut is broad and shallow, without obvious tactile clues about its boundaries, Bonnie could find herself in the street braving passing cars, unaware that she just walked through a curb cut. Therefore, even the curb cut—the quintessential symbol of accessibility—is unsafe for some people unless its designers consider all potential users. The solution is simple: narrow the curb cut or provide a small lip or other tactile demarcation at its base so that white cane users can identify the curb. In many communities, blind and low vision pedestrians have communicated this concern to city planners, demonstrating the value of involving diverse users in design. If I had not asked Bonnie about this issue, I would never have known.

Self-Management and Advocacy

I think that, more than the able-bodied community, we have to be very resourceful. We have to be problem-solvers because doctors don't solve problems for us very often. I've been nursing a rotator cuff injury, and I've decided not to seek any help for it. I'm thinking that I can reason it out—figure out what's aggravating it in my daily routine and see if I can do something differently.

—Marcia McDonough

Marcia McDonough, in her mid-thirties, has lived with spinal cord injury for a dozen years and has learned a lot about caring for herself. As happens to many long-term manual wheelchair users, Marcia's painful shoulder muscles (the so-called "rotator cuff" where her upper arm joint fits into her shoulder socket) present her newest challenge. A clinician's likely recommendation—rest—would leave Marcia stranded, unable to get around. Marcia feels she can best decide how to minimize stresses on her shoulders by altering her patterns of wheelchair use.

Since her injury, Marcia's attitudes about the role of clinicians have changed. Pre-injury, with few medical concerns, she thought little about health care services, holding standard "traditional" views that "regard physicians and other health professionals as experts, with patients bringing little to the table besides their illness" (Bodenheimer et al., 2002, p. 2470). Her post-injury experiences taught her to become her own diagnostician to the extent possible—unraveling the causes of problems and devising solutions that fit her daily life. Marcia's views thus gravitated toward a "new paradigm" of care, where people are "their own principal caregivers, and health care professionals—both in primary and specialty care—should be consultants supporting them in this role" (p. 2470).

For many persons, solutions to the difficulties with health care described in part II involve shifting their paradigm of care, as has Marcia McDonough—moving from traditional roles of clinicians and patients to a self-management and collaborative care approach (table 11.1). Although most care practiced in the United States still follows traditional patterns, increasing evidence suggests substantial benefits along many dimensions from self-management and collaborative care. Not only do patients feel more satisfied and in control of their care, but clinical outcomes can also improve. Furthermore, this new approach reflects the realities of living with chronic conditions. Hour by hour and day by day, people (and sometimes families) make countless decisions in their homes, workplaces, and communities that directly affect their health.

Self-management and collaborative care programs are well-developed for persons with chronic conditions such as diabetes, asthma, heart disease, depression, and arthritis. However, vision loss, hearing limitations, and physical functional impairments can pose significant challenges to self-management strategies. Depending on the nature of specific functional impairments, patients may not need to manage their impairments per se. For instance, persons who are born blind do not need to manage their blindness. But if they develop diabetes, they will need methods that do not require visual input for managing their diabetes—such as administering insulin, monitoring blood glucose levels, detecting wounds or injuries to their feet, exercising, and losing weight.[1] Working collaboratively with their clinicians,

Table 11.1. Comparison of Traditional and Collaborative Care

Question	Traditional Care	Collaborative Care
Relationships	Clinicians = experts; patients = passive	Clinicians and patients share expertise. Clinicians = experts about disease; patients = experts about their lives.
Principal caregiver	Clinicians	Clinicians and patients share responsibility for caregiving and solving problems.
Goals	Adherence to instructions	Patient sets goals; clinicians help patient achieve goals. If goals not achieved, change strategies.
Change behavior	External motivation	Internal motivation, as patients learn and develop confidence to change behaviors.
Identify problems	By clinicians	By patients and clinicians
Solve problems	By clinicians	Clinicians teach patients to solve problems and assist problem solving.

Adapted from: Bodenheimer et al. (2002, p. 2470).

patients must devise creative solutions that accommodate their limited vision.

This chapter addresses three topics. First, we highlight what interviewees like Marcia McDonough told us about what they want and need from their clinicians. Second, we briefly review approaches toward fostering self-management and collaborative care, then focus on how vision, hearing, and physical functional impairments—and clinicians' attitudes and knowledge about these conditions—might affect efforts to move to this new model of care. Third, we introduce examples of approaches and technologies that might accommodate certain functional impairments, giving patients opportunities to manage their own care independently and safely. Accurate and effective communication is obviously crucial to successful collaborative care; chapters 12 and 13 address ways to improve this aspect of the patient-clinician relationship.

What Persons with Disabilities Want

Several consistent themes emerged from our interviews, although most trace back to a single imperative—the need for clinicians to listen to and learn from patients. In this, individuals with disabilities share a common desire with other persons. But the possibility of clinicians' inadequate technical knowledge raises the stakes for persons with disabilities. Given the diversity of disabling conditions, most people do not expect primary care clinicians to know absolutely everything about their impairment. But they do expect clinicians to be honest about what they do not know and seek additional input—from clinical experts and, importantly, from patients themselves. Thus, informed patients would work together with clinicians, each contributing knowledge and expertise. In some instances, persons with disabilities have highly technical knowledge greater than that of clinicians, blurring the roles of patients and clinicians under even the collaborative care approach (table 11.1).

Patients as Experts

One message rang out loud and clear: some people know volumes about their sensory or physical impairments and every nuanced implication for their daily lives and activities. They want clinicians to treat them as experts in these functional domains and to hear and heed their cautions and advice. Unless clinical care plans and management goals accommodate patients' functional impairments, the plans cannot succeed.

Some persons with disabilities use their technical expertise to ensure they receive safe and effective care. For example, Marcia McDonough spent considerable time searching for an obstetrician to deliver her baby after being rejected by numerous obstetricians who said they knew nothing about women with spinal cord injuries (chapter 4). Marcia decided to educate the obstetrician who finally accepted her. As luck would have it, "when my delivery time came, that doctor wasn't available. So I was thrown back into a pool of doctors who really knew nothing." But Marcia had already laid the groundwork to educate the entire labor and delivery team.

"Before I went into labor, I sat down and wrote four pages of specifics that I wanted every delivery team person to read. It covered issues of [autonomic] dysreflexia, even though it wasn't a concern for my particular injury.[2] I talked about the IV [intravenous line]. I needed my IV in a place where I could still do transfers with my arms." If Marcia wanted to get out of bed independently while in labor, she would need her arms unencumbered by intravenous lines to transfer to her wheelchair.

"I'd had three appointments to discuss anesthesia. I thought it was all set. But then, just as I went into hard labor, they declared that I could not have an epidural because it was too close to my injury site, and I could risk an infection. No amount of pain was worth that. So I didn't have the epidural we'd planned." Nonetheless, Marcia safely—and painlessly—delivered a baby girl. Admittedly, some of Marcia's well laid plans went awry. Despite three prior visits, no anesthesiologist had objected to the epidural before she entered labor. Nevertheless, Marcia hopes that her efforts to educate the obstetrical team will help their next pregnant patient with spinal cord injury.

Focus on "Chief Complaints," Not Disabilities

Sometimes clinicians immediately focus on patients' functional impairments when patients seek care for completely unrelated reasons. Patients must then redirect clinicians' attention to why they sought care: their so-called "chief complaint." To obtain useful professional advice, patients must regain control of the clinical dialogue. Given clinicians' proclivity to control office visit discourse within seconds of its start (see chapter 8), this can require considerable effort and diplomacy on the patient's part. The obvious solution is for clinicians to start each encounter by listening fully to what worries patients—not to assume that all visits relate to underlying disabilities.

Carl Doubletree became blind from an injury in early adulthood, then later developed diabetes. Mr. Doubletree, a college graduate and African American, has visited many physicians. Over time he learned to get what he needs "by asking questions, being very knowledgeable about my own health. When we go to doctors, they assume the reason you're blind is that you're a diabetic or have glaucoma." Based on epidemiology, this assumption is reasonable: after refractive error and cataracts, diabetic retinopathy and glaucoma are the most common causes of adult vision loss, especially among black Americans (Rowe, MacLean, and Shekelle, 2004). Most importantly, clinical interventions can slow the progression of diabetic retinopathy and glaucoma, so physicians rightly wish to address these conditions. But his physicians' assumptions frustrate Mr. Doubletree.

> You have to be able to educate doctors and say, "Listen, I'm here for a headache; that has nothing to do with my blindness per se." I'm learning every day to do that. I try to educate doctors individually and say, "Listen, I appreciate you being concerned about my eyes, but I'm not here for my eyes. Just because you run into a lot of blindness caused by diabetes, that's not my problem. If you want, at some other time, I can explain why I lost my sight." And of course, they'll say, they don't mean to be offensive, but I don't need that. I don't want to be put in that mode.

Carl Doubletree wants his physician to discuss his acute problem—headache—not some incorrect conjecture about why he became blind. However, his comments highlight the complexities of negotiating who controls the agenda during clinical encounters. Although his blindness resulted from injury and not diabetes, Carl's doctor may have rightly worried about a link between diabetes and headache (e.g., through cerebrovascular complications of diabetes). If so, the physician obviously failed to explain this logic to Carl. The straightforward solution is better communication and exchange of information, after clinicians first listen to patients' chief complaints.

Educating Clinicians Can Pose Risks for Patients

Marcia McDonough and Carl Doubletree explicitly try to teach clinicians. Numerous other interviewees also describe efforts to educate clinicians—broadly on disability-related matters and narrowly on their specific needs. But patients' assuming the educator role runs counter to long-standing traditional relationships. This switch can raise complex and conflicting dynamics between patients and clinicians. According to Carl,

> If we educate medical professionals, they will have better knowledge. But a lot of times, we see things going on, and we don't say anything about it. We just sweep it under the rug instead of saying, "Listen, the next time you have someone here that has a handicap, wouldn't it be best if you do this? Wouldn't it make you a better practitioner in order to serve the next person?" But if we don't stop it, they're going to continue because they just don't know what to do.

A few interviewees worry about displaying "an attitude"—appearing confrontational, hostile, and narcissistic, thus potentially jeopardizing relationships with clinicians. Marta Redding, who is hard of hearing, finds that teaching doctors takes energy that she would otherwise spend coping with her constant anxieties about miscommunication. "I try to take responsibility to train people," Marta said, "and if I'm not too tired, I will start the whole spiel, 'I can only hear you if I can see you.'"

When clinicians fail to understand their basic concerns, patients must navigate complex interpersonal shoals as they respond. Steffie Giacommo, a nurse who has a spinal cord injury, views managing her own care as essential to preserving her health and even life. Several years ago after moving to a new city, she visited a local urologist. "I went to this physician who was supposed to be the best in town," Steffie recalled. "After talking to him, I realized that I knew more than he did about my neurogenic bladder. That really frightened me!" The urologist suggested that Steffie change her bladder management regimen from one that had worked well for her, minimizing urinary tract infections. She asked the urologist for scientific reasons why his proposed approach was better than hers, but he did not respond. Steffie refused to switch her bladder regimen.

Some time later, when Steffie needed a minor gynecologic procedure, her gynecologist "asked what I wanted to know about my surgery. I said that I wanted to know everything." The gynecologist had anticipated Steffie's assertive response and showed her what the urologist had written in her medical record—"that I was a demanding, aggressive woman, who wouldn't comply with his treatment."[3] The urologist obviously felt Steffie had committed an unacceptable transgression. "I went out of the role that the 'crippled' person is supposed to play—quiet, passive, and let people do anything to them." Fortunately, Steffie had not planned to return to that urologist.

Creating Their Own Plans for Care

Based on expertise about their disabilities and daily life, many persons with disabilities already manage their own care. As noted above, Marcia McDonough decided to handle her rotator cuff injury herself rather than seek medical attention. Presumably, Marcia can figure out ways to reduce her wheelchair excursions or the length of these trips. Perhaps Marcia can avoid developing such a severe injury that she must abandon her manual wheelchair for a power chair.

Sometimes, though, to manage their own health, people need their physicians' acquiescence or, at least, signature on an insurance referral form. Several women wheelchair users raised this issue when discussing worries about thinning bones. Osteoporosis results from many causes, including the inability to bear weight on one's legs. Compared with able-bodied women, women who no longer walk any distance can develop osteoporosis at younger ages, along with heightened risks of dangerous fractures. Some clinicians assume that since these women are seated, the likelihood of falls and fractures is low. This belief is false. People can fall, sustaining life-threatening fractures, while moving from their wheelchairs to beds, cars, shower seats, or other surfaces.

Some wheelchair users employ multiple strategies to avoid or minimize bone loss and fracture risks. Exercising they can do on their own. Candy Bonner, who had a low cervical spinal cord injury fifteen years ago, remains physically active. She belongs to a scuba diving club for wheelchair users, but because water is buoyant, swimming does not benefit bones. Candy has other risk factors for osteoporosis. Like many persons with spinal cord injury, to minimize risks of kidney stones, she limits her intake of dairy products and calcium supplements—the essential mineral for bone.[4] In addition, Candy strives to keep her slim figure.[5] Becoming heavier would mean pushing more weight in her manual wheelchair, stressing her shoulders and endurance. Candy doesn't actually know what she weighs: "I haven't been weighed in ten years because they don't have a wheelchair scale in my doctor's office—a brand new, multi-story building!"

Candy has heard that even the passive pull of gravity on vertical legs can reduce osteoporosis, so she regularly uses special equipment to hold her upright: "I stand up at the gym three days a week for fifteen minutes to a half-hour to increase bone density." Candy wanted objective evidence about the state of her bones, but to get it, she needed her physician's support.

"Last year, I turned forty. I said to my doctor that I'd like a bone density test. She goes, 'No, I won't do that until you're fifty.'" Candy's physician quoted standard guidelines from the time, failing to recognize Candy's increased risks. "She treated me the exact same way she treats everybody else." Without her physician's approval, Candy could not get the test. Despite her college degree, she is unemployed and doesn't have the money to pay for it herself. Her doctor's ill-informed refusal to approve bone density testing exacerbates Candy's anxiety about her bone health.

Self-Advocacy and Question Lists

Being assertive carries risks—of being judged uncooperative, obstreperous, or uncongenial (Olkin, 1999). Some interviewees nevertheless feel that when their health or health care is at stake, self-advocacy—or advocacy from family or friends—is essential to breaking down barriers to care. "Sometimes people have to be taught how to advocate with their doctor," said one man. "Some doctors don't want to hear it—they don't want to be told. But a good physician will learn and admit when they are wrong."

Asking questions and doing research supports self-advocacy. Some people bring written lists of questions to their clinician visits. Learning about their conditions (e.g., by searching the Internet, chapter 15), their health insurance benefits, legal rights under the Americans with Disabilities Act, and other topics empowers patients, preparing them to engage in productive dialogues with their clinicians. Centers for independent living (private, non-profit organizations located in communities throughout the United States and run by and for individuals with disabilities) advocate for community access and teach their clients general advocacy and empowerment skills. Certain independent living centers offer educational programs specifically about the health care system.

Some people bring family or friends to their clinical encounters—"another set of eyes" to ensure that he gets appropriate care, said one man. Dwight Eaton, who is blind, brings his wife, who has spent twenty years in nursing. "She can ask questions that I don't know how to ask." Dwight acknowledged that sometimes his physicians converse primarily with his wife, leaving him feeling excluded. "However, that might happen even if I weren't blind." His wife's bedside vigil was invaluable during Dwight's recent hospitalization for back surgery. "Especially at night, you can ring and ring and the nurses won't come." Inpatients without disabilities also face this shortfall—nursing staff cuts affect everybody—but "this is a particular problem of blindness. . . . If you're trying to get a simple thing like a glass of water, it's very, very difficult without somebody's help."

Sometimes, self-advocacy retreats before clinical necessity. Kate Cather, who is deaf, had a bicycle accident, and an ambulance rushed her to the emergency room, where she requested an American Sign Language (ASL) interpreter. "Here I am bleeding, on a stretcher, having to advocate for an interpreter, and they're telling me it's not important. I know a lot of deaf people will just give up, but I persisted." Kate wouldn't let clinicians treat her without an interpreter present so she would know what was happening. Finally, "a friend called my brother who is deaf. He said, 'Forget about the interpreter. Let them treat her.'" Her brother's command "led to my giving up. . . . Trying to advocate for yourself when you're injured is just not worth it." Not having an interpreter meant that Kate could not get information about her injuries that hearing persons would automatically expect.

Learning to advocate for oneself can take time and effort. Eleanor Peters, who contracted polio in early childhood, grew into the advocacy role:

> It's not like it happens overnight. I've been disabled forever, as far as I'm concerned. When I was younger and in the hospital, it wasn't peaches and cream. They definitely took advantage of me and my mother. My mother didn't understand a lot of what was happening, and whatever doctors said, she would agree with. My biggest thing was that when I turned eighteen, I could make my own decisions. My body is mine. I ask a lot of questions when they give me medication: What are the side effects? What happens if I mix this medication with another drug? We have to learn that. These are our bodies, whether they're disabled or not. I love my body, and I'm not going to let somebody mess around with it. We have to speak up for ourselves.

Nevertheless, persons with disabilities carry identical foibles and fallacies, as does everybody else. They also can lose perspective, hold unrealistic expectations, and deny problems that seemingly stare them in the face. "Magical thinking"—the common presumption that if you already have one disabling condition, you certainly won't get another—can have unfortunate consequences. Some women eschew mammograms believing they couldn't possibly get breast cancer on top of their disability.

Other personal attributes can impede self-advocacy for some persons with disabilities. Steffie Giacommo raised this caution. "I worked in a practice where they said, 'Make sure you teach all your clients to learn everything they can, so that when they go to their doctors they can teach their doctors.'" Steffie wonders about whether this exhortation is appropriate. "Nobody says to patients with a cardiac condition, 'You must learn about your disease so you can teach it to your doctor.' They don't expect that of any other type of disease," which physicians presumably already know about treating. "When you think about the population of people with disabilities—their educational background, socioeconomic backgrounds, their social skills, or their ability to communicate. . . . it just seems overwhelming to expect them to teach the doctor."

Steffie acknowledges that persons with disabilities vary widely in their emotional fortitude and knowledge base for self-management and advocacy. Poverty, low health literacy, isolation, unemployment, and myriad social disadvantages impede active partnerships with clinicians and patients' abilities to educate health care professionals. Steffie worries that "the population of people who are least skilled are the ones who have to deal with those barriers."

Self-Management and Collaborative Care

People with chronic health conditions and health-related sensory and physical disabilities make myriad decisions, day in and day out, that significantly affect their health and health care. Thus, they already manage their own care. The question then becomes whether people manage their conditions in ways geared toward achieving the best possible outcomes, however each individual defines their health goals.

The majority of people pursue self-management without explicitly collaborating with clinicians. Formalizing the collaborative care approach requires very different roles and expectations of clinicians and patients than those assumed under traditional care (table 11.1). In addition, the role of patient education differs substantially between traditional and collaborative care (table 11.2). Numerous resources exist to inform patients and assist self-management, including books, audiotapes, videotapes and DVDs, educational programs (at local settings or via the Internet), support groups, and Web sites and chat rooms. Many resources are condition-specific, such as those sponsored by particular disease advocacy organizations. Appendix 2

Table 11.2. Comparison of Traditional and Self-Management Patient Education

Issue	Traditional Education	Self-Management Education
Content	Information, technical skills about disease	Skills on responding to problems
Formulating problems	Problems reflect inadequate disease control	Patient identifies problems related and unrelated to disease
Education and disease	Education specific to disease and related technical skills	Education teaches problem-solving skills pertinent to chronic conditions generally, not specific diseases
Educational theory	Disease knowledge → behavior change → better clinical outcomes	Greater patient confidence in capacity to change behaviors (self-efficacy) → better clinical outcomes
Goal	Adherence with behavior change to improve clinical outcomes	Increased self-efficacy to improve clinical outcomes
Educator	Clinicians	Clinicians, peer, or other patients, often in group settings

Adapted from: Bodenheimer et al. (2002, p. 2471).

presents selected Internet resources relating to specific disabilities, diseases, or disorders. Here, we briefly review the broad principles and practices of self-management and collaborative care.[6]

The Chronic Care Model

As noted since chapter 1, the U.S. health care system is not structured to provide optimal—or perhaps even adequate care—for chronic medical conditions and persons with disabilities. Oriented primarily to addressing acute conditions, today's health care delivery system fails persons with chronic needs.

> Under a system designed for acute rather than chronic care, patients are not adequately taught to care for their own illnesses. Visits are brief and little planning takes place to ensure that acute and chronic needs are addressed. Lacking is a division of labor that would allow non-physician personnel to take greater responsibility in chronic care management. Too often, caring for chronic illness features an uninformed passive patient interacting with an unprepared practice team, resulting in frustrating, inadequate encounters. (Bodenheimer, Wagner, and Grumbach, 2002, p. 1775)

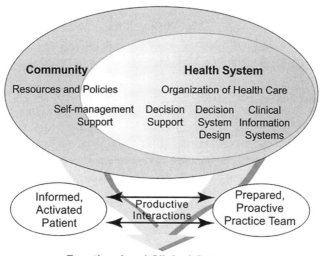

Functional and Clinical Outcomes

Figure 11.1. Chronic disease model. *Source:* E. H. Wagner, 1998, Chronic Disease Management: What Will It Take to Improve Care for Chronic Illness? *Effective Clinical Practice,* 1:2–4.

The "chronic care model," formulated by Edward H. Wagner, a physician in the MacColl Institute for Healthcare Innovation at Group Health Cooperative of Puget Sound, offers solutions to many of these problems (figure 11.1). The chronic care model builds upon six essential elements:

1. *Linking with community resources.* Health care providers must join with community-based organizations, such as exercise facilities, self-help and advocacy groups, senior centers, and centers for independent living, to offer programs and information.
2. *Reorienting the goals and structure of health care organizations.* Chronic care succeeds only if payment policies, quality monitoring and improvement programs, leadership goals, and other organizational initiatives all target chronic care as their guiding priority. Reimbursement is critical. Chronic care improvements will endure only if they increase revenues or lower costs.
3. *Restructuring health care delivery systems.* Teams of clinicians must divide responsibilities to efficiently address patients' diverse needs. Physicians' roles include treating acute problems, handling complex chronic concerns, and training the clinical team. Nonphysicians should assume responsibility for routine care tasks and assisting patients with self-management planning.

4. *Relying on medical evidence through practice guidelines.* To the extent possible, care should rest on strong clinical foundations and scientific evidence about effective interventions. Clinicians should integrate practice guidelines based on this evidence into daily clinical decisions.
5. *Using computerized information systems.* Computers can provide automated reminders to clinicians about practice guideline recommendations for individual patients and offer feedback to clinicians and health care organizations about how their patients are doing.
6. *Supporting patient self-management.* Clinicians must help patients, and sometimes their families, acquire skills, knowledge, and confidence to manage their own health care.

Informed patients actively engaged in self-management are the foundation of successful chronic care.

Overview of Self-Management

Self-management does not offer miracles or cures (Lorig et al., 2000, p. 1). Instead, its primary goal is to allow persons with chronic health conditions to live as well as possible—from both physical and emotional perspectives. Self-management represents a lifelong process, built upon the belief that patients' internal motivation sustains lifestyle change more powerfully than external exhortations. Over lifetimes, self-management strategies must bend and adapt as personal circumstances change.

Self-management requires patient education, but from a different perspective than traditional care (table 11.2). Traditional patient education focuses on teaching disease-specific information and skills, such as methods for controlling glucose and preventing complications of diabetes. In contrast, self-management patient education emphasizes training patients to recognize their own health problems and flag new concerns. Then this training teaches patients skills to find solutions that fit within evolving realities of their daily lives. These skills fall into three primary categories:

- Skills concerning specific needs related to underlying medical conditions
- Skills allowing patients to continue normal daily activities and relationships with family, friends, and colleagues
- Skills addressing emotional concerns, especially anger, fear, depression, and isolation (Bodenheimer et al., 2002, p. 2471)

Self-management programs start with persons setting their own goals for what they want to accomplish relating to their health and health care, then identifying alternative options for achieving these goals (Lorig et al., 2000). Experts recommend that goals be specific and realistic—definite and demonstrable behaviors or actions that individuals can reasonably accomplish within days, weeks, or months. Goals could address a spectrum of outcomes. For example, Marcia McDonough might aim to reduce stresses on her shoulders and rotator cuff by altering her patterns of wheelchair use, while Marta Redding may strive to socialize more with friends, employing strategies to handle anxiety about her hearing deficit.

Seeking resources in communities or more broadly (e.g., via the Internet), soliciting advice from family and friends, and getting input from clinicians may yield critical advice about achieving various goals. For example, to rest her shoulders, Marcia might aim temporarily to reduce her daily excursions from home. She could investigate whether local grocery stores, pharmacies, dry cleaners, and other services offer home delivery. She could seek shops, banks, post offices, and other services that are easily accessible to wheelchair users (e.g., have nearby parking or public transportation, are located on level terrain with well-maintained sidewalks). Marcia could investigate temporarily renting a power wheelchair or hiring an in-home personal assistant to help her with transfers and performing other shoulder-stressing tasks.

Specifying an "action plan" to reach the identified goal is the next step. Drawing upon identified resources and notions about what would work well within their daily routines, persons should lay out specific behaviors or actions along several dimensions: exactly what they will do, how much, how often, and when. Action plans should set realistic expectations and time frames, recognizing that persons may occasionally need some time off. People must honestly assess whether their action plan is something *they* want to do for themselves (rather than satisfying someone else's objectives) and gauge their confidence that they can actually accomplish the plan.

Even well-considered action plans generally need periodic adjustments to accommodate unanticipated occurrences or barriers. "If something doesn't work, don't give up. Try something else" (Lorig et al., 2000, p. 21). The self-management approach views successful achievement of a practical and realistic action plan as more important than the plans themselves.[7] Modest success can breed self-confidence, motivating people to persist in managing their own health.

To inform and support self-management activities, clinicians join collaborative care as partners with patients, not directors. "The partnership paradigm credits patients with an expertise similar in importance to the expertise of professionals. This paradigm implies that while professionals are experts about diseases, patients are experts about their own lives" (Bodenheimer et al., 2002, p. 2470). As suggested above, this paradigm may not fit precisely for some persons with disabilities who possess superior technical understanding of their health conditions and risks than do clinicians. Nonetheless, this paradigm explicitly recognizes the primacy of patients in the critical sphere for ongoing self-management—daily life.

The collaborative care paradigm moves away from the traditional approach of blaming patients for failing to comply with clinicians' recommendations as did Steffie Giacommo's urologist—clearly a traditionalist. He viewed her as noncompliant and aggressive when she refused to accept his advice and continued her own bladder control regimen. From Steffie's viewpoint, the urologist had not provided sufficient scientific justification for her to abandon an approach that had successfully controlled urinary tract infections for years. Under the collaborative approach, Steffie's urologist would have accepted the validity of her rationale for not adhering to his proposed regimen. In urging Steffie to follow his recommendation, the urologist would need to argue the merits of his approach along the dimensions that she finds important.

Does Self-Management Work?

Dozens of studies have explored the effects of self-management for various outcomes, including clinical endpoints (e.g., glucose control in diabetes), patients' sense of well-being and symptom control, emotions and ability to "cope" with conditions, and health care utilization and costs. The effects of self-management vary across conditions and outcomes of interest. Self-management does not always produce better health; nor does it uniformly lower health care costs. But it can make important and positive differences in the lives of many patients and their attitudes about their health. Even when disability increases, persons engaged in self-management report fewer declines in their physical activity and social roles and better emotional well-being (Lorig et al., 2001). These effects can persist over years, along with reduced use of emergency rooms and outpatient visits.

Bodenheimer and colleagues (2002) extensively reviewed research about the effects of self-management programs.[8] Most studies address specific health conditions—notably asthma, diabetes, and arthritis—while some explore chronic conditions in general. Their review produced two major conclusions. First, teaching self-management skills improves clinical outcomes more than simply providing information about health conditions. Second, in some circumstances, self-management programs both enhance clinical outcomes and lower health care costs. Studies that examined overall health status, emotional distress, and sense of control over one's health generally found benefits from self-management programs.

Given these potentially helpful results, why haven't self-management programs spread more widely throughout the health care system (Reuben, 2002)? This question echoes the broader concern about the failure of the U.S. health care system to implement broadly new and better ways of managing chronic health conditions. Explanations run deep within the health care system and professional mores. Substantial changes will require leadership from health care payers and clinical professionals. Today, Medicare, Medicaid, and private health insurers typically do not reimburse self-management training.[9] Thus, such programs are generally available only to those who are willing and able to pay for them. Relatively few professionals have received training to teach self-management skills. Although books and other educational materials are widely available (e.g., on the Internet; see appendix 2), the best results occur when patients receive formal self-management training rather than trying to teach themselves. Another impediment is attitudinal. "People with chronic conditions have been socialized into the medical model, fostering dependence on professionals, rather than a patient-physician partnership model; this barrier hinders recruitment of patients to self-management education programs" (Bodenheimer et al., 2002, p. 2474).

Despite these challenges, improving health nationwide requires enhancing the ability of persons with chronic conditions to manage their own health—a core component of patient-centered care. Many factors contribute to poorer health among socially and economically disadvantaged populations in the United States, including poor education, low incomes, and ineffective self-management of chronic conditions. Such socioeconomic and cultural attributes likely contribute more to poor population health than limited access to traditional health care services. These observations, supported by numerous studies, raise the specter of "blaming the victim"—casting fault on poor or uneducated persons for their faulty health behaviors or on clinicians for failing to teach patients self-management skills (Pincus et al., 1998). Assigning blame, however, neglects the continuing dominance of the traditional medical model both in paying for care and training health professionals. Adopting self-management principles and supporting partnerships with patients will require shifts in practice paradigms throughout the health care system.

Implications of Sensory and Physical Disabilities

Many persons with sensory and physical disabilities already surmount barriers to daily activities and navigate inaccessible spaces and communities—skills that might serve them well in managing health conditions. As noted earlier, various disabilities carry different implications for self-management of health conditions. In some circumstances, persons with disabilities already perform major self-management roles virtually independently, while in others, collaboration with clinicians is essential.

In certain instances, managing impairments per se is unnecessary: fixed or constant conditions, like congenital blindness or deafness, do not require management. Instead, these conditions shape persons' needs for accommodations and adaptations throughout many aspects of daily functioning. When, later in life, individuals develop the chronic conditions that many experience (e.g., hypertension, diabetes, heart or lung disease, arthritis), limited vision or hearing could affect strategies for managing these disorders.

In contrast, other disabling conditions require that patients actively manage basic bodily functions—day in and day out—or risk life-threatening complications. For instance, persons with spinal cord injury or neurological conditions affecting bladder and bowel function must attend closely to urination and bowel evacuation to avoid dangerous infections or intestinal impaction and possible bowel rupture. This can involve continual self-management decisions, ranging from diet and drinking patterns to medication use. Such strategies become part of the fabric of daily life. Patients typically know much more than their clinicians about how best to handle these basic concerns.

Some sensory or physical disabilities progress or change over time. In certain instances, clinical interventions and patients' behaviors could slow or alter this progression. Such diseases as diabetes, heart disease, and emphysema exemplify this situation. Each requires explicit medical interventions—insulin injections, medications, and supplemental oxygen—aiming both to prevent acute complications (such as diabetic coma, heart attack, or respiratory failure) and to slow long-term progression of disability and organ damage. Each might also respond to lifestyle or behavioral factors, such as exercise, diet, and stress reduction. Patients remain the experts in fitting both medical interventions and behavioral changes into their daily routines and in judging how their bodies respond, while collaborative clinicians provide essential guidance on safety and potential effectiveness.

Self-management programs with specific recommendations exist for common conditions, such as diabetes, asthma, chronic heart and lung diseases, stroke, arthritis, depression, and multiple sclerosis (appendix 2). Disabilities related to less common causes may not yet have their own self-management program. Nonetheless, "generic" recommendations cut across chronic conditions, representing basic principles and practices regardless of underlying disease or disorder. Some issues, such as the need for physical activity and questions about emotional health, are almost universal.

Given how they already live their daily lives, many persons with disabilities could welcome and benefit from self-management along with collaborative clinicians. Marcia McDonough might say, "I'm already doing that!" Nonetheless, formal training in self-management skills might aid Marcia in formulating future self-care plans. Three major concerns remain: inadequate technical knowledge among clinicians to fulfill their side of the educational bargain; the effect of boundaries circumscribing what falls inside and outside health care (see chapter 9); and questions about the accessibility of information, facilities, and technologies required for self-management.

Addressing Clinicians' Technical Knowledge

Most primary care physicians probably possess ample technical knowledge about common disabling conditions—arthritis, diabetes, and so on—to function as educational partners with patient self-managers. But the average primary care clinician sees relatively few patients with rarer disabling disorders, such as spinal cord injuries, spina bifida, and major neurological diseases. Many technical issues fall outside basic primary care training into such specialized areas as neurology, ophthalmology, otolaryngology, physiatry, and urology.

Inadequate technical knowledge potentially compromises interactions between patients and clinicians, as well as threatening quality of care (see chapter 8). Given the explosion of medical knowledge in recent decades, primary care clinicians could never realistically learn about all technical topics. Therefore, clinicians should comfortably acknowledge up front when they have inadequate technical understanding. Furthermore, when facing patients with unfamiliar disorders, clinicians should anticipate that they may not know enough to treat the patient appropriately.

Except in unusual circumstances, clinicians without explicit technical knowledge should not conduct even seemingly minor therapeutic interventions based on assumptions or clinical hunches. Instead, they should seek necessary information or refer patients to experienced specialists. Within the context of individual clinical encounters, clinicians could start by asking patients, "Is there anything about your condition that you want me to know about or that especially worries you?" Referring to appropriate specialists does not mean relinquishing responsibility for patients. Primary care clinicians should follow up referrals with both patients and specialists to ensure that patients' needs are met and to learn specialists' opinions and therapeutic plans. This follow-up offers primary care clinicians opportunities to learn more about disabling conditions, both from specialist colleagues and patients.

In certain situations, primary care physicians and specialists must collaborate with each other, as well as with patients. For instance, if a patient with substantial impairments from multiple sclerosis develops cancer, oncologists—who may have few experiences treating patients with such deficits—might need to consult with the patient's neurologist, urologist, and other clinicians when making technical decisions about surgery, chemotherapy, or radiation. Cancer interventions, regardless of whether patients have disabilities, can hugely alter quality of life. Certain physical impairments may magnify some effects. With the patient as the central decision-maker, multiple clinicians may need to gather round in a multifaceted collaboration.

Clinicians' Roles at Health Care Boundaries

Sometimes, the best self-management tools for persons with disabilities bump up against that perimeter circumscribing the standard health care delivery system (see chapter 9). For instance, hearing aids, prescription eyeglasses, bath chairs, certain wheelchairs, and home modifications to improve safety and accessibility generally fall outside that boundary, and health insurers refuse to pay for them. If patients do not have the resources to purchase these aids or services themselves, patients—along with families and clinicians—must consider ways to compensate for this absence. In today's health care system, stark reality holds that some people will have lower quality of life than they otherwise might because they cannot afford potentially helpful items or services. As one physical therapist matter-of-factly observed, "People need a rich uncle."

Other times, tools that could aid self-management sit uncertainly astride that boundary. For example, as described in chapter 9, Marcia McDonough believes that an ultra-lightweight wheelchair could substantially ameliorate her rotator cuff problem. Her health insurer covers wheelchairs, but not this particular model. The insurer views ultra-lightweight wheelchairs as a "convenience item" rather than a "medical necessity." All Marcia's arguments and self-advocacy are powerless against her insurer's refusal. Could her clinicians help?

As noted in chapter 3, before reimbursing covered services, health insurers generally review each case to establish the "medical necessity" of specific items or services. They rely largely upon written documentation—so-called "certificates of medical necessity"—from patients' physicians. Physicians receive little training about writing effective medical necessity justifications. Furthermore, since denials frequently ensue, these forms represent thankless paperwork. Dr. Johnny Baker was the primary care physician of Erna Dodd, a woman denied a scooter by Medicare (chapter 3). He dreads the time consumed by applying for equipment and appealing denials. "When this sort of thing comes along, I immediately get hold of a social worker and ask for help," said Dr. Baker, who works in a large practice. Other physicians might not have such support.

Sometimes, battles with health insurers can wrench collaborations between patients and clinicians. Some interviewees describe physicians refusing to aggressively fight denials from health insurers for assistive technologies or other services. Other times, physicians seem ineffective at framing compelling clinical arguments to persuade health insurers. The idiosyncratic nature of medical necessity decisions poses major challenges: rarely do health insurers clearly state their explicit rationales for refuting the medical justifications offered by clinicians (Singer and Bergthold, 2001). "I will write a lengthy justification if a wheelchair prescription is denied," said one occupational therapist who often argues that special equipment will save money by preventing expensive complications, such as pressure ulcers or other injuries. "If I persevere, it really does pay off, but the process can extend for months. It means I have to spend a lot of time on the phone and paperwork rather than treating patients" (Karp, 1999, p. 214).

Medical necessity requirements can stymie patients' efforts at self-advocacy. However, sometimes people's persistence mobilizes their clinicians and ultimately achieves success—albeit at the cost of considerable time, energy, and aggravation. One woman severely disabled by multiple sclerosis got Medicare to purchase her scooter based on her neurologist's well-crafted prescription and medical necessity justification. She believes that her training as a social worker also helped: "It's being educated in how things work. I always have worked with people who are cowed by the system before they'd even try it. They say that it can't be done, and they're afraid to ask."

Accessibility of Facilities and Services

Community resources play essential roles in the chronic care model and self-management activities. After all, virtually by definition, self-management occurs outside health care settings, in homes and communities. All the issues raised in chapter 5 about physical access recur in this context: just as patients face barriers to access within health care facilities, homes and community-based facilities can pose equal or greater impediments.

Especially when discussing self-management ideas with persons with disabilities, clinicians should inquire about their home environments. After all, many homes pose substantial physical barriers, such as absent handrails and inaccessible bathrooms (chapter 9). Depending on patients' self-management goals, homes therefore could pose significant obstacles, as well as safety hazards. Inaccessible entryways could impede self-management plans calling for daily walks outside the home. Home evaluations by skilled occupational therapists could identify such problems and help patients devise strategies to circumvent or eliminate them.

Whenever possible, before referring patients to specific community resources, clinicians should be aware of their accessibility, such as ease of physical entry, parking, availability of public transportation, and TTY use. In large practices and clinics, social workers or community resource specialists often serve this informational role. Providers could also request pamphlets containing specific accessibility information from sites where they refer patients. Accessibility of community-based facilities can determine whether or not patients accomplish key self-management goals. As Marcia McDonough suggested:

> I got some good advice early on. Right after my spinal cord injury, when I was in rehab, they emphasized that if we did not keep the parts of our body that were not paralyzed fit, we would end up having more injuries and a lower quality of life. I really believe that is true. Not that I do a great job at exercising, but the habit started early. They had pool therapy at rehab, and to this day I do the pool exercises that they taught me.
>
> Not all health clubs are accessible even if they're supposed to be. The club I currently belong to couldn't be more wonderful. They

gave me a locker at my height. They have a shower I can pull the wheelchair into, with a great big bench and a handheld shower.

Marcia says that her physiatrist thinks improving access to exercise facilities could potentially lower overall health care costs. But he acknowledges "the lack of access to exercise equipment for people in wheelchairs. There's no quad-friendly gym." Marcia's physiatrist might consider advocating within his community for more accessible gyms. As providers move toward a chronic care model—where linking with community resources is key—creating partnerships with local developers of health-related settings, like exercise and recreational facilities, could pay off for all sides (see chapter 16). Health care professionals would have appropriate sites to refer their patients, developers would open doors to new potential customers, and persons with disabilities would have more opportunities to improve or maintain their health.

Tools to Improve Shared Clinical Decision-Making

Many medical decisions—about diagnosis, treatment, and prevention of disease—require nuanced judgments among competing approaches. Collecting and sorting through the pros and cons of various options present challenges to clinicians and patients. Traditionally, clinicians weigh the strength and weakness of scientific evidence, while patients interject their values and preferences. Under collaborative care, optimal choices balance not only the science but also patients' goals, hopes, and expectations through a process of "shared decision-making" between clinicians and patients.

A growing number of products and information tools aim to assist shared decision-making for very specific clinical decisions, such as therapy for breast, lung, ovarian, and prostate cancers; treatments for benign prostate disease, heart disease, back pain, knee osteoarthritis, rheumatoid arthritis, and osteoporosis; screening for the breast cancer gene or prostate cancer using prostate-specific antigen (PSA); and vaccination for hepatitis B.[10] These tools come in various formats, including written brochures or booklets, audiotapes, videotapes, DVDs, and interactive videos (where patients choose how much and what type of information they receive by responding to prompts during the presentation). Video presentations generally include observations from patients with the particular condition, describing their experiences with specific treatment choices. Consumers with disabilities should check first to ensure that particular shared decision-making products accommodate sensory or physical impairments: these tools are not universally accessible.

Although shared decision-making tools vary in content and format, they all follow one basic outline: they present two or more reasonable options for the specific clinical decision, and then review potential pros and cons of each choice. Discussions between clinicians and patients build upon this information. More than two dozen research studies have examined how shared decision-making tools affect patients' choices (Barry, 2002). When major surgery is a treatment option, use of decision aids generally leads to selection of more conservative nonsurgical treatments. Several studies find that persons who use decision aids participate more actively in making therapeutic choices than other patients. Patients using decision tools appear better informed but no more satisfied than other patients.

Some shared decision-making tools directly address disabling conditions, such as arthritis, back pain, osteoporosis, and heart disease. Nonetheless, questions arise about how well these tools apply to persons with sensory and physical disabilities. These tools use scientific evidence to build cases for and against different decision options. However, the clinical trials that comprise this evidence base generally explicitly exclude persons with certain types of disabilities. This leaves important gaps in the scientific evidence about clinical decisions for persons with disabilities, holes that patients using the tools—and even their clinicians—may not appreciate fully.

Thus, existing tools for shared medical decision-making offer the potential to delineate different clinical options and begin discussions between patients and clinicians about choices to maximize health benefits and meet patients' goals. Specific details of the information contained in these tools may not apply to persons with certain disabilities. Both patients and clinicians should therefore employ these tools cautiously, only as starting points for their decision-making. Given the paucity of scientific evidence relevant to persons with certain disabilities, most medical decisions will likely involve considerable uncertainty and rely largely on patients' and clinicians' judgments.

Technologies to Aid Self-Management

Sensory and physical impairments can impede basic self-management tasks (e.g., taking pills, using inhalers), as well as more complex activities, such as testing glucose levels and injecting medications. Numerous technologies exist to help patients with sensory and physical impairments accomplish self-management activities. For instance, insulin delivery equipment and glucose monitoring devices are available for patients who are blind or low vision, as are talking watches, various magnification devices, and computers with voice capabilities (Goldzweig et al., 2004). Physical and occupational therapists who specialize in visual disabilities can work with persons who are blind or low vision to devise ways to perform care-related tasks. Web sites listed in appendix 2 offer information about some of these technologies; medical supply vendors and various manufacturers provide additional product information.

Technologies offer many advantages, but they do not eliminate all barriers to self-management for everyone with disabilities. One core task—taking medications—highlights the potential complexities (Logue, 2002). Some patients with disabilities and chronic conditions must take multiple medications, following complicated daily schedules. Persons who are blind or have low vision face difficulties identifying different drugs and reading instructions, typically printed in tiny type on bottles or small slips of paper (see chapter 8). Similarly, clinicians may not provide information about medication administration or side effects in accessible formats to persons who are deaf or hard of hearing, leaving these individuals with inaccurate impressions about how to proceed. Arthritis, tremors, and other manual dexterity problems can impede persons from opening and closing medication bottles, especially vials with childproof caps. Hand problems also increase the likelihood that patients will drop and lose pills.

Companies now market diverse technologies to assist pill taking, including prompting devices (e.g., watches, beeping key chains, pagers, programmable human voice reminders, telephone-computer services) that alert persons when they have missed medication doses; electronic pill containers, dispensers, and organizers; monitoring devices (e.g., electronic medication vials); and data management systems using personal digital assistants. The complexity of this gadgetry appeals to some persons but daunts others. In addition, sensory and physical impairments pose challenges to operating these technologies similar to those raised by the ordinary pill bottle. Little research has been conducted to document the pros and cons of various devices for different groups of patients. Nonetheless, anecdotal evidence suggests that people must carefully choose devices that best match their needs, capabilities, and preferences. Otherwise, persons will reject these technologies as more burdensome than helpful, and the latest gizmos will sit unused.

The good news is that manufacturers are responding aggressively to the needs precipitated by the aging U.S. population, producing new technologies to assist persons with vision, hearing, and various physical difficulties to perform routine, daily, self-management tasks independently and safely. Consumers now have multiple options to meet various needs, and the number and variety of products are growing. Health insurance currently covers few of these devices, so only people wealthy enough to purchase this equipment now benefit. Prices for various medication devices vary widely, from less than $20 to close to $1,000. The coming decades should offer even more technologies to assist persons in managing their own health and health care.

12

Improving Patient-Clinician Communication

Patricia Fielding, who is hard of hearing, offers a suggestion to health care professionals:

> The ideal thing in all health care—whether it's a receptionist or the doctor, nurses or the hospital—is to ask me, "How can I best communicate with you?" That's what I want to hear. We're all a little different. We all hear a bit differently and have slightly different needs. One thing isn't going to work for everybody. So they should ask me, "What do *I* need?"

Effective health care requires open and effective patient-clinician communication. However, as part II suggests, communication between clinicians and persons with disabilities can break down. Sometimes, inaccessible communication techniques or formats cause these failures. Other times, communication problems result from clinicians' erroneous assumptions about patients' experiences, perspectives, preferences, and needs. Complex interpersonal factors can complicate communication, as patients worry about offending clinicians or make incorrect presumptions about their clinician's attitudes, and as clinicians dismiss, misinterpret, or ignore patients' views. Short appointment times and economic pressures exacerbate the problems.

Given these complexities, finding workable strategies to enhance patient-clinician communication and interactions with office staff for persons with disabilities requires careful thought and planning. Certain solutions are easy, such as selecting a large font before printing medication prescriptions and instructions for patients with low vision. In this situation, reminding clinicians and office staff to make this simple change presents the greatest challenge. Finding a systems solution, such as by adding "large print" to computer menu options for printing medication information, could help. In contrast, confronting the complicated interpersonal dynamics and erroneous assumptions that can derail communication eludes quick technological fixes.

Drawing upon the collaborative care approach described in chapter 11, persons with disabilities and their clinicians ideally should discuss communication shortfalls together and devise practical solutions. Optimally, each would assume partial ownership of the communication process. "It's a mutual responsibility between the patient and the health care provider to make sure that communication is successful—it takes two to tango," observed one woman who is hard of hearing. She feels responsible for acknowledging her hearing loss and speaking up when she can't hear; then she expects her clinician to make appropriate accommodations. "If you're going to be an effective physician, you should recognize when someone has a hearing loss and adjust your communication style."

However, this ideal of patients and clinicians sharing "mutual responsibility" for communication can falter against interpersonal realities. Many patients shy away from self-revelations and advocacy about communication needs in health care settings. "Most people are not going to speak up and be assertive in the doctor's office," Patricia Fielding observed. "I've learned how to do it, but, boy, it takes everything I've got! Sometimes I shrivel up." Ms. Fielding's clinicians bear professional, ethical, and legal responsibility for identifying communication lapses and ensuring she understands critical aspects of her health care. However, clinicians require patients' help to appreciate fully their needs and devise effective communication solutions.

Chapter 12 explores strategies to improve communication between clinicians and patients. This topic is complex and multidimensional, requiring numerous and varied solutions, and we cover only highlights. This chapter examines interpersonal issues—training clinicians to recognize and remedy communication lapses. Chapter 13 looks at legal requirements for accessible information, then addresses accommodations for ensuring this access using human (e.g., sign language interpreters) and technological means (e.g., computers with synthetic speech systems). Appendix 2 lists selected Web sites, such as the American Foundation for the Blind (www.afb.org) and the Gallaudet University Technology Access Program (tap.gallaudet.edu), containing voluminous information about communication services and assistive technologies. Appendix 3 offers specific recommendations proposed by the interviewees for many communication problems they have encountered.

Recognizing Communication Barriers

Clinicians sometimes fail to recognize that communication barriers exist— many clinicians simply don't think about this possibility, and some patients don't raise the issue. As Ms. Fielding suggests, one obvious solution is to start clinical encounters with a straightforward question: "How can I best communicate with you?" Later on, to ensure that patients understand critical information, Ms. Fielding recommends that clinicians "ask you to repeat it back to them. I've gotten medicine wrong because I heard it wrong." If

Ms. Fielding had verbalized her understanding, her clinician could have identified and remedied her misconception.

To protect patients' safety and well-being, clinicians must take time to ensure that patients like Patricia Fielding understand their medications and other critical information. Time pressures and multitasking demands can impede this ideal. As encounters begin, clinicians may not pause to determine each patient's communication preferences. Asking office staff to assist in gathering patients' communication preferences and setting up "communication-sensitive" systems within offices and clinics could speed this process. Several interviewees suggested posting brief notes about communication needs and preferences in bright colors and bold print on the front of each patient's medical chart or another obvious place.

Clinicians, hospitals, and other health care providers should invite persons with disabilities to identify points where communication breaks down and to suggest communication-sensitive systems to resolve these problems. Organizations that advocate for persons with particular disabilities can provide helpful insight, such as those suggested by the American Foundation for the Blind (box 12.1). Although well-meaning clinicians believe they understand patients' needs, they may not appreciate fully critical details.

Teaching office staff to recognize and overcome communication barriers is essential. Training should involve everyone in the organization, from leadership to front-line office assistants. Many interviewees recommend approaches similar to that proposed by one woman who is deaf:

> Every year, everyone could spend one day on awareness training for staff to remember what they've learned, reinforce old information, and have a refresher about how to deal with different languages and cultures, different disability groups. . . . New employees in job orientation would see a training video. [This would] include training about who they might see at the job, and when deaf patients come in, how to communicate with them. How do you make them comfortable? That's partly a cultural issue and partly a communication issue and applies pretty well to everyone, not just deaf people.

When designing new office systems for accommodating communication, staff should involve persons with disabilities (see chapter 15). For instance, many organizations use automated telephone menus to route calls efficiently to their desired locations. Designers must consider all potential users when developing these systems. Telephone menus are "very stressful for a hard of hearing person," said a woman who has trouble hearing the menu instructions within allotted time frames. "If you're hard of hearing, you really need to talk to a person right away—a person who is trained to speak clearly."

Box 12.1. Selected Ways to Accommodate Communication and Mobility for Persons Who Are Blind or Have Low Vision

- Do not make assumptions about a person's visual acuity or its functional effects
- Speak in normal conversational tones; do not raise voice
- Routinely ask, "How can I be of assistance to you, Mr. A?"
- Address persons by name and identify yourself to persons by name, explaining your role. Persons may not see name badges or uniforms
- Do not touch or remove mobility aids, such as white canes, unless asked by persons
- Do not touch or interfere with guide dogs
- If patients accept assistance with mobility, offer your arm to them; people generally will hold your arm lightly above the elbow; relax and walk at a comfortable pace, allowing the person to walk a step or two behind; indicate changes in terrain or obstacles by slowing briefly as you approach and describe the situation
- Describe verbally or demonstrate procedures before performing them; as appropriate and feasible, allow patients to inspect equipment
- Be very specific when giving verbal directions; provide accessible signage, including braille and raised character signs, as well as audible direction and floor indicators in elevators
- Staff should read aloud, upon request, all written forms and documents and assist persons, in confidential settings, to complete paperwork
- Provide instruction materials in patients' preferred accessible formats, including large print, braille, audiotape, and computer diskette. Consider allowing patients to audiotape discussions with clinician, if patients wish to do so
- Reading aloud may not provide effective communication for some patients
- When handing paper currency to persons, individually identify and count each bill. Persons who are blind usually develop their own method for identifying different denominations of bills in their wallets. Hand credit cards to patients after making the imprint; do not simply place on a countertop
- The Americans with Disabilities Act (ADA) does not require organizations to undertake self-evaluations about their ADA compliance. Nonetheless, self-evaluations can help identify barriers to their facilities and services

Source: These suggestions draw upon recommendations in a pamphlet prepared by the Governmental Relations Department, American Foundation for the Blind, *Self-Evaluation Checklist for Health Care Facilities and Service Providers to Ensure Access to Services and Facilities by Patients Who Are Blind, Deaf-Blind, or Visually Impaired* (Washington, DC: undated).

Interviewees recommend formally evaluating providers' communication performance. One deaf man suggested surveying patients after each health care visit, asking ways to improve communication and the overall experience. Providers would use this feedback to implement improvements and then track the results. Such feedback forms would themselves need to accommodate all potential users, including persons with limited vision, difficulty writing, and low English proficiency. Although many health care settings already survey patients about their experiences with care, not all questionnaires use accessible formats. For instance, forms designed for optical scanning—with tiny ovals or circles that respondents must blacken with a pen or number 2 pencil—are difficult for some persons to complete (e.g., because of visual disabilities or manual dexterity problems). Without ready and confidential assistance, people may not fill out inaccessible forms.

Training Clinicians to Improve Communication

"When I meet a disabled person I have to keep reminding myself that I must not try to guess what their difficulties and concerns will be," wrote a physician who has become deaf over the past fifteen years. "To someone with medical training, this goes very much against the grain. Doctors are supposed either to know these things, or to be able to make an educated guess" (Kvalsvig, 2003, p. 2079). Clinicians may need explicit training to learn how to ask patients about their specific concerns.

During the past decade, health care educators have increasingly recognized communication skills—and, in particular, cultural understanding—as keys to providing high-quality, patient-centered care. Training programs for health care professionals now address these topics and require trainees to demonstrate proficiency. In 1999, the Accreditation Council for Graduate Medical Education (ACGME), the organization that accredits post–medical degree residency and fellowship training programs, specified six areas that they considered "core competencies":

- *Patient care:* compassionate, appropriate, and effective for treating health problems and promoting health
- *Medical knowledge:* biomedical, clinical, social-behavioral, and epidemiological, and applications to clinical care
- *Practice-based learning and improvement:* evaluation and enhancement of their own patient care against scientific evidence and standards
- *Interpersonal and communication skills:* "effective information exchange and teaming with patients, their families, and other health professionals"
- *Professionalism:* "adherence to ethical principles, and sensitivity to a diverse patient population"

- *Systems-based practice:* recognition of larger health care context and effective use of resources (ACGME, 1999)

The ACGME does not specify exactly how training programs should test trainees for these core competencies, leaving that up to individual institutions. Cultural and communication training programs typically emphasize race, ethnicity, non-English oral languages, and social factors, including income, education, health literacy, sexual preference, gender, and age (Betancourt, Green, and Carrillo, 2002; Green, Betancourt, and Carrillo, 2002). Training young health care professionals about cultural competence along these dimensions *is* hugely important. In its report, *Unequal Treatment,* documenting racial and ethnic disparities in health care services, the Institute of Medicine (Committee on Understanding, 2002) speculates that prejudicial attitudes could contribute to these discrepancies.

Rarely do training programs about cultural competence explicitly mention disability. However, negative attitudes may be more overt and affect clinical decision-making more directly in the context of disability than in minority race, ethnicity, and other patient attributes. Some clinicians hold openly negative views of disability—and expressly act upon them in clinical decision-making—justifying their actions based on perceived poor quality of life (see chapter 6). One study surveyed 153 emergency care providers about their attitudes toward spinal cord injury and found that 41 percent felt that efforts to resuscitate newly injured persons are too aggressive; imagining themselves living with spinal cord injury, 83 percent anticipated they would sometimes feel they are "no good at all" (Gerhart et al., 1994, p. 810).[1] These attitudes contrasted sharply with views of 128 individuals with actual tetraplegia, only 39 percent of whom reported sometimes feeling "no good at all." Furthermore, while only 44 percent of emergency care providers believe that persons with tetraplegia leave their homes for activities at least three or more days per week, 68.5 percent of people with tetraplegia actually do.

Communication training must begin with better understanding by clinicians of how disability affects persons' daily lives and expectations. Persons with disabilities could help teach these lessons. Caroline Patrick, who is tetraplegic, teaches medical students about interacting with persons with physical disabilities. "At first, they're really afraid," Caroline observed. "To them it's a new thing. They're like, 'What do I say? Do I shake their hand?' They throw all these questions out there. Then at the end of the session, they say, 'It's really great, we want more.' But there's no funding for it." Without resources, Caroline knows her brief efforts barely make a dent.[2]

Teaching could take many forms, from people with disabilities simply telling trainees about their lives to "role playing" exercises about common clinical scenarios. "I've participated in emergency training for paramedics," Helen Corrigan reported. "One part of the paramedic workshop was a hard of hearing spouse whose husband was having a heart attack. This hard of hearing woman played the wife. She was a great actress—she seemed in a panic. One paramedic talked to her one-on-one while the other paramedic helped her husband." Mrs. Corrigan felt that seeing actors—including one who was hard of hearing—role play a common clinical scenario offered compelling lessons about effective communication. "If you show students a situation they can relate to, then they'll know how to respond when the situation occurs."

A growing number of documentary films and television programs examine various aspects of disability and offer useful teaching points. In 2005, the World Institute on Disability (WID; www.wid.org) released a twenty-minute educational video with its companion "Training Curriculum for Medical Professionals on Improving the Quality of Care for People with Disabilities." Directed by persons with disabilities, the video focuses on improving access and communication in health care settings. Among others, including a practicing physician with a spinal cord injury, it features persons who are blind, deaf, or wheelchair users discussing barriers they have experienced while obtaining health care and interacting with clinicians and office staff. The film eloquently highlights the full and varied lives of its featured speakers and their desires for health care services to enhance their wellness and quality of life.

Medical students told us that they learn immensely from persons with disabilities who come into classrooms to describe living with specific conditions (Iezzoni, Ramanan, and Drews, 2005).[3] Such visits must avoid putting persons with disabilities "on display," a troubling practice dating back to "freak shows" of the early nineteenth century (Thomson, 1997). Persons with disabilities can be remarkably effective teachers, and years later, students vividly remember lessons taught by them. "A man with Parkinson's disease came to our neuroscience class two years ago," said Carly, a fourth-year medical student. "He had not taken his medication that morning." His wife rolled him into the medical school classroom in his wheelchair, his body virtually frozen by Parkinson's disease. He then took levodopa and later rose from his chair, walking across the classroom, commenting to the students about his physical experiences.[4] "Just having him actually be there and seeing how difficult it was for him to get started walking was incredibly meaningful." His wife spoke movingly about how her husband's Parkinson's disease had affected their entire family. The man relished teaching, having been a high school teacher for twenty-five years before retiring because of his disease.

Another training method commonly used in medical schools is "standardized patients"—actors or persons with actual health conditions specifically trained to interact with students during mock office visits and to critique the students' performance after their interview. Tufts University School of Medicine employs persons with disabilities trained as standardized patients to teach students interview skills (Kahn, 2003; Minihan et al., 2004). One standardized patient scenario involves evaluation of shoulder pain similar to that of Marcia McDonough. Instructors do not warn students beforehand that the patient uses a manual wheelchair. During the interview, the standardized patient follows a preset clinical script, adding details from her own life to lend reality. She simultaneously judges students' comfort with the interview and ability to understand not only how shoulder pain affects her daily activities but also the implications for treatment. After the interview, the standardized patient switches roles and becomes the educator, carefully crafting criticism to guide the student toward insight into how to do better.

Videotaping interactions between trainees and actual patients (or standardized patients) offers important opportunities to assess technical interviewing skills (e.g., abilities to elicit specific information) but also more complex aspects of interpersonal communication (Markakis et al., 2000). Afterward, trainees review these videotapes in small groups or with an individual instructor expert in communication skills. In addition to recording language, videotapes also capture physical interactions and thus reveal whether trainees appear awkward around patients with certain sensory or physical impairments (e.g., during interviews or physical examinations). Sometimes, trainees are completely unaware of their awkwardness and simply seeing their actions captured on videotape leads to substantial improvements.

Making home visits offers important opportunities for students to understand how disabilities affect patients' abilities to carry out prescribed therapies, as well as persons' attitudes toward their disability and daily life. Alan attended a medical school that requires fourth-year students to spend one month with a multidisciplinary team that does home care. He described an especially memorable patient:

> This gentleman lives a block from the medical center. He's eighty-something, African American, this little guy with really severe scoliosis.[5] When you go to his apartment, the whole place is damp because the radiator leaks. He hasn't taken his pills that morning. He goes to the faucet, and little drips of water come out of the rusty pipe. He's stumbling around, and you wonder why he hasn't fallen a billion times—there's stuff all over the place. The cup he uses is dirty, and there's piles of dirty dishes. When I reach down to get something from the bottom of our supply bag, it's wet because his carpet was soaking wet.

Overwhelmed by the patient's dilapidated apartment, Alan admitted thinking, "How does this guy stay here by himself? But he does, and I'm sure he's much happier there than being stuck in a nursing home. . . . You learn visiting him that he's able to do a lot. Now I think about those things."

Marcia McDonough concurs that home visits offer critical opportunities to appreciate the totality of people's lives. "See us in our own environment," urged Marcia. "Go to the home of a couple of disabled people. Seeing how people live helps you understand how to treat them." Marcia thinks that "doctors anticipate a much lower quality of life than we actually have."

One program does exactly what Marcia suggests—pairing residents in physical medicine and rehabilitation with persons with spinal cord injury living in the community (Siebens et al., 2004). In the PoWER Program, "People with Disabilities Educating Residents," these "consumer-trainers" let physiatry residents visit them in their homes and at workplaces. Residents arrive at the trainer's home between 6 and 7 o'clock in the morning and spend the next six hours observing activities of daily living, home adaptations, personal assistant services, assistive technologies, and activities at work, including transportation. Trainers uniformly enjoy the sessions, making such comments as, "It's great to have the ear of doctors in a non-rehab setting and a chance for doctors to see the real daily life of someone with a disability" (Siebens et al., 2004, p. 205). Residents typically use such terms as "excellent," "outstanding," and "invaluable" to describe their experiences.

To make persons without disabilities more sensitive to physical and attitudinal barriers, some educators advocate "disability simulations"—for several hours or a day, mimicking impairments by such means as wearing blindfolds, smearing eyeglass lenses with petroleum jelly, inserting ear plugs, binding legs or arms so they cannot move, or using wheelchairs. Several interviewees with disabilities advocated this approach: "Put a blindfold on [medical students] and let them experience for themselves what we go through," urged one blind man.

Other interviewees with disabilities, as well as fourth-year medical students we spoke to, voice concerns that simulating disability can reinforce negative attitudes. Several years earlier, Colleen had joined a disability simulation exercise at her college:

> It was fun. I was in a wheelchair. My college campus is very accessible to wheelchairs, so I didn't have all that many obstacles. I had a lot of people pushing me in my wheelchair, whipping me around. I had to write a paper about it. But I wrote the paper not really on the experience of my day but on what I was supposed to have experienced. It's artificial, so I don't know that it has the right effect.

Other students also questioned the value and lessons of simulation exercises. Lynne worried that such programs "end up trivializing disabilities. Maybe you have some superficial sense of the inconveniences by being blindfolded for one day or being wheelchair bound. But you don't lose the autonomy or independence. At the end of the day, you can still walk out of the wheelchair or take off the blindfold."

Several interviewees with disabilities articulated the most compelling rationale against disability simulations. Unlike the medical students, who felt that simulation exercises could never convey the "profundity" or "isolation" or "dependence" of disability, the interviewees with disabilities framed a diametrically opposing argument: that brief stints with simulated impairments do not let participants appreciate how good life can be once persons, over time, find ways to accommodate their disabilities. Dwight Eaton, who is blind, strongly opposes disability simulations, leading him directly to a broader plea to clinicians:

> Day-in-the-life exercises are not very valuable because most people who go through them just get scared to hell. They think, oh my God, I can't do this. From a few hours in the dark, they don't understand that you can acquire techniques for living a successful life as a blind person, that it takes time and perseverance and planning.
>
> What doctors have to be told, first and foremost, is to accept the blind person as another human being. We're not accepted as that, over and over again. We have got to be seen as persons of worth and intelligence who actually can contribute to our own care and recovery. Then, most important, doctors should ask us what we need, ask us if there's anything in particular—anything special, anything different—than for other people.

Bonnie and I also believe that disability simulations seldom convey the right educational message and therefore have little role in clinical training. Dwight Eaton's suggestion—just asking people what they might need as accommodations—offers much more useful input directed to the ultimate goal of improving communication and quality of care.

Finally, although this discussion focuses on patient-clinician communication, training to improve interdisciplinary communication among diverse health care professionals is also essential. Some persons with disabilities, especially those with significant physical impairments, require input from professionals cutting across clinical disciplines. Although certain specialties explicitly school their trainees in interdisciplinary collaboration, other training programs do not. Primary care physicians, in particular, may know little about rehabilitation professionals: as one general internist asked me, "Isn't a physiatrist like a physical therapist?" Primary care physicians are often uncertain when to refer patients to rehabilitation specialists (Hoenig, 1993). Health care professionals in training must learn "about the contributions which other disciplines can make to the assessment and care and to meeting the complex needs of persons with disabilities. . . . They need to learn to recognize when they have reached the limits of their own ability and expertise and need to refer to or consult with another discipline for needed care and services" (Center for Health Policy Research, 1996, p. 31).

Questions to Ask

Some clinicians communicate naturally and effectively with patients, just as certain people have more outgoing personalities than do others. Yet, clinical training—and the continuing education that accompanies years of practice—can instill specific skills to improve communication techniques. Knowing the goal of communication is essential to crafting the optimal communication process.

As clinicians move to collaborative care partnerships with patients (chapter 11), they may need new communication skills. In particular, to motivate patients to change their behaviors—such as to begin exercising, stop smoking, reduce drinking, or lose weight—patient-clinician communication can play an important role. New interviewing techniques have emerged, identifying specific skills that can help clinicians encourage patients to make important behavior changes to improve their health (Miller and Rollnick, 1991; Rollnick, Mason, and Butler, 1999).[6] Little research on these interviewing approaches specifically targets patients with sensory or physical disabilities, although most studies do address chronic diseases or conditions like obesity. While interviewing techniques to motivate behavior change likely generalize well to persons with disabilities, one particular aspect of clinical interviews may prove different in this context: information exchange.

"A large part of the practitioner's job is giving information to the patient. A large part of the patient's job is giving information to the practitioner" (Rollnick, Mason, and Butler, 1999, p. 106). In traditional care, clinicians are the experts, conveying information to patients (see table 11.1). When information exchanges involve expert clinicians "talking at" patients, this process leaves patients as passive observers, unlikely to find the information useful in changing their daily behaviors or improving their health. Persons with sensory impairments might be especially susceptible to one-sided information exchange if clinicians fail proactively to make accommodations to ensure effective communication. Especially when writing notes or communicating through interpreters, clinicians may feel that this one-sided tactic is more efficient for them—although it may compromise patients' knowledge and thus quality of care. More effective ways of conveying information involve skillful listening and careful questioning by clinicians:

> Instead, we view the process in terms of the following circular *elicit-provide-elicit process:* first, patients are encouraged to describe their behavior, ask questions, indicate what they would most like to know, or disclose what they do and do not know about a particular topic (*elicit*). Unlike the more traditional approach, the practitioner is encouraged to adopt a curious and eliciting interviewing style during this phase, and the patient will do most of the talking. . . . Second, the practitioner is active in conveying clear, non-judgmental in-

formation (*provide*) which, crucially, in the third phase, the patient is given an opportunity to absorb and reflect upon (*elicit*). (Rollnick, Mason, and Butler, 1999, p. 109)

Although this process works well in contexts where clinicians *do* have useful knowledge to impart, it remains unclear how well it would work in settings where patients may have more technical understanding of their impairments than do clinicians (see chapter 11). In these settings, presumably the circular interviewing technique, with a back-and-forth exchange between patients and clinicians, could establish the boundaries of the technical expertise of both patients and clinicians. For some patient-clinician pairs, it may ultimately produce more collaborative dialogues. Clinicians could ask patients open-ended questions, such as:

- How much do you know about (*fill in the blank*)?
- Would you like to know more about (*fill in the blank*)?
- Would you like to know how to (*fill in the blank*)?

Even if clinicians do not themselves know the answers to these questions, patients' responses would indicate what patients want to know and do know. Collaboratively, patients and clinicians could develop strategies for filling in the gaps of knowledge.

Asking patients about their "typical day" offers a patient-centered technique for clinicians to gather volumes of important information about patients' health, the role of their disability in their daily life, and any health behaviors that might offer targets for change. This approach, in the form of a conversation led by the patient, not only provides crucial clinical details, but also builds rapport between patients and clinicians. Rollnick, Mason, and Butler (1999, pp. 112–114) suggest that clinicians launch directly into the typical day query once they have established the particular health or behavior topic patients wish to address. This process ideally takes six to eight minutes, although three to five minutes sometimes suffice; longer periods become tiresome for both patients and clinicians.[7]

Clinicians should start the typical day inquiry by appearing interested and relaxed, asking: "Can you take me through a typical day in your life, so that I can understand in more detail what happens?" As patients talk, clinicians should listen carefully and interrupt as little as possible, asking only simple questions like: "What happened then? How did you feel? What exactly made you feel that way?" Even if, as patients speak, clinicians develop clinical hypotheses they would like to explore, clinicians should allow patients to continue their stories. Speeding things up is sometimes appropriate: "Can you take us forward a bit more quickly?" Overall, clinicians should do only 10 to 15 percent of the talking (Rollnick, Mason, and Butler, 1999, p. 114). As patients wrap up, a summary question helps: "Is there anything else about your typical day that you would like to tell me?"

This typical day scenario was not developed specifically for persons with disabilities, but it seems especially valuable in this context. Knowing how patients' disabilities affect daily life is crucial for clinicians to recommend therapeutic plans that have the greatest chance for success—and for patients to demonstrate their own understanding of their conditions and what interventions might work best for them. Describing a typical day might take longer for persons with disabilities than for other patients, but the detailed insight could prove extremely valuable.

Clinician Peers with Disabilities

Vera, a fourth-year medical student, offered a novel idea for training clinicians to communicate better with persons with disabilities. She knows of a deaf woman "who started medical school two years ago. Her classmates must be so much more educated just by having her there. One of the best educational things we could do would be to look at our [professional school] admissions policies and open the door"—let persons with disabilities into clinical training programs.

No one knows how many clinical trainees and health care professionals in the United States have sensory or physical impairments. Although the Association of American Medical Colleges annually tracks the numbers of entering medical students by sex, race, and ethnicity, persons with disabilities remain uncounted. Occasionally, stories of specific medical students with disabilities make the news, painting seemingly heroic tales of overcoming enormous odds (Villarosa, 2003), but their admission seems more noteworthy than routine. Health care practitioners and students with disabilities remain largely invisible, and their experiences generally escape notice.

Certainly physicians with disabilities do attract attention and sometimes consternation, although with familiarity can come comfort and routine. A rehabilitation physician who is blind told Bonnie that when he first appeared in his hospital with his white coat and white cane, "Everybody almost fell over. They couldn't understand how it's possible for me to practice. When I'd walk down the hallway, I'd hear these mutterings behind me, 'There goes the blind doctor.' But over time, those observations changed, and now people say instead, 'There goes the rehab doctor.' There's an incredible amount of ignorance among my colleagues—they don't know too many blind guys. They don't realize that a person with vision impairment functions with various kinds of accommodations. . . . They know mostly about what people can't do rather than what people can do."

In its report on redressing racial and ethnic disparities in health care services, the Institute of Medicine (Committee on Understanding, 2002) recommended increasing the proportion of underrepresented racial and ethnic minorities in the health professions. This recommendation draws from studies suggesting that greater racial and ethnic diversity among providers strengthens relationships with patients and improves care (see chapter 6). Parallel arguments concerning physicians with disabilities may prove imperfect. Nevertheless, clinicians with disabilities could appreciate, with acute and immediate insight, myriad issues confronting patients with similar impairments.

Some practicing physicians with disabilities believe their conditions enhance rapport with many patients, increasing patients' responsiveness to clinical recommendations, and sometimes offering patients hope by their example (Steinberg et al., 2002). Even patients' negative responses can provide important therapeutic insight, such as patients' fears about what might happen to them. Deaf clinicians fluent in American Sign Language offer dual advantages of shared language and culture with Deaf patients. "Some of the most gratifying patients I see come to me with arthritis," the rehabilitation physician who is blind told Bonnie, "and they turn out to have some vision problems. I may or may not make their arthritis better, but I tell them about Talking Books, News Line for the Blind, magnifiers, or whatever else. And it makes a big difference in their lives."

Clinicians with specific disabilities do not necessarily have superior insight about other impairments. As a physician who became deaf wrote:

> The single most important insight I have gained from being a disabled doctor is that I really have no idea what life is like for my patients. . . . The disability I know best is deafness. The profession I know best is medicine. So I accept that I've no idea how life is for, say, an accountant with cerebral palsy. But I do at least know what not to do if I should meet such a person. I won't automatically assume that they can't do certain things—nor will I blithely reassure them that they can. I'll . . . try to build up a picture of a more complex reality. Above all, I will let them tell me how it is. (Kvalsvig, 2003, pp. 2079–2080)

This physician with a disability doesn't need to be taught to avoid making assumptions and just ask her patients.

Admitting persons with sensory and physical disabilities to health care professional schools raises important questions about required technical skills and ethical obligations. In medicine, the Hippocratic tradition and "do no harm" ethos hold patient well-being sacrosanct. Patients' health and safety must always come before the needs of students or practitioners with disabilities. Certain physical, sensory, cognitive, and emotional impairments may legitimately preclude persons from specific types of practice. However, given increasing specialization within medical fields, the precise sensory and physical abilities required to practice within specific areas vary widely. Although most medical school admission guidelines still require students to demonstrate technical sensory and physical proficiencies, some skills no longer apply to the vast majority of daily clinical practice.[8]

New technologies and approaches can accommodate certain sensory or physical impairments. For example, a special blood pressure cuff speaks diastolic and systolic readings out loud. Electronic stethoscopes, priced under $500, offer many features that accommodate hearing deficits. Sound analysis software picks up sounds from these stethoscopes, storing it on computers and letting users display and print pictures of soundwaves (phonocardiograms). Some stethoscopes substantially amplify sounds and contain special filter circuitry to magnify particular types of sounds. The Web site of the Association of Medical Professionals with Hearing Loss, a nonprofit organization representing various clinical disciplines (www.AMPHL.org), provides links to equipment and communication services to accommodate practitioners with hearing impairments.[9]

Nonetheless, anecdotal information suggests that clinicians hesitate to reveal potentially disabling conditions (Steinberg et al., 2002). Most people want respect, approbation, and acceptance from their peers. Being surrounded by other physicians, who often believe their medical training gives them special insight, poses a hefty impediment to admitting disability. These colleagues can harbor misconceptions and faulty knowledge about specific diseases and disorders, stoking overt and hidden biases. For instance, a senior surgeon described serving on an examination committee for a young surgeon, a rising star at a prestigious institution but recently diagnosed with multiple sclerosis (MS). The examinee tripped while entering the room and briefly joked about it, then answered the questions flawlessly. The committee's deliberations, however, focused on whether the joke signaled emotional lability from MS, making the young surgeon unfit to practice. Many years later, the examinee, now using a wheelchair, is a respected teacher and role model in a nonsurgical practice.

Medical school faculty with visible and known disabilities report mixed attitudes among their peers and supervisors. Typically, medical schools show little interest in disability accommodations and meeting Americans with Disabilities Act (ADA) mandates. Neither medical school faculty nor students are expected to have disabilities, so improving this situation seems unlikely. Faculty committees addressing gender, racial, and ethnic diversity do not discuss disability. Some faculty believe that they must work harder than their nondisabled colleagues to gain recognition, describing their experiences as "a silent and lonely tenacity" (Steinberg et al., 2002, p. 3150).

When I attended Harvard Medical School more than twenty years ago, the institution was ill-equipped to respond to students with potentially disabling conditions. As I describe in the preface to *When Walking Fails* (2003), being diagnosed with MS during my first year carried consequences on many levels. Confronting the physical limitations and uncertainty of MS was only one step. I also had to deal with people's reactions to me—the "me" they equated with my disease. Early on, I received frequent hints that my medical career was in jeopardy. For instance, on my first day in the operating room during my surgical rotation, the attending surgeon let me hold a finger retractor during a delicate procedure. Once the concentrated silence broke and closing the surgical wound began, the surgeon turned to me, saying, "You will make a *terrible* doctor. You lack the most important quality in a good doctor—accessibility."

Late in my third year, I began thinking about applying for an internal medicine residency. At a student dinner, I sat next to a top leader at a Harvard teaching hospital and decided to ask his advice. I would not be able to stay up all night; perhaps I could share a residency with someone else. Few other accommodations seemed necessary. "What would your hospital think of my situation?" I asked.

"Frankly," he replied in a conversational tone, "there are too many doctors in the country right now for us to worry about training handicapped physicians. If that means certain people get left by the wayside, that's too bad."

Over the next months, after a wrenching internal debate (joined by my husband, caring but realistic) and with little medical school support, I decided not to battle for an internship but to go straight into research. I never became a practicing physician. From four years at medical school, I left with one overwhelming lesson: never, ever, talk about IT, the MS! It can't be cured, so don't mention it. For fifteen years, I almost never did.

My experiences occurred in the early 1980s, prior to the ADA, and certainly experiences have improved substantially for medical students now newly diagnosed with disabling conditions. Nonetheless, Vera's proposal for increasing the number of practicing clinicians with sensory and physical disabilities must still await fundamental changes at many levels, including admission, testing, board certification, licensure, and credentialing policies and procedures. Sweeping changes are unlikely anytime soon, although the American Association of Medical Colleges plans to update guidance it gives to medical schools about admitting students with disabilities (Cohen, 2004). At this time, persons with disabilities cannot yet obtain clinical training without considerable extra effort.

Communicating Patient to Patient

This chapter has addressed patient-clinician communication. But as the interviewees told us, conversations with other persons with similar disabilities can offer insight and support, both practical and emotional, surpassing that provided by clinicians. Communities of patients—and their families—can immediately convey relevant advice and understanding born of shared experiences. Tight-knit networks already exist. "In the Deaf community, our grapevine is extremely well established," asserted Kate Cather. "The word gets out very quickly." If a doctor makes special efforts to communicate better with deaf persons "the entire Deaf community would hear about it." Some supportive communities build slowly, person by person, as newly disabled individuals join their ranks. Todd Paulson recalls the time of his spinal cord injury more than twenty years ago:

> When I got injured way back when, there was a really active informal network of people and families of people that had spinal cord injuries. That informal network was extremely important. We had it set up at the hospital where I went. A number of us would get called by the trauma team if somebody came in with a spinal cord injury. We'd go talk to the patient. My mother used to get calls from mothers of other kids that got injured who wanted to talk about it.
>
> It became very apparent that the social work teams, the neurologists, and neurosurgeons knew absolutely nothing of the community services that you needed. Could you expect them to? There are a hell of a lot of things that physicians have to learn about acute care; they can't even think about subacute care and rehab issues unless they're a rehab specialist. Yet if you don't set up community services until you're in the rehab unit, you're never going to have those services in place when your insurance kicks you out and you need to go home. The place to start getting all the community services organized is the acute care unit. Since the acute care unit isn't set up to tell you about rehab, personal care attendants, or community services, the families did it.

Years later, Mr. Paulson tried to obtain funding from the hospital to organize formal channels for providing timely and practical advice to newly injured persons. The money never materialized. Nevertheless, an informal family support network continues today—people with disabilities and their families helping other people.

Accessible Communication and Information

Many options—human and technological—now exist to make information accessible to persons with impaired vision and hearing. When individuals need communication accommodations, the Americans with Disabilities Act (ADA) expects *them* to request specific formats or assistance. But some interviewees believe that health care providers should proactively anticipate patients' needs and offer information in accessible formats up front. As one woman accurately observed, "It's the doctor's obligation to make sure that I understand what's going on."

Given continuing technological advances and the breadth of approaches for making information accessible, this chapter offers only a brief overview. The ADA and its regulations contain fairly specific requirements and suggestions, so we start there. Appendix 2 lists selected Web sites that offer information about communication services and assistive technologies for specific disabling conditions.

Legal Responsibilities

The ADA sets a legal "floor"—what the law requires to ensure "effective communication," unless doing so poses an undue burden on providers. ADA regulations list possible procedural and technological options (box 13.1). Accommodating communication for persons who are deaf or hard of hearing could involve such "auxiliary aids and services" as qualified interpreters, note-takers, computer-aided transcription services, written materials, assistive listening devices, closed captioning, telephone handset amplifiers, and teletypewriters or TTYs (figure 13.1) [28 CFR Sec. 36.303(b)]. For persons with limited vision, communication accommodations include qualified readers, taped texts, audio recordings, braille and large-print reading materials, and braille and raised-print signs (figure 13.2). Providing information on computer diskette or directing persons to accessible Web sites also meets access requirements.

Box 13.1.   Americans with Disabilities Act Title III
                 Regulations 28 CFR Part 36. Subpart C—Specific
                 Requirements Sec. 36.303 Auxiliary Aids and Services

(a) General. A public accommodation shall take those steps that may
    be necessary to ensure that no individual with a disability is ex-
    cluded, denied services, segregated or otherwise treated differently
    than other individuals because of the absence of auxiliary aids and
    services, unless the public accommodation can demonstrate that
    taking those steps would fundamentally alter the nature of the
    [service] . . . or accommodations being offered or would result in
    an undue burden, i.e., significant difficulty or expense.

(b) Examples. The term "auxiliary aids and services" includes—

    (1) Qualified interpreters, notetakers, computer-aided transcription
        services, written materials, telephone handset amplifiers, assis-
        tive listening devices, assistive listening systems, telephones
        compatible with hearing aids, closed caption decoders, open
        and closed captioning, telecommunications devices for deaf
        persons (TDDs), videotext displays, or other effective methods
        of making aurally delivered materials available to individuals
        with hearing impairments;

    (2) Qualified readers, taped texts, audio recordings, Brailled mate-
        rials, large print materials, or other effective methods of mak-
        ing visually delivered materials available to individuals with
        visual impairments;

    (3) Acquisition or modification of equipment or devices; and

    (4) Other similar services and actions.

(c) Effective communication. A public accommodation shall furnish
    appropriate auxiliary aids and services where necessary to ensure
    effective communication with individuals with disabilities. . . .

All private and public health care providers must fulfill ADA requirements, ensuring effective communication with every person who seeks or
receives their services.[1] These obligations extend beyond "patients." For example, a prenatal class serving prospective parents must offer communication accommodations to both mothers and fathers who need them (National
Association of the Deaf Law Center, 2004). The basic goal of the ADA is to
build communication accommodations into routine practices, to avoid segregating persons who might require accommodations.[2] To decide which auxiliary aid or service would effectively facilitate communication, the Department of Justice expects health care providers to consult with patients or

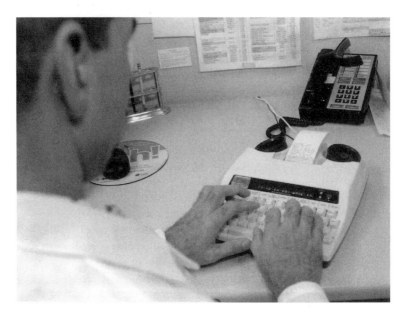

Figure 13.1. Teletypewriter (TTY). Ned, who works as an ASL interpreter, plugs his TTY directly into the telephone jack so he does not need to place the handset of his regular telephone into the TTY's couplers to make a connection. As he types, Ned's message appears on the lighted display over the keyboard, and it prints out on the rolled strip of paper. Ned's Deaf client is reading the typed message on his own TTY, wherever he is.

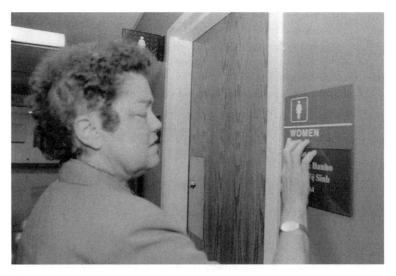

Figure 13.2. Reading by fingertip. Doris, who is blind, reads the braille sign to locate the women's restroom. "WOMEN," written above the braille, is in raised print. Below the braille, "women" is repeated in five languages (Spanish, Portuguese, Vietnamese, Russian, and Chinese).

clients, weighing carefully their preferred approach. Providers have the ultimate authority to decide which aid or service to employ.

Federal analyses of disability regulations, including evaluations by the Office for Civil Rights in the Department of Health and Human Services, have identified "critical points" during which crucial medical information is communicated. This list includes eliciting medical histories; obtaining informed consents or permissions; explaining diagnoses, prognoses, and treatments; instructing patients on medication use and side effects; communicating before and after major procedures; conducting psychotherapy; explaining care following hospital discharge; and discussing medical costs and insurance coverage. Basically, these critical points encompass most communication between clinicians and patients. Nonetheless, the list underscores when clinicians should make extra efforts to consider patients' communication preferences, for instance, by hiring sign language interpreters for deaf individuals who want them.[3] Clinicians could face legal liabilities for failing to adequately accommodate communication needs if complications arise because of faulty or inadequate communication.

The ADA also requires health care providers to ensure effective communication in other services and materials they provide. For instance, educational videotapes and DVDs should contain captions and audio descriptions of visual images. Wherever patients watch television (e.g., in waiting rooms, patient care rooms), the caption display feature on television sets must be activated so that viewers can access captions of programs that contain them. Health education programs and conferences open to the general public must provide oral and written information in formats accessible to persons with disabilities.

As noted throughout part II, the persons we interviewed—all more than ten years following the ADA's enactment—report that their clinicians and health care facilities frequently violate these mandates, denying individuals accommodations for effective communication. Clinicians refuse to obtain sign language interpreters for deaf patients and fail to give blind persons information in accessible formats; educational videos or DVDs (e.g., about breast self-examinations) do not contain captions or verbal descriptions of the examinations. These denials can compromise safety, leaving patients unaware of critical information about their health conditions and care. The interviewees attribute many of these lapses to clinicians' fears about the costs of providing accommodations.

Some communication accommodations—such as choosing a large font for the printer or activating captioning on the waiting room television— cost little or nothing. By law, telephone relay and video relay services are "free" to the users. Certainly, purchasing and servicing communication equipment will generate some expense, although costs are often relatively modest. For example, depending on specific features, TTYs today typically range from less than $200 to near $500; software priced under $100 allows computers to function as TTYs; and amplified telephones cost roughly $150. Health care providers should remember that such equipment can benefit not only patients but also employees with sensory or physical impairments.

Some health care providers fear burdensome personnel costs, such as salary expenses for staff time and training and hourly charges for sign language interpreters. In my state, the Massachusetts Commission for the Deaf and Hard of Hearing provides interpreters qualified by the Registry of Interpreters for the Deaf (RID) at hourly charges from $33 to $50, depending on the interpreter's qualifications and years since RID certification (price list from July 1, 2003, through June 30, 2005). Interpreting for clients who are deaf-blind costs $3 more per hour.

Health care providers cannot charge patients for costs of providing auxiliary aids or services, either directly or indirectly through the patient's health insurer [28 CFR, Sec. 36.301(c)]. The ADA does not require provision of specific accommodations that pose an "undue burden" on providers (i.e., present significant difficulties or expense[4]). Instead, providers should offer less burdensome accommodations that achieve the same goal. However, hourly rates charged by interpreters are unlikely to be judged excessively burdensome in most settings. Admittedly, sometimes costs of interpreters or other reasonable accommodations could exceed the provider's reimbursement for the health care service. In these situations, the government expects providers to treat these expenses as routine costs of operating their business.

Recognizing these expenses, alongside the ADA's passage in 1990, the Internal Revenue Code created two types of tax incentives for improving accessibility:

- Tax credits for various expenditures, such as producing accessible formats for printed materials (e.g., large print, braille, audiotape); hiring sign language interpreters; making architectural modifications; and acquiring equipment (e.g., TTYs, automatically adjustable examination tables)
- Tax deductions for architectural and transportation adaptations

At this time, tax credits apply only to businesses that, in the previous tax year, either had revenues of $1,000,000 or less or had thirty or fewer employees; businesses of any size can claim tax deductions. The Department of Justice Internet Web site and the Internal Revenue Service offer current information about these tax incentives.[5]

Decisions in lawsuits to enforce the ADA suggest helpful ways health care providers could respond to mandates for accessible communication. For instance, the 1998 Consent Decree from the case of *Janet DeVinney and the United States of America v. Maine Medical Center* itemizes steps hospitals should take to ensure "effective communication" for persons with hearing impairments (box

13.2). These requirements start with "initial intake": the hospital must initiate "proactive assessment" of the communication needs of patients who are deaf upon their first contact with the facility [Civil No. 97-276-P-C, Paragraph 5(a)]. Recognizing potential communication barriers is the first step.

Box 13.2.   Selected Steps for Hospitals to Accommodate Communication with Patients Who Are Deaf or Hard of Hearing

- Proactively assess patients' communication needs and preferences during first contact with hospital personnel
- Place information about patients' communication needs and preferences prominently in medical chart
- Prepare easy-to-read pamphlet to inform persons identified as deaf or hard of hearing about their rights and the communication services offered by the hospital
- Once need for interpreter or other communication service is identified, request service promptly (within fifteen minutes)
- To ensure effective communication, provide appropriate auxiliary aids and services, including sign language interpreters and Communication Access Realtime Translation (CART) providers with the skills, training, and experience necessary in medical settings
- Provide text telephones (TTYs) and telephones with amplified sound at prominent locations where telephones are available
- Post signs using international symbols at prominent locations about TTY locations and sign language interpreter and other communication services
- For hospitalized inpatients, provide appropriate telephone equipment, with visual flashers if needed; activate television caption display feature
- Obtain flash cards and pictographs to communicate routine needs that do not involve complex medical or legal decisions in emergency departments and other locations
- Develop a written hospital policy about ensuring effective communication with persons who are deaf or hard of hearing and distribute to all clinicians and hospital employees
- Require all senior hospital staff and all emergency department personnel to attend in-service training about communicating with patients who are deaf or hard of hearing. Training must include basic communication skills, such as looking at patients rather than interpreters and fundamental differences between sign language and English grammar and syntax

(continued)

Box 13.2. *(continued)*

- Survey patients who are deaf or hard of hearing, using easily understandable language, about their communication experiences at the hospital and recommendations for improvement; follow up to rectify problem
- Assign an Americans with Disabilities Act Communications Services Coordinator with responsibility for meeting and monitoring all communications-related activities

Source: These recommendations are based partially upon recommendations in the 1998 consent decree in *Janet DeVinney and the United States of America v. Maine Medical Center* (Civil No. 97-276-P-C), available on the National Association for the Deaf Web site at www.nad.org/infocenter/infotogo/legal/devinney.html, accessed May 13, 2004.

Information Technologies for People with Visual Disabilities

Andrew Potok, a writer and painter, became blind from retinitis pigmentosa. He kept writing and painting and says

> Even though I'm an anxious and naive user of computers, I can now, not seeing the screen, log on to the Internet every morning and have my computer read me whatever I want to read in the *New York Times*. It's only my technological inadequacy, not my lack of eyesight, that keeps me from going further, from doing absolutely anything a sighted user can do to find relevant texts, research material, games or chat rooms. . . .
>
> Nevertheless, for several years I've been using and taking for granted an earlier innovation, a more simply devised screen-reading computer whose voice reads the words that appear on the screen. Even that less complex technology had brought me into the mainstream in a way that had not been possible for blind people previously. (Potok, 2002, p. 129)

Indeed, as the American Foundation for the Blind Web site proclaims, although computer technologies have revolutionized daily life for virtually everyone in developed nations, the transformation for persons with visual disabilities has been breathtaking.[6] Note-takers that provide speech or braille output, Web access by telephone, well-designed Web pages (see chapter 15), and other technical innovations enable ready access for users who are blind or low vision to the same information available to sighted persons. Such dramatic technological advances will likely continue apace for the foreseeable future.

Health care seems a logical place to use new technologies to improve communication access for persons with visual disabilities. Some large health plans offer telephone information hotlines that provide recorded messages containing general information about health problems or conditions. Web sites designed to be fully accessible to all users, such as those of various agencies within the U.S. Department of Health and Human Services, offer growing volumes of useful health information.

Unfortunately, however, many basic information exchanges between individual patients and various health care providers remain a technological backwater. As noted in part II, clinicians rarely provide routine information, such as prescription drug or post-discharge instructions, test results, and appointment slips, in accessible formats to patients with visual disabilities. At home, patients can sometimes use technologies to access this information, for example, by magnifying tiny print using video magnifiers or closed circuit television systems. Depending on individual preferences, giving patients information in large print, braille, audiotape, or digital formats (such as sending appointment reminders, test results, and other information through secure Internet portals, chapter 15) could readily improve the accessibility of information. If high-tech formats are unavailable, clinicians should discuss with patients who are blind or have low vision alternative ways of conveying critical information, even by such low-tech means as telephone calls (e.g., to make sure patients understand medication instructions, provide visit reminders).

Web sites of the American Foundation for the Blind, the National Federation of the Blind, and other organizations provide up-to-date and comprehensive information about various assistive technologies. Today, key components of these adaptive devices fit into broad categories. Synthetic speech systems—in which a synthesizer does the speaking and a screen reader tells the synthesizer what to say—allow persons with visual disabilities to "hear" texts that appear on computer screens. Text-to-speech software contains all the phonemes and grammatical rules of the designated language, producing fairly natural pronunciations; speech synthesizer sounds range from robotic to nearly human (prices from $150 to $1,300). Keyboard commands instruct these systems to perform various functions, such as reading specific portions of texts, identifying the cursor location, and finding strings of text.

Optical character recognition technologies scan printed texts and then speak the words using synthetic speech or save it on a computer. Technology does not yet exist that conveys graphic or pictorial information into accessible formats for persons with impaired vision. But current optical character recognition programs contain logic to identify and correct errors, such as major grammatical or spelling snafus, before speaking the texts. Prices of optical character recognition systems that hook up to a customer's personal computer range from $2,000 to $3,000.

For persons with low vision who can see enlarged images, screen magnification programs offer access without speech. With screen magnification, however, users can focus only on one part of the screen at a time. They could thus lose track of relationships among snippets of images. Web site designers must ensure that their pages interface well with such technologies as screen readers and magnification programs (see chapter 15). Web pages designed with universal access in mind give users flexibility to make accommodations that meet their individual needs.

Interpreters and Services to Accommodate Hearing Needs

Clinicians should never assume they know what will best accommodate each patient's communication needs. Instead, clinicians must ask individual patients what strategy works for them. Although many deaf persons use American Sign Language (ASL), others do not, especially persons who lose their hearing in middle or old age. The varied needs and preferences of individual patients demand different communication accommodations. ASL users might require interpreters fluent in ASL, a language with fundamentally different grammar and syntax than English (see box 4.1). In contrast, other persons use signed English, which employs identical word usage as English. Since sign languages can vary across populations, patients from abroad may not understand ASL. Some persons do not know sign language and prefer "oral interpreters" (who carefully articulate spoken words) or "cued speech interpreters" (who provide visual cues to assist lip reading). English-proficient persons who are deaf or hard of hearing may desire written information, such as through typing on a TTY, text messaging device, or computer or using a Communication Access Realtime Translation (CART) reporter.

The availability of communication services varies across locales nationwide. By law, all states must provide basic telephone relay services (box 13.3). However, states differ in other telecommunications services they offer. For instance, the telephone company serving Massachusetts provides free or discounted TTY equipment, amplified telephones, and alerting devices to qualified state residents. The state also offers video relay services (VRS): a video camera mounted on a box where a call originates, such as persons' homes and offices, captures real-time pictures of sign language speakers; through the relay video link, they communicate directly with a communications assistant who speaks the signed message to the person being called; the communications assistant then signs spoken return messages to the caller, who sees the image on their video screen.[7] To use VRS, per-

Box 13.3. Telecommunications Relay Services Definitions
from the Federal Communications Commission

Telecommunications Relay Services (TRS)

Enable standard voice telephone users to talk to people who have difficulty hearing or speaking on the telephone. Under Title IV of the Americans with Disabilities Act, all telephone companies must provide free relay services . . . throughout the 50 states . . .

How Does TRS Work?

TRS uses operators, called "communications assistants" (CAs), to facilitate telephone calls for people who have difficulty hearing or speaking. . . . Telephone companies [must] provide TRS nationwide on a 24 hour-a-day, 7 day a week basis, at no extra cost to callers. Conversations are relayed in real-time and CAs are not permitted to disclose the content of any conversation. Relay callers are not limited in the type, length, or nature of their calls.

What is a TTY (Text Telephone)?

TTYs are also called [teletypewriters or telecommunications devices for the deaf, TDD]. TTYs have a typewriter keyboard and allow persons to type the telephone conversation via two-way text. The conversation is read on a lighted display screen and/or paper printout on the TTY. . . . Text-to-Voice TRS . . . uses a CA who speaks what a TTY user types, and types what a voice telephone user replies.

Video Relay Services

The caller signs to the CA with the use of videoequipment [such as computer cameras with broadband connections] and the CA voices what is said to the called party and signs back to the caller. This type of relay service is not required by the FCC, but is offered on a voluntary basis by certain TRS programs.

7-1-1 Access to TRS

Just as you can call 4-1-1 for information, as of October, 2001, you can dial 7-1-1 to connect to relay service anywhere in the United States.

Source: Text taken verbatim from Consumer & Government Affairs Bureau, Federal Communications Commission, www.fcc.gov/cgb/consumerfacts/trs.html, accessed December 17, 2004.

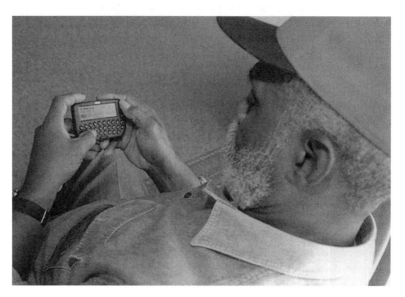

Figure 13.3. Handheld communication. Tom, who is Deaf, uses a handheld text messaging device instead of a TTY for much of his remote communication.

sons must obtain the necessary equipment—more affordable for some persons than others. Hand-held text messaging devices are replacing TTYs as the preferred communication technology in some Deaf communities. Tom, who is deaf and prefers to use an ASL interpreter to accommodate communication during physician visits, uses text messaging in many other situations—even communicating face-to-face with a hearing person (figure 13.3).

The availability of sign language interpreter services varies across communities. Many rural regions have few if any professional interpreters. In large urban areas, requests for services can overwhelm the small cadre of highly skilled interpreters, forcing patients to delay nonurgent health care visits for days or weeks. Some health care providers, such as hospital emergency departments, use teleconferencing or video relay interpreting to link with remote locations staffed round-the-clock with sign language interpreters. Video relay interpreting (VRI) is especially suited to emergency departments, where the need for sign language interpreters is immediate, unpredictable, and sporadic. Kate Cather, who is deaf, would rather have remote video interpreting than someone in person: "You have an extremely skilled signer. And since you're on TV, there's nothing personal. They're not going to be able to break the [interpreter] code of ethics." Kate believes this approach better protects patient privacy.

Technical aspects of remote teleconferencing for VRI, specifically the bandwidth of the digital telephone connections, can affect the accuracy of sign language interpretation. One medical center compared sign language interpretation of a sentence (containing a doctor's name and giving a telephone number patients could call with questions) presented first using one integrated services digital network (ISDN) line then again using three ISDN line bandwidths.[8] In the one ISDN line transmission, frames periodically froze, while others dropped from view, resulting in missing segments of the doctor's name and the telephone number. The evaluators concluded that three ISDN lines are required to ensure accurate sign language transmissions. Even if wide bandwidths are available, teleconferencing remains very expensive, limiting its use.

Training and Qualifications of Sign Language Interpreters

Clinicians sometimes assume that interpreters already know "what is wrong" with a patient who is deaf and start interviews by turning to the interpreter, asking his or her assessment. This approach is wrong on multiple levels.

> Speak with deaf people directly. The interpreter is a professional who shows up for the job and meets the deaf person at the time of the appointment. Interpreters are bound by a professional code of ethics that prohibits them from becoming involved in the content of the conversation. Their job is to facilitate the flow of communication between the deaf person and the doctor. Let the interpreters interpret. That is why you are paying them. (San Augustin, Atchison, and Gracer, 2004, p. 34)

Legal guidelines underscore the need for "qualified interpreters" rather than relying on family or friends. According to the Department of Justice, even if family members or friends are certified interpreters, they may be unable to interpret "effectively, accurately, and impartially" because of "emotional or personal involvement or considerations of confidentiality" (56 Fed. Reg. at 35553). Clinicians who do not know sign language would likely remain unaware when complex interpersonal dynamics compromise communication. If clinicians sense that an informal interpreter brought by a patient is biased or giving inaccurate information, clinicians can insist on bringing in a professional interpreter to ensure their words are interpreted impartially.

RID, the National Association for the Deaf, and other state and local agencies certify or credential interpreters based on their training and experience. Because certain regions have few certified interpreters, neither the Department of Justice nor the Department of Health and Human Services mandates specific certification for sign language interpreters in health care settings. Medical interpretation generally requires formal training and experience to handle the specialized technical vocabulary. The departments strongly advise hospitals to employ skilled interpreters to minimize risks of diagnosis or treatment errors arising from faulty communication.

The RID Web site provides detailed information about sign language interpreter training, testing, and credentialing (www.rid.org). Obtaining RID certification generally takes three to five years and requires rigorous written examinations and skills testing. Numerous educational institutions and recreational programs offer sign language training, but with varying quality. Candidates should carefully research different programs to determine which will best meet their goals. Native ASL speakers from local Deaf communities can provide valuable insight into which programs train the best interpreters. Simply completing an interpreter training program does not ensure RID certification. RID currently provides several different types of certifications, each requiring specific skills and testing.[9]

RID's eight-point Code of Ethics applies to all RID members and certified non-members (box 13.4). Maintaining confidentiality appears first on the list and is especially critical in medical contexts. Interpreters must not interject personal comments, including counseling or advising patients. An interpreter with extensive experience in medical settings tells me that this ethical precept sometimes poses a dilemma: "Suppose the doctor says to the patient, 'Take this pill three times a day,' and nothing more. What does that

---

Box 13.4. Code of Ethics, Registry of Interpreters for the Deaf

Interpreters/transliterators shall:

- Keep all assignment-related information strictly confidential
- Render the message faithfully, always conveying the content and spirit of the speaker using language most readily understood by the person(s) whom they serve
- Not counsel, advise, or interject personal opinions
- Accept assignments using discretion with regard to skill, setting, and the consumers involved
- Request compensation for services in a professional and judicious manner
- Function in a manner appropriate to the situation
- Strive to further knowledge and skills . . .
- Strive to maintain high professional standards . . .

Adapted from: Registry of Interpreters for the Deaf, *RID's Code of Ethics*, www.rid. org/coe.html, accessed May 19, 2004.

mean? Take three pills a day? One pill every eight hours? One pill with each meal? If the patient doesn't ask the doctor, the patient may not know what to do." The RID Code of Ethics prevents interpreters from asking physicians to clarify this issue, as if asking on the patient's behalf. To avoid this appearance, the interpreter might therefore ask the physician, "Could you please clarify—for the interpreter's benefit—what you mean by 'three times a day'?" The response would give the patient essential information for safely and effectively taking the medication.

Accommodating Persons Who Are Hard of Hearing

Persons who become hard of hearing or deaf during later childhood or adulthood often employ different strategies to assist communication as their hearing loss progresses. Therefore, their preferences for accommodations to ensure effective communication may change over time. The most basic accommodations involve facing the person while speaking, keeping the mouth visible; speaking naturally but clearly, without shouting or rushing; ensuring adequate lighting, especially of the face; and eliminating background noise. When clinicians must wear surgical masks, choosing clear, or transparent, fog-free masks could assist lip readers.[10] Persons who are hard of hearing also make their own accommodations, such as by using hearing aids, assistive listening devices, or (as appropriate and desired) cochlear implants. However, many people who are hard of hearing require additional accommodations especially when communicating important information. As a physician who became deaf observed:

> Hearing aids are very useful in some kinds of deafness, but not in mine. The best I can expect from a hearing aid these days is a huge amount of non-specific noise. It's very tiring, but not half as tiring as lip reading. You can only see a small fraction of the vowels and consonants by watching someone's mouth. The rest is done by following the cadence of speech, watching facial expression, matching possible words to the context—it's like solving crossword puzzles at break-neck speed, and it is exhausting. (Kvalsvig, 2003, p. 2080)

Numerous technologies exist to assist persons who are hard of hearing, most costing under $500. These technologies fall into two basic categories: those to facilitate written communication; and others to assist hearing. TTYs, for instance, offer the dual benefits of permitting telephone communication as well as providing paper records of typed conversations. Some persons carry their TTYs with them (the equipment is lightweight and can come with sturdy carrier bags); special TTY equipment even produces braille texts, facilitating communication with persons who are deaf and blind. Sitting nearby, clinicians and patients can sequentially type on the TTY keyboard, while words appear on the small screen above the keyboard and print off rolled paper at the top of the TTY. Clinicians can review important information (e.g., about prescribed medications) on this printed record to ensure clarity and accuracy, and then patients can keep the typed record for future reference. Clinicians and patients could also type messages back and forth on text messaging devices or on standard computers.

Assistive listening devices (ALDs) aim to improve the "signal to noise ratio," thus allowing listeners to hear better: the process is technically equivalent to putting listeners' ears closer to the sound source. ALDs come in four types—personal amplified, infrared, FM, and loop systems—differing by their mechanisms for enhancing sound.[11] These technologies are widely used in public settings, such as theaters and concert halls. Personal amplified ALDs represent the most basic technology, consisting of a pocket-sized, lightweight amplifier with a microphone, either attached to the unit or connected by a wire. During conversations, users place the microphone near the speaker's mouth and hear the amplified sounds via earphones or headphones. Infrared, FM, and loop systems eliminate the cord but are slightly more expensive and require more planning, although all methods would fit easily into most medical office settings. Having one or more ALD units available could assist people with hearing loss and may be acceptable even to patients who generally hesitate to admit difficulty hearing.

CART is sometimes used in health care settings, generally by late-deafened persons who speak English. CART providers employ court stenography machines with phonetic keyboards to type proceedings verbatim at conversational speeds (200–250 words/minute). Laptop computers translate this phonetic output realtime into English and display the texts on screens for persons to read; texts can also be printed onto paper for persons to retain. In my state, CART services are available through the Massachusetts Commission for the Deaf and Hard of Hearing—the same office that provides sign language interpreters. As for interpreters, health care settings cannot charge patients for CART services, but persons typically use CART only for particularly important meetings with their physicians. The CART provider requires space to set up the court stenography machine and position the text display for the patient to read easily.

Communicating by Teletypewriter and Relay Services

As noted earlier, all states must offer free telephone relay services round-the-clock (see box 13.2). TTYs have a typewriter keyboard for persons to type their messages; the typed text appears on a lighted display screen on the TTY and/or paper printout. Two-way text conversations involve two TTY users typing messages to each other. Text-to-voice telephone relay services (TRS) use a "communications assistant" (CA) who speaks to the hearing person what the TTY user types, and types to the deaf person what a voice telephone user replies. To connect with a TRS anywhere in the United States, users dial 7-1-1.

Deaf users of TTYs use abbreviations and slang to speed typed communication. "GA," for "go ahead," indicates when the speaker has completed his or her thought and wants the other person to respond. When conversations are ending, both parties type "SK," for "stop keying." Because ASL has fundamentally different grammar and syntax than English, translations between the two languages do not match word for word. Many ASL speakers type in short, efficient phrases—called "ASL gloss"—that do not follow standard English constructions, aiming for brevity and quickness. Hearing recipients of such typed messages may erroneously equate nonstandard grammar and English usage with limited intellect or poor academic achievement of the Deaf individual. At the end of messages, users often type "smile" aiming to convey the same friendly sign off as when concluding positive face-to-face interactions.

The following brief example of a two-way text conversation involves Mr. C, who is feeling ill, contacting Dr. A's office to see if he can visit the physician. "Q" represents a question mark.

Office: THIS IS DR A'S OFFICE. HOW MAY WE HELP U Q GA[12]
Mr. C: hi. sick need see dr ga
Office: WHAT IS UR NAME PLS Q GA
Mr. C: chris cook ga
Office: DO U NEED SEE DR TODAY Q GA
Mr. C: cough 2 weeks. better see dr tmw off work ga
Office: OK CAN U COM TMW AT 2 PM Q GA
Mr. C: yes fine. thx ga or sk
Office: SEE U TMW BUT IF WORSE CALL AGAIN OR GO TO ER.
        GA OR SK
Mr. C: ok thx. have a nice day smile sksk

Quick-paced ASL gloss is especially efficient for text messaging—the coming technology—with the limited screen space on most handheld devices.

Designing Accessible Health Care Settings

Eleanor Peters's doctor recently moved to a new clinic, designed explicitly to accommodate the needs of all patients, their clinicians, and other users of the facility. Because she cannot lift her arms, Eleanor must use her mouth stick to press the automatic door opener (figure 14.1). The door instantly swings open but away from Eleanor, thus avoiding collisions with her. The clinic's designers eliminated the doorway threshold, allowing Eleanor to roll smoothly into the reception area without even a bump. The clinic flooring is smooth and durable, made of materials engineered to minimize slips and falls but also with low enough friction for easy wheelchair movement. Now Eleanor can enter and leave her doctor's office independently as she chooses, and clinic staff no longer need to interrupt their activities to open the door for her.

Making health care facilities accessible to persons with sensory and physical disabilities requires three straightforward steps. The first is simply to think about it. When designing or renovating health care settings, remember the full breadth of persons who might use the facility and commit to making spaces and equipment accessible, welcoming, and comfortable to all. An overarching goal is to maximize opportunities for all persons to navigate spaces as freely and independently as possible. The principles of universal design (chapter 10) offer a broad conceptual framework for considering all potential users. Second, involve persons with disabilities in generating ideas, making plans, and assessing results. From years or lifetimes confronting and negotiating barriers in built environments, persons with disabilities can readily identify potential problems often overlooked by others and suggest practical solutions. Third, be creative and seek new ideas and wide-ranging options. A vibrant universal design movement worldwide is generating innovative architectural approaches, furnishings, lighting, equipment, and other products to address consumers with diverse needs. Ideas likely already exist somewhere that will inspire solutions for most design dilemmas.

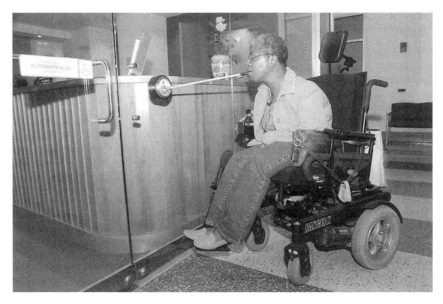

Figure 14.1. Independent entry. Using her mouthstick, Eleanor Peters presses the automatic door opener to independently enter a clinic. The entryway has no raised threshold, so Eleanor's wheelchair easily rolls through without even a bump.

These three steps are straightforward, but carrying them out can prove daunting. Although designing for all is an overarching goal, some people may find their specific needs unmet by broadly inclusive designs. Identifying appropriate persons with various disabilities to assist in planning requires thought and outreach, and obtaining the comprehensive input takes time and willingness to listen. Researching accessible and feasible designs and equipment demands persistence and openness to new ideas. Nevertheless, addressing each of these steps should prove informative, interesting, and even fun. Remembering that health care settings ultimately exist to help people, this exercise goes to the heart of the matter. As health care delivery systems strive to provide patient-centered care, patient-centered design should guide decisions about where that care takes place.

Growing evidence suggests that aspects of design significantly affect—and most importantly improve—physical and emotional health outcomes for hospitalized patients. One review of 600 studies, drawn from the scientific literature, found compelling evidence that the physical environment can enhance patient safety and comfort, reduce fatigue and stress among staff, decrease certain complications (e.g., hospital-acquired infections, medication errors, depression), and improve health care quality (Ulrich et al., 2004). This extensive review, which focused on inpatient settings, did not mention universal design or improving access for persons with disabilities. Although a natural fit for health care environments, the universal design philosophy is only now seeping into the mainstream of design within health care settings.

This chapter briefly reviews an overall approach for making all health care settings accessible and welcoming to persons with sensory and physical disabilities. Patient-centered architectural, lighting, flooring, furnishing, and numerous other aspects of design can enhance the experiences of all patients, as well as their families, visitors, and staff. However, accommodating persons with disabilities demands specific attention. Each setting is unique, and "one size fits all" solutions do not exist. Addressing accessibility in a systematic and comprehensive fashion could benefit most design projects, large and small.

We start by reviewing the Americans with Disabilities Act (ADA) and other regulations, but do so with trepidation. Metaphorically, the ADA represents a floor, not a ceiling. Meeting ADA standards, as well as state and local accessibility requirements and building codes, often produces space that falls short of welcoming persons with disabilities or even being easy to navigate. Yet people constructing or renovating space often implore designers, "Just tell me what I need to do to fulfill the law." Sometimes, people make appropriate accommodations but then fail to maintain accessibility, such as by not clearing snow adequately from exterior ramps or keeping automatic door openers in working order. Design teams must reach beyond regulations to create truly accessible, patient-centered health care environments, and then owners must commit to maintaining access.

Accessibility Rules

"Unfortunately, planning health facilities that meet the needs of patients and visitors with physical [sensory and other] impairments is not a simple matter of following relevant building codes" (Carpman and Grant, 1993, p. 218). In the past four decades, federal, state, and local governments, as well as standards-setting and other regulatory organizations, have established a complex labyrinth of rules and codes governing physical access to structures. Often calibrated to the inch or centimeter, these myriad instructions address such topics as the width of doorways, depth and rise of stair treads, positioning of grab bars in bathrooms, and pitch of ramps. Despite their volume and detail, taken together these regulations represent only a starting point for ensuring comfortable and safe accessibility.

Health care providers bear responsibility for ensuring adherence to accessibility rules when building, buying, remodeling, or equipping their facilities. In addition, practitioners who rent their office space are generally responsible for ensuring accessibility (Duprey, 2004, p. 21), although typically, property owners and tenants share the obligation for required renovations or modifications. Unlike other aspects of construction projects, such as plumbing and electrical wiring, governmental agencies generally do not demand plan reviews, approvals, and permit processes specifically to determine if accessibility standards are met (Mace, 1998, p. 4).[1] Health care providers contemplating building projects should learn at least enough to ask informed questions about federal and local access requirements.

ADA Regulations

The earliest legislative victories of disabilities rights advocates targeted physical access, aiming to integrate persons with disabilities more fully into community life (see chapter 2). Section 504 of the Rehabilitation Act of 1973 opened physical access to federally funded programs and facilities, and the ADA extended access requirements to other public facilities and the private sector. Some states and localities promulgate accessibility standards going beyond the ADA.[2]

ADA regulations address physical access within both new construction and existing structures. Appendix A of 28 CFR Part 36 details ADA accessibility standards generally, while Section 6 of Appendix A specifically addresses medical care facilities (see www.usdoj.gov/crt/ada.stdspdf.htm).[3] Provisions for new construction are fairly straightforward. With limited exceptions, new facilities must be "readily accessible to and useable by individuals with disabilities" [Title III, Sec. 303(a)(1)]. Health care settings carry somewhat stricter access mandates than do other buildings. For instance, bowing to cost concerns, the ADA does not require elevators in all new buildings with fewer than three stories or less than 3,000 square feet per story. However, "the professional office of a health care provider" cannot claim this exemption and must install an elevator, as must shopping centers [Sec. 303(b)].

Delineating ADA requirements for existing structures generated heated congressional debate. Anticipating high costs and structural difficulties retrofitting old buildings, business constituents lobbied against initial drafts of the legislation. Supporters substantially rewrote the ADA to avoid defeat:[4]

> The original bill, S. [Senate] 2345, required that nearly every place of public accommodation had to remove all barriers within five years. This provision earned S. 2345 the nickname of the "flat earth" bill. Drafters of S. 933, however, dispensed with the idea of wholesale retrofitting. Instead they required that all *new* construction be accessible. Nevertheless, they did not want to leave existing structures untouched. Consequently, drafters created a new legal term. S. 933 required that businesses make changes to existing structures where accessibility was "readily achievable." (Young, 1997, p. 101)

Box 14.1 presents the ADA's broad definition of readily achievable renovations—changes that are structurally feasible and not unduly costly.

Box 14.1. Definition of Readily Achievable: Americans
with Disabilities Act Title III, Sec. 301(9)

The term "readily achievable" means easily accomplishable and able to be
carried out without much difficulty or expense. In determining whether an
action is readily achievable, factors to be considered include —:

(A) the nature and cost of the action needed under this Act;
(B) the overall financial resources of the facility . . . ; the number of
persons employed at such facility; the effect on expenses and resources, or the impact otherwise of such action upon the operation
of the facility; . . . and
[. . .]
(D) the type of operation or operations of the covered entity, including the composition, structure, and functions of the workforce of
such entity; the geographic separateness, administrative or fiscal
relationship of the facility . . . to the covered entity.

ADA regulations list examples of "steps to remove barriers" (box 14.2)
that are generally readily achievable. Some steps, such as repositioning paper towel and cup dispensers and installing raised toilet seats, cost little.
Others, including widening doorways, repositioning toilet partitions, and
installing new carpeting, could cost hundreds or thousands of dollars depending on the extent of remodeling required. Neither the ADA nor its regulations delineate precisely what constitutes readily achievable, with some
exceptions.[5] In conciliatory language, the regulations state, a "public accommodation is urged to comply with the barrier removal" along the following order of priorities: (a) access into buildings from streets and sidewalks, (b) access within public spaces of buildings where goods and services
are provided, and (c) access to restrooms [28 CFR Part 36, Sec. 36.304(c)].
The Internal Revenue Code offers two types of tax incentives for making
ADA accessibility improvements and renovations to existing structures (see
chapter 13).

As a concession to political and practical realities, the ADA explicitly acknowledges that accessibility sometimes is not readily achieved. In such situations, providers must offer goods or services to persons with disabilities
"through alternative methods, if those methods are readily achievable" [28
CFR Part 36, Sec. 36.305(a)]. Alternatives to barrier removal include providing curb services or home delivery, retrieving merchandise from inaccessible shelves or racks, and relocating activities to accessible locations [28
CFR Part 36, Sec. 36.305(b)]. What constitutes acceptable alternatives is an
especially sensitive issue in health care.

Box 14.2. Examples of Steps to Remove Barriers: Americans with Disabilities Act Title III Regulations, 28 CFR Part 36, Sec. 36.304(b)

---

1. Installing ramps
2. Making curb cuts in sidewalks and entrances
3. Repositioning shelves
4. Rearranging tables, chairs, vending machines, display racks, and other furniture
5. Repositioning telephones
6. Adding raised markings on elevator control buttons
7. Installing flashing alarm lights
8. Widening doors
9. Installing offset hinges to widen doorways
10. Eliminating a turnstile or providing an alternative accessible path
11. Installing accessible door hardware
12. Installing grab bars in toilet stalls
13. Rearranging toilet partitions to increase maneuvering space
14. Insulating lavatory pipes under sinks to prevent burns
15. Installing a raised toilet seat
16. Installing a full-length bathroom mirror
17. Repositioning the paper towel dispenser in a bathroom
18. Creating designated accessible parking spaces
19. Installing an accessible paper cup dispenser at an existing inaccessible water fountain
20. Removing high-pile, low-density carpeting
21. Installing vehicle hand controls

Enforcement

"No civil rights law, including the ADA, is self-executing. . . . Enforcement can only be triggered if people with disabilities are aware of their legal rights and act on that information" (Reis et al., 2004, p. 20). To enforce ADA accessibility requirements, persons with disabilities must file complaints or bring legal actions when they confront physical barriers that providers refuse to remedy. This demand imposes huge burdens on persons with disabilities, especially when they might feel most vulnerable—when they are sick, seek the goodwill of their clinicians, and need access to health care services *now* (i.e., not once facilities are finally renovated). Furthermore, some persons may believe it is their own fault, not the provider's, when they cannot climb unaided onto high examining tables, mount stairs at the only entrance, or otherwise physically access services.

The U.S. Department of Justice has the primary authority to uphold most disability civil rights laws, although the U.S. Department of Health and Human Services also enforces these statutes in health care settings.[6] The Disability Rights Section in the Civil Rights Division within the Justice Department takes lead responsibility, either initiating actions when it learns of persistent problems or joining private lawsuits filed by individuals or organizations. Whenever possible, the Disability Rights Section aims to avoid litigation by mediation and resolving disputes out of court.

In recent years, lawsuits brought by persons with disabilities have forced the federal courts to consider how far ADA mandates can go in requiring access to buildings and services for persons with disabilities. The most prominent federal case thus far about physical access—*Tennessee v. Lane*—occurred outside health care and concerned access to courtrooms. In this case, the U.S. Supreme Court considered whether Congress had overreached by letting private citizens, such as George Lane, sue states for ADA violations under Title II (National Council on Disability, 2003).[7] Lane, who used a wheelchair, had appeared at the Polk County Courthouse in Benton, Tennessee, for hearings about misdemeanor traffic violations.[8] Because the courthouse had no elevator, Lane left his wheelchair and crawled up two flights of stairs for his morning arraignment in a second-story courtroom. When Lane refused to repeat this climb for his afternoon hearing and declined to be carried by court officers, who had laughed as he made his morning ascent, the court arrested and jailed him for failing to appear. Lane sued Tennessee for damages and relief; Tennessee argued "states rights" protected it from ADA lawsuits from private citizens.

On May 17, 2004, a closely divided Supreme Court decided in favor of Lane. Writing for the five-to-four majority, Associate Justice John Paul Stevens stated that Congress had the authority to enforce the constitutional right of access specifically to courts, arguing that "Title II does not require States to employ any and all means to make judicial services accessible to persons with disabilities. . . . It requires only 'reasonable modifications'" (*Tennessee v. Lane*, 2004, p. 20). In this narrow ruling asserting a "fundamental right of access to the courts" (p. 23), Stevens did not extend this right to other services offered by states. In his dissenting opinion, the late Chief Justice William Rehnquist appeared to condone carrying wheelchair users up stairs.[9]

After *Tennessee v. Lane*, questions remain about whether Title II guarantees independent access to buildings offering public services beyond the courtroom, such as the county building in Distant Dunes where people apply for Medicaid. Although Medicaid serves many persons with disabilities, its offices are on the second floor, and the building has no elevator. Medicaid staff meet applicants who cannot climb stairs on the first floor and conduct their interviews in public waiting rooms. "There's no confidentiality whatsoever," said one woman. "None. I've heard entire interviews sitting in the waiting room." A Medicaid client handled this way could potentially bring a lawsuit complaining about the lack of physical access, but the state would likely claim that the person did get the desired service—a meeting with Medicaid officials—even if in a public setting.

With limited resources and huge numbers of inaccessible structures nationwide, the Department of Justice Disability Rights Section must set enforcement priorities. In health care, efforts currently focus on two areas: providing auxiliary aids and sign language interpreters to deaf patients in hospitals, and ensuring that individuals receive services in integrated settings rather than being separated from other patients.[10] Nonetheless, the Department has resolved other physical access actions brought primarily by health care consumers. A review of quarterly ADA status reports between April 1994 and March 2003 posted on the Department of Justice Web site found 114 health care cases (Reis et al., 2004, p. 15). Thirty-five addressed mobility access to health care facilities; two cases involved access for persons who are blind or low vision; and three cases related to inaccessible examining tables.[11] The mobility access cases considered such basic topics as barriers to entering buildings, inaccessible restrooms, inadequate parking, and difficulties navigating corridors, doorways, laboratories, offices, and examining rooms.

The 2001 settlement to the lawsuit filed against Kaiser Permanente by three wheelchair users (see chapter 5) offers a comprehensive template for making health care settings accessible.[12] The settlement requires Kaiser to eliminate architectural barriers, replace inaccessible medical equipment, revise policies and procedures that had discriminated against persons with disabilities, and train staff at all levels about disability rights and staff responsibilities. In addition, at the request of parties to this lawsuit, a medical equipment manufacturer and rehabilitation design engineers collaborated to design examining tables that accommodate multiple different physical needs and raise and lower automatically. The new power examining tables lower farther than previous models and have contouring and various attachments that improve safety and comfort of patients. All of Kaiser Permanente's California sites are installing these accessible examining tables.

The Kaiser settlement broke new ground by demonstrating the value of ADA litigation as a springboard to comprehensive rethinking of health care environments in ways that should benefit all patients. However, as noted earlier, although they offer a valuable start, ADA standards do not guarantee easy access to facilities for persons with disabilities. Eleanor Peters's clinic did not violate the ADA by failing to install an automatic opener on its door. ADA regulations do not require health care providers to install railings along corridors, provide accessible examining tables, or make other environmental accommodations to maximize patients' sense of safety, comfort, confidence, and independence. Nonetheless, "The potential and intent of the ADA . . . goes far beyond bricks and mortar. The law's core principles—nondiscrimination, inclusion, and accommodation—set the stage for examining and reshaping the way healthcare [*sic*] is delivered" (Reis et al., 2004, p. 12). Thus, the philosophy underlying the ADA offers strong moral guideposts to patient-centered design, even if its specific regulations remain insufficient to accomplish the job alone.

Other Accessibility Oversight

In addition to governmental agencies, some private oversight and purchaser organizations are interested in ensuring physical accessibility of health care settings. The Joint Commission on Accreditation of Healthcare Organizations (JCAHO) evaluates and accredits approximately 16,000 health care providers nationwide that apply voluntarily for its review, including general and specialty hospitals, health plans, group practices, nursing homes, home care agencies, and clinical laboratories (but not individual physician offices; see www.jcaho.org). The JCAHO accreditation manual for hospitals indicates that facilities must comply with the ADA and other applicable laws and regulations, going on to require that "the built environment supports the development and maintenance of the patient's interests, skills, and opportunities for personal growth" (Reis et al., 2004, p. 27). Presumably, this comment encompasses notions of physical access. The JCAHO accreditation manual contains more explicit instructions relating to communication accommodations.[13]

Some health insurers explicitly require that their designated providers meet ADA standards, including physical access. The most notable example is Medicaid, which covers care for millions of persons with disabilities, often through contracts with specific provider organizations. The Office of Civil Rights in the U.S. Department of Health and Human Services offers technical assistance to states to ensure that Medicaid managed care organizations and their contracted providers meet ADA specifications. Much of this advice addresses clinical expertise and accessible communication, but some considers physical access issues, including access to physicians' offices and transportation services. Pennsylvania Medicaid, for example, inspects providers' offices for accessibility and requires reasonable efforts to make offices "architecturally accessible to persons with mobility impairments" (Shalala, 2000, p. 136). Nevada requires that Medicaid health maintenance organizations demonstrate that their facilities "will not present architectural barriers to aged and handicapped individuals."

Designing Accessible Health Care Settings

Designers aiming to create accessible health care environments must often overcome entrenched biases and attitudes. One widely held assumption is

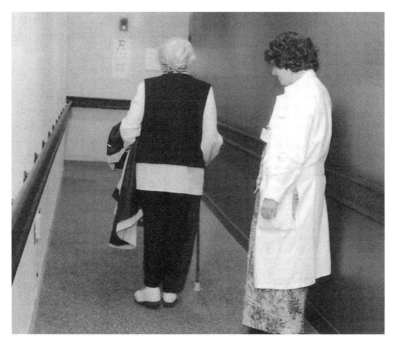

Figure 14.2. Handrails for safety. In their decorating scheme, designers chose railing colors to contrast with the wall colors. To maximize
safety and convenience for patients, they installed railings on either
side of the hallway. The corridor thus offers a secure environment for
this physician to watch her elderly patient walk, a critical component
of the clinical evaluation.

that creating accessible settings is exorbitantly expensive. This perception is
often erroneous. "In new construction, accessibility features generally do not
increase costs. In fact, even in existing facilities, necessary modifications are
not always expensive" (Mace, 1998, p. 4). Another assumption is that accessible fixtures, equipment, furnishings, and structural features (such as
ramps) are ugly. An architect told me she had not installed railings along
lengthy corridors in a renovated clinic because the clinic's managers thought
railings would be unattractive. This assumption is also untrue: Many cre-
ators of accessibility products, including railings, strive for designs that are
both appealing and practical (e.g., railings in natural wood or colored finishes, figure 14.2). However, perhaps the biggest barrier is failure to even
think about accessibility. As a physician friend with disabling arthritis recently told me:

> My rheumatologist just completely renovated his office. I asked him
> whether he had installed an automatically adjustable examining
> table, and he said, "What? I never heard of such a thing. Do they

exist?" Even though he sees a lot of people with disabilities, he hadn't even thought of the most basic thing—making it easy for patients to get onto his examining table.

Growing numbers of universities, nonprofit organizations, companies, and private consultants help design accessible health care settings. In this chapter, we draw upon what our interviewees told us, as well as various other sources.[14] New ideas and products pop up every day. Therefore, instead of making specific suggestions, we sketch overarching goals and principles, along with some basic design essentials that are unlikely to change anytime soon. The universal design principles (Story, Mueller, and Mace, 1998) outlined in chapter 10 guide our thinking. Appendix 3 contains more detailed suggestions from interviewees and our own experiences, intended to start readers thinking about approaches that may work in their own settings.

Involve Persons with Disabilities

Design projects almost always require a team effort, with each member bringing essential expertise to the table. With some exceptions, architects, construction engineers, builders, and other technical designers are not routinely taught about accommodating the full range of human abilities. Their technical knowledge alone does not ensure that these experts will create accessible and welcoming designs. Different projects demand design teams appropriate to the specific task: redecorating waiting rooms requires much less technical expertise than planning new multistory medical centers. Nonetheless, even efforts as modest as redecorating (e.g., selecting new waiting room furniture) could benefit from discussions with persons with disabilities. "Involving persons with a variety of disabilities as part of a team . . . is essential. The lived experience of disability is an excellent resource" (Mace, 1998, p. 12).

The persons with disabilities whom we interviewed have definite ideas about designing clinical settings that they would happily convey—"just ask us!" Health care providers initiating design projects of any size will likely find willing partners with disabilities among their own patients. Depending on the setting, patients' family members may also yield valuable advice. Of course, designers must obtain extensive input from the clinicians who work in the space—but primarily to address the clinicians' own activities and perceptions. Even sincere and well-meaning clinicians cannot fully represent the views and preferences of persons with disabilities. If clinicians were effective proxies, health care facilities today would be completely accessible!

Eliciting input from various "customer groups"—such as patients, clinicians, and managers—could involve different tactics, depending on the available resources and scope of the project. Meetings of small groups may produce more insight than discussions with individual customers. Through encouraging participants to interact, skilled moderators can prompt people to generate plentiful new ideas and constructively evaluate potential options. Small group discussions typically work best when all participants share important traits (Krueger, 1994): For example, one group could include patients, while another involves clinicians. Design teams would need to identify key ideas from each group, noting commonalities and discrepancies, and then decide how to address differences within the context of each project.

As another strategy, members of the design team could spend time observing specific groups of potential customers—including patients, visitors, clinicians, office assistants, and housekeeping staff—in their current environments to understand what works well and what should change. One approach involves mapping how patients arrive at the facility and then proceeding, step by step, through each destination and activity along the way.[15] On a parallel track, office staff, clinicians, and other occupants of the eventual space should look at their various tasks and conceptualize designs to optimize their performance.

To obtain insight beyond their own patients with disabilities, health care providers can also seek advice in their communities from disability advocacy groups. Specific resources vary across locales. Many communities, including rural regions, have centers for independent living, overseen by persons with disabilities, that perform support, educational, and advocacy activities.[16] Some centers for independent living consult with businesses and other organizations to address regional access issues for local residents with disabilities. Governmental and nonprofit groups specializing in services for elderly persons can also provide valuable input.

As noted earlier, sometimes design preferences of different customers diverge. Reconciling these discrepancies requires both discussion and comprehensive consideration of different design options. Sophisticated computerized software allows people to explore the implications of various design decisions by taking "virtual" tours through three-dimensional architectural drawings. With relatively little effort these computerized tools can alter specific aspects of the design to examine the effects of different structural and aesthetic choices. Admittedly, virtual tours cannot give a complete sense of how the actual "bricks and mortar" space will function. Especially for massive projects, such as constructing new hospitals, design teams (including persons with disabilities) should consider visiting other facilities and meeting with their staff. Touring real buildings can highlight how design decisions affect not only work-related activities but also the essential qualities of the space—whether it welcomes and offers easy access to patients.

In creating health care settings, final design decisions must sometimes balance patients' interests against competing demands. As in other specialized settings, very specific technical needs may stipulate certain structural or environmental attributes. An obvious example is the operating room, where patients, with or without disabilities, rarely move independently.

Operating suite design must maximize safety and the technical performance of practitioners.

> Technical design considerations, however . . . are of remote concern for many users of a health care facility. Of immediate concern is the availability of a comfortable place to wait, the accessibility of rest rooms for someone in a wheelchair, or the ability to find a particular destination easily. The design, therefore, must balance technological needs and human needs. (Carpman and Grant, 1993, p. 7)

An excellent way to find out about those human needs is just to ask patients, including persons with disabilities, and their families.

Design Basics

Core human functions raise design demands cutting across all spaces and settings. Although abilities and approaches vary, most people see, hear, speak, move through spaces, breath ambient air, and like staying safe and warm and knowing where they are going. Therefore, at every point, designers must consider such items as

- Lighting, including overhead and surface lighting
- Acoustics and level of ambient noise
- Floor or ground surface smoothness, flatness, and friction
- Air quality, circulation, and filtration
- Heating and cooling systems and local temperature controls
- Emergency notification alarms and exit routes
- Signs and other signals indicating locations and directions

Although these topics represent bread-and-butter design basics critical for everyone, introducing sensory and physical impairments raises myriad issues. Researchers in design constantly learn more about these relationships, especially the interactions of aging-related vision, hearing, and mobility changes with lighting, acoustics, and physical spaces. Several examples underscore the need to consider sensory and physical impairments even for these design fundamentals.

Lighting raises critical issues across visual, hearing, and physical disabilities. Some persons with impaired vision, especially elderly individuals, are acutely sensitive to glare, have difficulty transitioning quickly between darkness and light, require more light to discriminate small details, and lose the ability to differentiate certain color ranges (e.g., distinguishing green-blue tones). For facilities serving this population, lighting designs should reduce glare, avoid abrupt transitions in brightness, use indirect and warm-toned lighting when possible, and provide adequate lighting for tasks such as reading and filling out forms. Many persons with hearing impairments rely heavily on their vision to communicate and orient them in space. For this population, suggestions include using natural light whenever possible and avoiding backlighting (i.e., illuminating from behind) conversational partners and interpreters. Persons with mobility problems, especially from neurologic causes, rely on their vision to maintain balance and sense of space. They also need well-illuminated environments, free from glare.

Acoustics and level of ambient noise are especially important for persons with sensory disabilities. "Hard surfaces on the floors, ceilings, and walls . . . should be avoided, because these surfaces reflect and redirect sounds that are particularly important spatial location cues for blind persons. Such hard surfaces can cause a . . . conversation to appear to be on one side of the corridor when it is really on the other, resulting in disorientation" (Carpman and Grant, 1993, p. 221). Hearing loss impairs the ability to distinguish among multiple competing sounds. Minimizing background noises, especially within particularly disruptive soundwave frequencies, accommodates persons who are hard of hearing or who use hearing aids. Strategies include installing baffling materials, such as acoustic panels and wall hangings, as well as wall, ceiling, and floor products designed to attenuate sounds. Avoiding blaring televisions in waiting rooms and "canned" background music also helps.

Flooring should minimize glare and attenuate sounds, in addition to being durable, easy to clean, and reducing risks of slips and falls. The coefficient of friction (COF), an industry-wide rating system for commercial products, quantifies the extent to which flooring products are "nonslip": COFs of 0.6 or greater offer the best slip resistance (Bakker, 1997, p. 105). Vinyl flooring is generally preferable to ceramic tiles, because it is softer and has higher COF ratings; nonglazed small ceramic tiles have higher COFs than large glazed tiles. Carpeting should be unpadded and have a pile height of less than one-half inch (Carpman and Grant, 1993, p. 228): rolling wheelchairs against plush or thickly padded carpets consumes considerable energy. Loose seams and curled edges pose hazards of tripping. Colors, prints, and textures of flooring also affect safety. Broad stripes, large geometric designs, and wavy patterns can prompt misperceptions and mirages in persons with impaired vision, increasing risks of falls and disorientation.

Good design, alone, cannot solve all physical access issues: sometimes humans must intervene. Emergency preparedness presents one critical example. Alerting and safely evacuating persons with disabilities requires not only structural attention but also careful planning with key personnel assigned specific roles. Alarms must provide visual signals (e.g., flashing lights, strobes) in addition to auditory cues (e.g., sirens, beeps). Tactile signage can direct persons with visual disabilities to exit routes.[17] Depending on their patient populations, providers should purchase appropriate equipment, such as light-weight frames for carrying persons with mobility impairments down stairs. The federal Jobs Accommodation Network provides general information and consultation on designing evacuation plans for persons with disabilities (Batiste and Loy, 2004), as does the National Organization on Disability (www.nod.org). Local laws and safety codes generally stipulate the evacuation protocols required for large health care institutions.

An ultimate goal of accessible design is to allow persons with disabilities to function within spaces as freely and independently as possible. So-called "way finding" (i.e., finding one's way around facilities) provides a case in point. Signage should be clear and simply presented in accessible formats—including graphics, large print, braille, raised letters or engravings, and audible signals—so that people can easily find their own ways without having to ask (see figure 13.2). Sometimes designers forget the obvious. Last year, I attended a conference at an immense hotel complex, recently built, that hung all signs indicating wheelchair-accessible routes high upon ceiling rafters. I, far below, could barely locate the signs and needed to ask staff about accessible routes. Builders should post such directions, with their universal wheelchair logo, at wheelchair level, where users can readily see them.

Transferring to Beds, Tables, and Chairs—and Other Equipment

In medical settings, complex medical equipment fills various spaces, but from patients' points of view much of it functions essentially as furniture—like beds, tables, or chairs. In all instances, such as examining tables, weighing scales, magnetic resonance imaging scanners, and dental chairs, identical issues arise. Patients must be able to safely, comfortably, and, to the greatest extent possible, independently get on or off—or into or out of—this equipment.

As noted earlier, in certain clinical situations (e.g., operating rooms, intensive care units), patients are typically unable to move independently or without considerable assistance. In these settings, designing beds, tables, and other equipment to maximize easy and safe movement for staff makes sense. Among different jobs, nursing aides and orderlies have the second highest numbers of nonfatal occupational injuries requiring time off from work (79,000 nationally in 2002; Bureau of Labor Statistics, 2004a), and many of these injuries result from transferring patients.[18] Poor ergonomic design of patient beds and other equipment contributes to back stress, fatigue, and injuries among staff. In one study, a nursing home reduced staff injuries by 50 percent by installing patient-transferring devices and redesigning toilets and shower rooms (Ulrich et al., 2004, p. 5). Equipment designs that make transferring patients less difficult and risky for staff also likely maximize patients' safety and comfort.

Some persons with physical disabilities will need assistance transferring (e.g., onto beds, examining tables, toilets) even in the most accessible surroundings. Devices, such as Hoyer and other automated lifts (figure 14.3) and simple transfer boards, can minimize risks to both patients and staff. In these situations, staff should ask persons with disabilities for guidance about

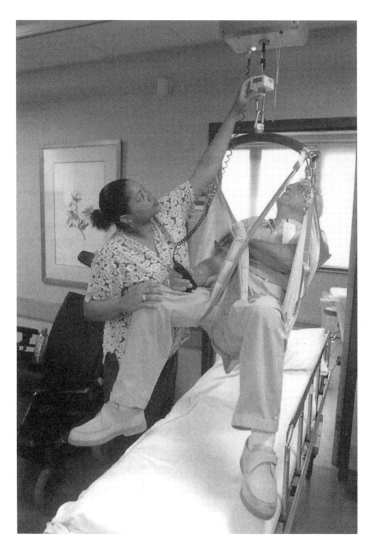

Figure 14.3. Getting a lift. Gary, who is tetraplegic, helps the clinic practice assistant secure the lift's straps around his legs while he sits in his power wheelchair. Then, with the assistant's guidance, the device automatically lifts Gary from his chair, positioning him over the gurney. Here, Gary and the assistant pause to note Gary's weight, measured by the lift. Gary drives three hours to this clinic. Providers closer to home do not have such lifts or the facilities to examine him fully.

what approach works best and communicate actively with them during the move (Ferreyra and Hughes, 1984). For instance, Gary (figure 14.3) has long experience helping clinic staff secure the straps for the automated lift devices, which make the transfer from his power wheelchair safe and easy both for Gary and the practice assistant. Methodical training in safe transferring practices can help staff avoid back injuries. Typically, staff should use their legs instead of backs, rely on large muscle groups, keep their spines aligned, position themselves as close to patients as possible, minimize twisting and bending, and enlist the assistance of another staff member when necessary.

Having accessible equipment does make transfers easier, both for persons with disabilities and clinical staff. Accessible equipment offers three critical advantages: maximizing safety and comfort for patients with disabilities, demonstrating recognition of their needs, and easing demands on clinical staff and possibly reducing occupational injuries and days lost from work. Adjustable-height examining tables that lower automatically to eighteen to twenty-two inches from the floor maximize opportunities for easy and independent movement from wheelchairs (figure 14.4). Power tables come in two basic styles: flat surfaces much like regular examining tables, sometimes with head or foot sections that clinicians can elevate; and chair-like configurations, where once patients are safely seated, the chair automatically stretches out (the back rest lowering and foot rest raising) to become a flat surface. Accessible examining tables address the universal design goal of assisting everybody. They can accommodate not only persons with physical disabilities but also women late in pregnancy, persons of short stature, those temporarily disabled by injury, and persons weakened by frailty or illness.

All sorts of medical technologies—ranging from mammography machines to radiographic imaging equipment to examining chairs for ophthalmology or dental examinations—now offer accessible models. Wheelchair-accessible platform scales allow patients to roll easily on and off (figure 14.5).[19] When purchasing new equipment, health care providers should search for models that maximize physical access and, when options seem inadequate, advocate for new designs. Accessible equipment does sometimes cost more than other models, and financial considerations may overwhelm motivations when selecting among options. However, providers should recall potential savings in staff time and risks. Furthermore, with the aging population, growing numbers of patients may benefit from accessible equipment and seek providers that offer greater comfort and ease.

One final observation involves chairs at their most basic—the seats patients occupy, sometimes for hours, in waiting and reception rooms. Choosing safe and comfortable seating requires careful thought, especially if the patient population includes many elderly individuals, persons who are overweight or obese, or ambulatory persons with upper and lower extremity mobility or strength difficulties. For some persons, sitting (rather than falling)

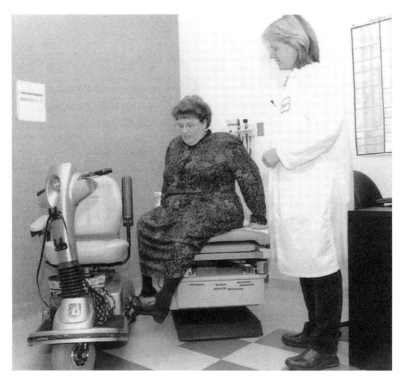

Figure 14.4. Independent transfer. This flat table automatically lowers to twenty-four inches from the floor, roughly the height of the seat on Penny's scooter wheelchair. The physician stands by, ready to help if needed, but with the lowered table, Penny independently moves onto the examining table. Once Penny is securely positioned, the physician automatically raises the table to thirty-one inches, a height convenient for her to conduct the physical examination. Other tables lower even closer to the ground—eighteen to twenty inches—for easy transfers from lower wheelchairs.

down on chairs, as well as getting up, poses significant challenges that thoughtful chair design can accommodate.

Especially for providers with diverse populations, one single style of chair will not meet all patients' needs. For instance, chair arms, positioned with their front edge in the same vertical plane as the front of the seat, minimize the strength required to sit down and stand up (Carpman and Grant, 1993, p. 229). However, chair arms may prevent persons who are obese from sitting comfortably in chairs of standard widths. A seat height of seventeen inches from the floor works well for many elderly persons, who tend to be shorter than younger adults. Seat angle, crossbars, and upholstery material also affect com-

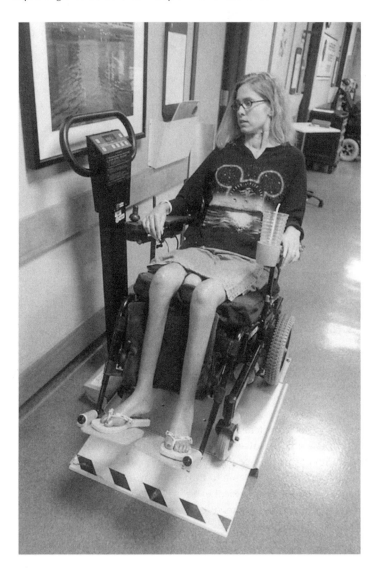

Figure 14.5.   Rolling onto the scale. Gretchen rolls her power wheelchair onto a scale to determine her weight. Clinic staff had previously weighed Gretchen's wheelchair. To determine her weight, Gretchen simply subtracts the wheelchair's weight from the total recorded on the scale.

fort and safety.[20] Finally, countless color and style options can make choice of even this ordinary item seem daunting. We mention this most basic of decisions to highlight again the value of involving one's own patients in discussing options. They will likely spend more time in these chairs than the providers ever will and might have useful ideas about the optimal selection.

Even after giving these myriad design questions careful thought, one must remember that design only sets the stage. In all spaces, creating truly patient-centered environments also demands caring and respectful interpersonal interactions with clinicians and office staff. Creating settings that maximize everyone's comfort—from patients to staff—should make these positive interactions more likely. Therefore, all the topics discussed in part III come into play when thinking about designing health care environments.

15

The Internet and Information Technologies

We're told we live in the Information Age, and nowhere is information more crucial than in health care. But as in previous epochs, the Information Age has its "haves" and "have nots"—persons on either side of the so-called "digital divide," users and non-users of the Internet and information technologies. The women living in rural Distant Dunes starkly demonstrated this digital divide. "I'm addicted to computers," admitted Christine, while other avid users agreed. Mary eagerly surfs the World Wide Web. "The doctors in Distant Dunes aren't up with the latest news about cerebral palsy, the latest technologies, the latest medications. Just through the Internet, I've shared things with my doctor about cerebral palsy—things that he'd never heard of."

Bonnie turned to those who'd remained silent. "I don't have a computer," Roxanne confessed. "I can't afford one." Others, also computerless, concurred. A few go online at local public libraries, but most have no access to computers or the Internet.

Persons who search for health care information on the Internet can find hope, validation, and a new sense of power and control over their health and health care, with 73 percent saying that the Internet improves the medical information and services they receive (Fox and Fallows, 2003, p. 24).[1] The Internet and other computer-based technologies offer enormous potential to enhance the knowledge, understanding, and interpersonal connections of persons with disabilities on multiple levels: from providing information in more accessible formats to facilitating access to reports about new treatments and assistive technologies to fostering "virtual" peer support groups. Thus, the transformative power of information technologies could prove especially profound for users with disabilities.

However, substantial barriers impede widespread use of information technologies among persons with disabilities. As for Roxanne, money poses a fundamental obstacle. Other common hurdles include disadvantages in education, literacy, income, employment, and access to technological expertise and support. Accommodating specific sensory and physical functional impairments also presents challenges, as designers fail to make computer operating systems, hardware, and Internet sites adaptable and easily accessible to persons with disabilities. Section 508 of the Rehabilitation Act Amendments of 1998 requires that most federal agency Web sites be accessible to individuals with disabilities (see www.section508.gov).[2] But many public and private Internet sites remain challenging to access and navigate.

Information technologies thus offer critical tools to enhance communication and knowledge of health and health care that could prove especially accessible to persons with sensory and physical disabilities. To achieve this promise, designers of computerized information resources and technologies must consider ways to accommodate persons with differing functional abilities. This chapter explores the potential of information technologies and addresses special challenges and benefits for users with sensory and physical disabilities.

Information Technology Opportunities and Obstacles

Cynthia Walker, in her mid-thirties with two preschool children, never expected her diagnosis. "It was June four years ago, and I was literally doing cartwheels in the yard teaching my daughter," Cynthia recalled (Iezzoni, 2003, p. 67). "That's when the sensations all began. I was diagnosed in October with rheumatoid arthritis, and by December I had difficulty walking." Her arthritis primarily affected her ankles, knees, and wrists. "I was foolish enough to believe that arthritis only happens to older people." Cynthia felt alone and unsure what to do, without friends her age to share ideas and experiences. Her health insurer narrowed her choice of rheumatologists, and she worries that her current physician doesn't understand how rheumatoid arthritis compounds the hectic demands of her daily life:

> In short, I feel sometimes that I'm the doctor in practice, and he's the patient who's learning. Truly, I am comfortable with him on many levels. However, I don't feel heard as a patient sometimes. . . . To find specific things that would be helpful to me, I have to do my own homework. I recently found the Arthritis Foundation on the Internet with the help of a friend. I was so excited. . . . You get up-to-date information at your fingertips. You see what they have and say, "My God, I never knew they invented all these different things! This could have helped me, or that could have helped me."
>
> You go back to your rheumatologist and say, "This device is really cool." And he says, "Okay, we'll get you one." Well, why didn't you tell me that a year ago when I could have used it? I had no idea that these very helpful products were out there. This is the age we live in. You have to take on the information yourself and learn as much about your own condition as you can. You can't expect your doctor to do it for you.

Just over 60 percent of Americans now use the Internet.[3] The most popular online activity is e-mail (93 percent of users), followed by researching products or services prior to purchase (83 percent). Searching for health information is a close third—80 percent of Internet users or roughly 93 million Americans (Fox and Fallows, 2003, p. i).[4] Cynthia Walker fits the profile of Internet users who search for health information: she is middle aged, female, white, college educated, not poor, and lives with a chronic condition.[5] The most common topic of health-related searches involves specific diseases or medical problems (63 percent), followed by medical treatments or procedures (47 percent); diet, nutrition, vitamins, or nutrition supplements (44 percent); exercise or fitness (36 percent); and prescription or over-the-counter medications (34 percent). Frequent seekers of electronic health information fall into three broad groups: persons conducting Internet searches to assist someone else; home caregivers desiring information about treatments and ways to ease the demands of care; and persons with disabilities.[6]

Internet Use by Persons with Disabilities

Americans with disabilities report relatively low levels of Internet use. Only 38 percent of persons with disabilities use the Internet, and about 19 percent of them say that disability impedes their use (Horrigan et al., 2003, p. 30).[7] Among the 62 percent of persons with disabilities who do not go online, 28 percent report their impairments hamper or prevent them entirely from using the Internet.

Several barriers block persons with disabilities from Internet access, starting with money. Many persons with disabilities cannot afford computers and monthly fees for Internet connections, let alone essential adaptive hardware or software for accessing computers and navigating the Web. Adaptive technologies—such as magnified or large computer monitors, a hands-free mouse, hands-free keyboards, and speech synthesizers—can total thousands of dollars. A head-mounted mouse often costs ten times the price of a usual mouse; prices of some large button keyboards are five-fold those of usual keyboards; braille interface machines run more than $3,000; and magnified screens sell for almost $2,000 (Horrigan et al., 2003, p. 32).

Persons with disabilities also confront difficulties obtaining Internet access at local facilities, such as libraries, community centers, and Internet cafes: 24 percent of persons with disabilities say that accessing the Internet in community settings is difficult compared with 15 percent of those without disabilities (Horrigan et al., 2003, p. 31). Physical barriers sometimes block persons from entering public and private buildings or rooms offering computer access to the public. Computer work stations at public locations often lack appropriate seating, tables, and other equipment to facilitate computer use. Internet users with disabilities have access *only* at home more often than others, although high unemployment among disabled persons may contribute to this pattern.

In addition, large numbers of persons with disabilities are age sixty-five or older—the least likely age group to use the Internet regardless of disability (see note 3). Only 22 percent of elderly persons—primarily white, well educated, wealthy individuals, with slightly higher percentages of men than women—go online (Fox, 2004). Older users display equal enthusiasm for the Internet as their younger counterparts, but roughly 80 percent of offline elderly persons say they will never go online. Some have few peers surfing the Web and wonder why they should purchase computers and spend time learning to use them. Previously employed elderly individuals generally left the workforce before computers became ubiquitous, so digital technologies seem unfamiliar and daunting. Many elderly persons are satisfied with the health information they already receive and therefore feel no compunction to search online.

Furthermore, persons age sixty-five and older often have visual, manual dexterity, or other impairments that impede their ability to access and use the Internet. Small print, low-contrast colors, and pull-down menus pose substantial challenges to navigating Web sites for many elderly persons. One small study found that, when performing routine Internet tasks (e.g., fact finding, making purchases, retrieving information), 53 percent of persons age sixty-five and older completed tasks successfully, compared with 78 percent of persons age twenty-one to fifty-five (Nielsen, 2002).[8] Older persons averaged 12:33 minutes:seconds to complete each task, compared with 7:14 minutes:seconds for younger individuals; older persons performed almost five erroneous actions per task, compared with 0.6 errors for younger subjects.

Regardless of age, persons with disabilities who currently lack Internet access face considerable barriers to gaining connections. Nonetheless, "the Internet can be an important resource for people who have difficulty leaving their homes. With information, shopping, and social resources available in their households, this lifeline can make the world more accessible for people with disabilities" (Horrigan et al., 2003, p. 32). Tina DiNatale, midforties with multiple sclerosis (MS), exemplifies these important benefits, as well as potential cautions (Iezzoni, 2003). Every day, from the moment she arises, Mrs. DiNatale constantly monitors her energy level, calculating what she can feasibly do. She makes trade-offs: on days she does laundry, she can't possibly visit friends. Alone at home for countless hours as her husband works overtime, Tina finds information she needs on the Internet.

All my books are in the basement, but sometimes I'm afraid to walk down the stairs. If I go down there to get a book, it's a major effort. You never know when your leg could give out or something else could happen. So I say, "Should I bother to do that? I don't think so!

I'll just look it up on the Web instead of in the book." I look up all sorts of things. I looked up my primary care doctor. I looked up my neurologist. I look up different types of wheelchairs—I'm trying to find a light-weight one, titanium.

The one thing Tina can't find on the Internet is the immediacy of human presence. Her husband and friends do rally round her. Nonetheless, Tina worries about becoming a "shut in. With CNN, CNBC, and the Internet, I have so much knowledge and no one to share it with."

Making the Web Accessible

"The power of the Web is in its universality. Access by everyone regardless of disability is an essential aspect," observed Tim Berners-Lee, credited with inventing the World Wide Web (Web Accessibility Initiative, 2004). However, ensuring this universal access requires careful attention to the needs of diverse users. Different impairments demand different solutions. For example, persons with visual disabilities need oral descriptions of graphics or video; persons who use American Sign Language as their primary language could benefit from video inserts depicting persons signing the content of written material appearing on the screen.

Various organizations, including the federal Architectural and Transportation Barriers Compliance Board (the so-called Access Board), specify electronic and information technology accessibility standards for persons with disabilities (see note 2). Many of these provisions ensure access for people with vision impairments who rely on assistive products to access computer-based information. Examples of such products include screen readers, which translate information or images on computer screens into automated audible output, and refreshable braille displays. Certain conventions, such as verbal tags or identification of graphics and format devices (e.g., frames), allows users to "read" computer screen content in a sensible way. The standards do not prohibit the use of Web site graphics or animation, instead aiming to ensure this information is also available in accessible formats. Generally, this means use of text labels or descriptors for graphics and certain format elements. (HTML code already provides an "Alt Text" tag for graphics, which can serve as verbal descriptors.)

The World Wide Web Consortium (W3C), an international collaboration among 400 member organizations, strives to facilitate universal access. In addition to host sites in Europe and Asia, the Massachusetts Institute of Technology in Boston serves as the W3C's North American home base for launching initiatives worldwide, including the Web Accessibility Initiative (WAI).[9] Working with experts, its member organizations, and disability advocacy groups, the WAI has developed extensive technical guidelines for universal design of new Web sites and evaluating the accessibility of existing sites. Various companies and organizations use WAI and other guidelines to assess

Web site accessibility, leaving an imprimatur when sites pass their tests. Web sites that meet WAI accessibility criteria should suit most users.

As elsewhere in universal design, what works well for persons with disabilities can facilitate Internet use by other people, too. Examples include guidelines suggested by the National Institute on Aging and the National Library of Medicine (2004) for "making your Web site senior friendly." Aging-related vision changes—such as the loss of contrast sensitivity and ability to discriminate fine details—make reading texts on computer screens more difficult. Recommendations are easy and straightforward. For instance, strategies for improving readability include the following:

- Use sans serif typefaces, such as Helvetica, Arial, and Univers. Avoid serif, novelty, and display typefaces, such as Times New Roman and Old English Text.
- Use 12- or 14-point type sizes for body text.
- Use medium or boldface type.
- Double space all body text.
- Present body text in upper and lowercase letters, reserving use of all capital letters and italic for headlines. Left justify text.
- Underline links only.
- Avoid placing yellow, blue, and green close together, since these colors when juxtaposed are difficult for older eyes to discriminate.
- Use dark type or graphics against light backgrounds or white lettering against black or dark backgrounds. Avoid patterned backgrounds.

Making Web sites easy to navigate and understand will certainly help all users.

E-Health

So-called "e-health"—a global term describing digital creation, sharing, searches, and storage of health information—offers tremendous potential to enhance and streamline health care delivery for everyone, especially persons with disabilities. Two particular benefits loom large: facilitating easy, rapid, and accurate communication between clinicians and patients; and helping patients better understand their conditions and options for interventions—especially strategies outside the standard clinical mainstream, such as assistive technologies, home modifications, and transportation.[10]

E-Mail

While telephones and pagers dramatically improved communication in prior eras, computer technologies could revolutionize clinician-patient communication. "Many interactions—informing patients of test results, arranging specialty referrals, receiving data on home glucose levels, and adjusting medication doses accordingly—can be handled by e-mail, bypassing the frustrating telephone system plaguing many medical facilities." Continuity of care could improve as patients "interact with their personal physician asynchronously via e-mail" (Bodenheimer and Grumbach, 2003, p. 260). E-mail follow-up to office visits allows patients to ask the important questions they may have forgotten or did not have time to raise and offers opportunities to clarify instructions. "E-mail creates a written record that removes doubt as to what information was conveyed" (Kane and Sands, 1998, p. 105).

Electronic communication could also improve correspondence among clinicians caring for individual patients, such as between primary care clinicians and specialists. Not only can clinicians share consultation notes via e-mail, but they can also send electronic attachments containing laboratory test results, digital images (e.g., of radiographs), and other reports. Through e-mail, patients could perhaps prompt their various clinicians to communicate with each other electronically or at least share the same information.

Because routine e-mail is generally not encrypted and is susceptible to interception by third parties, it fails to comply with the privacy standards of current Health Insurance Portability and Accountability Act of 1996 regulations (Katz and Moyer, 2004). Thus, going beyond simple e-mail, secure Web sites provide even more protected, comprehensive, and structured communication opportunities between patients and clinicians. Some health care organizations have created patient Internet portals, surrounded by electronic "firewalls" to protect the privacy of information and communication. These Web pages support e-mail as well as customized information accessible to individual patients, such as lists of diagnoses, allergies, prescribed medications, test results, and reminders about appointments and recommended routine screening and preventive services. Some Web pages allow patients to enter data about their health (such as blood glucose levels from home monitoring for diabetes), access various screening questionnaires, link to other health information sources, post reviews of specific health topics, and access Web sites of affiliated health care organizations. Certain providers allow patients access to their entire online medical records via a secure Web portal (Slack, 2004).

Electronic communication offers particular advantages to persons with sensory and physical disabilities. E-mail effectively removes communication barriers between deaf or hard of hearing persons and their clinicians by enabling them to communicate without an interpreter, teletypewriter (TTY), or other intermediary. Furthermore, e-mail transcends geographic distance: from the convenience of their own homes, people can obtain important information about their health and answers to routine questions from their own clinicians. Persons with chronic health conditions, like diabetes or hypertension, that require periodic monitoring could conveniently e-mail crucial data to their clinicians. Furthermore, the technology provides information in accessible formats and allows persons to electronically accomplish basic tasks, such as making appointments, which otherwise cause tremendous frustration. Computers with voice synthesizers can read e-mail and electronic attachments aloud, giving persons with visual disabilities critical information previously inaccessible.

However, unlike the e-mail explosion elsewhere in cyberspace, electronic correspondence between clinicians and patients has spread very slowly. "I've found one doctor who has agreed to let me e-mail him, which has been wonderful," said Marta Redding, who is hard of hearing. "But not everybody will do that. Doctors don't want to give their e-mail addresses to you and have you e-mailing them all the time." As of 2002, only 7 percent of persons have exchanged e-mail with their physicians (Fox and Fallows, 2003, p. 17). Barriers to online communication between patients and clinicians arise on numerous levels.

For patients, the digital divide poses a large barrier, but even persons who actively use the Web admit reluctance to e-mail their clinicians. Some patients worry legitimately about threats to their privacy with routine e-mail. Although communicating through secure patient Internet portals largely eliminates these risks, patients may remain leery, uncertain who may have access to their messages. Sensory and physical impairments that impede access to other Web sites may complicate navigation of patient Internet portals that contain complex modules and options (e.g., for entering or accessing detailed personal health information).

Clinicians' resistance also reflects multiple factors. Already juggling substantial workloads, physicians worry that e-mailing patients will precipitate "incessant, unreasonable, round-the-clock demands of patients with uncensored access to them" (Blumenthal, 2002, p. 536). Some clinicians anticipate that patients' messages may prove clinically irrelevant or inappropriate. Apart from several demonstration projects, health insurers do not yet pay for online communication. Thus, the time spent answering e-mails is typically uncompensated.

Early reports find that answering e-mails in a primary care practice *does* consume more time than that saved on returning telephone calls and office visits (Bodenheimer and Grumbach, 2003). The first patients to use e-mail are generally healthier than others, so their e-mails typically increase communication rather than substitute for office visits. Once more patients with chronic conditions use e-mail as substitutes for routine face-to-face visits, physicians' workload may decrease. However, when e-mails replace in-person visits, physicians in fee-for-service practices could lose money if they divert time away from "paying" patients.

Some clinicians also express professional discomfort with e-mail. Online communication can never substitute entirely for face-to-face encounters. Clinicians must develop skills for sorting "the wheat from the chaff"—

identifying clues within potentially voluminous e-mails of acute clinical needs demanding urgent in-person attention. Heavy reliance on e-mail could hamper growth of clinician-patient relationships. Clinicians carry an ethical and legal obligation to guard the confidentiality of health information, but protecting privacy of e-mail correspondence raises additional technical requirements, as noted previously. Encrypting e-mail messages best ensures their privacy but could complicate electronic correspondence. Because of privacy concerns, clinicians should routinely inform patients about the risks and benefits of e-mail exchanges.

Legal liability questions also arise. E-mails between clinicians and patients constitute part of the medical record and thus require appropriate handling.

> E-mail provides direct evidence of a patient-physician conversation.
> . . . The e-mail message is itself a medical record; it should be stored electronically or printed in hard copy and placed in a patient's medical record. From a liability standpoint, this is necessary for the physician, because it accurately documents the communication; additionally, the patient may retain these communications. . . . Indeed, there is no advantage to simply deleting e-mail messages, as even deleted messages are recoverable (and legally discoverable). (Spielberg, 1998, p. 1357)

E-mail users often treat online correspondence as transitory, immediate, and erasable, using casual language, quickly typed, rarely proofread. But with ever-present threats of medicolegal liability, correspondents should craft their prose with identical care as for other written records.

Clinicians' personal reservations generally reflect moral imponderables, such as how to handle a digital divide that further perpetuates potential inequities in the American health care delivery system. Even if persons have e-mail access, functional illiteracy endemic among vulnerable populations impedes complete and open written communication. For some clinicians, moving communication from direct person-to-person encounters to seemingly sterile and solitary computer screens severs a core pleasure from clinical practice—the "hands-on care that produces much of the therapeutic benefit and professional satisfaction of primary care practice" (Bodenheimer and Grumbach, 2003, p. 259).

Despite these reservations, clinician enthusiasts of e-mailing patients exist today. They say that e-mail substitutes efficiently for time-consuming telephone calls and gives them opportunities to respond thoughtfully and carefully to patients' queries. They deny being deluged by e-mail messages and report feeling greater control over their time, since they decide when to reply (Spielberg, 2003). In 1997, the Board of Directors of the American Medical Informatics Association endorsed guidelines "to guide clinicians and health care delivery organizations in . . . e-mail communication with patients . . . [to] enhance the value of, rather than introduce complications into, the provider-

Box 15.1. Guidelines for Clinicians Concerning Online
Communication with Patients

- Discuss privacy and security issues with patients. Encourage use of most secure online communication option (e.g., secure Internet portal, encryption)
- Never forward patient-identifiable information to a third party without the patient's explicit permission; double-check all "To" fields before sending messages
- Place or back-up all online communication into long-term storage (e.g., print off and place in patient's paper record, upload into patient's electronic medical record)
- Establish and inform patients of standard turnaround time for online communication; do not use e-mail for urgent communication
- Establish types of transactions and ask patient to type transaction type into subject line (e.g., prescription refill, medical advice, billing question, appointment)
- Configure automatic reply to acknowledge receipt of patients' messages
- After completing a patient's request (e.g., refill), send a confirmation message
- Request that patients reply to acknowledge reading the clinician's message
- Avoid language that is angry, sarcastic, harsh, critical, or libelous to third parties

Adapted from: Kane and Sands (1998, p. 106) which lists additional guidelines relating to communication, medicolegal, and administrative issues. Electronic communication of personal health information must also comply with provisions of the Health Insurance Portability and Accountability Act of 1996 regulations, which were implemented in 2003. More information is available at www.hhs.gov/ocr/hipaa/.

patient relationship" (Kane and Sands, 1998, p. 104; box 15.1). Patients' demands will likely push more clinicians into digital discourse with their patients—a practice that could especially benefit persons with disabilities.

Online Searches for Health-Related Information

Persons with disabilities often know volumes about their clinical conditions (see chapter 11). Increasingly, this information comes off the World Wide Web. By making health information readily available, round-the-clock, the

Internet is now an important self-management tool. Online patients, such as Cynthia Walker searching for devices to accommodate her arthritis, can find assistance beyond their clinicians' expertise and knowledge.

As noted above, 80 percent of Internet users search for health-related information. Most seek technical medical information about diseases, scientific evidence, and treatments. Some explore the Web systematically, as does Lester Goodall—mid-fifties with MS, a mid-level manager at a Fortune 500 company (Iezzoni, 2003). From his managerial vantage, Lester quips that "the Internet's probably most busy from nine to five when people are at work."[11] But he peruses the Web methodically, typically on his own time.

> I have my [Web] pages bookmarked. I have about three different Web sites for MS. I'll go on there and just look to see if anything's new. I look for experiments. They give you updates. Like there was an experiment about myelin [the fatty sheath around nerves, eroded in MS]. I remember when they first started it off. I read about it again maybe last month. They got the results in, and they haven't been that encouraging.
>
> Then I move onto something else. I need to look up the new drugs that are out there. I did a lot of research on Avonex [interferon beta-1a] when I first found out about that. And there are two or three more drugs that were out there. One was doing well; one wasn't doing too well.
>
> Then I sit and look in one of those little chat lounges [rooms] where people write in about their comments. A lot of people use them as a basis of comparison, although there are no two cases of MS alike. So it's really hard to benchmark where you are versus someone else. . . . But I think you need to have that support group out there.

Lester Goodall proceeds sequentially, scanning his bookmarked MS Web sites for information and updates about clinical trials and new medications, but also popping into chat rooms to see what other persons with MS are doing, experiencing, and learning. However, when it comes to deciding what to do, Mr. Goodall relies on his neurologist, Dr. Graham. "I like her very much; I see her twice a year," Lester reported. After complete physical examinations, Lester and Dr. Graham settle down to talk about interventions. "We've had a lot of good conversations about the beta interferon or the Avonex. I'm willing to help advance the research, but I would rather have Dr. Graham say, 'I think this is a good move,' or 'Lester, I wouldn't want you to do that.' I have a lot of faith in her judgment."

Thus, Lester Goodall's attitudes parallel those of many others who search the Internet for health information: He seeks information to inform himself, then brings that knowledge to his physician visits. With this background, persons feel better able to discuss treatment options and other related topics with their clinicians. "For the most part, [people] report that their use of the Internet makes them feel more independent of their doctors, empowers them to ask more informed questions during appointments, and allows them to have less fear of the unknown because of what they learn during their online health research" (Fox and Fallows, 2003, p. 16).

The Internet nevertheless can complicate interactions between patients and clinicians. Informed patients challenge the heart of professional authority—the supremacy of professionals in specialized technical knowledge and skills. Thus, the ability of patients to easily, quickly, and unobtrusively acquire voluminous health and health care knowledge via the Internet

> may affect the asymmetry of technical competence between physician and patient, thus reducing the value that physicians add in their interactions with patients. Patients with rare and chronic illnesses have always collected information about their conditions that rivaled or exceeded that of many physicians, but the information revolution will dramatically reduce the cost of acquiring such knowledge and open unprecedented new sources. As a result, a much larger fraction of the patient population will have a knowledge of their problems that matches all but that of the most specialized physicians. (Blumenthal, 2002, p. 533)

Additional problems arise when patients latch onto information that clinicians view as outdated or inaccurate, or when patients appear unable to understand fully the implications of information they retrieve online. Clinicians must then carefully but effectively challenge the veracity of the information without antagonizing or offending patients. Relatively little is known about the quality of health information available online or the ability of patients to comprehend the strengths and limitations of these materials. From July to December 2000, thirty-four physicians examined health information found through English and Spanish language search engines and Web sites (Berland et al., 2001).[12] They found that search engines with simple search terms frequently fail to efficiently identify useful Web sites. Neither English nor Spanish language Web sites generally provide complete clinical information. Posted information is usually accurate, although Web sites often contain contradictory statements. Importantly, most Web sites require relatively high reading levels to comprehend the information.

The most useful online health-related searches require time, care, and skepticism. To assess the credibility of given Web sites, searchers must determine the site's sponsor, check the date and source of the information, and visit four to six Web sites. This rarely happens. Although Internet users typically question sources that clearly appear commercial, about 75 percent of persons do not follow recommended guidelines for vetting online health information every time they search (Fox and Fallows, 2003, p. 32). Persons tend to feel reassured when they find information that agrees with their preconceived notions.

Not surprisingly, patients report that physicians exhibit mixed responses when they introduce Internet-derived health information. Some physicians take extra time to review and discuss the information with patients. Others react dismissively, defensively, or with irritation. Physicians may perceive patients' enthusiasm for Web searches as questioning their professional knowledge or judgment. Negative reactions cause some patients to avoid mentioning their online research or to change doctors.

Some clinicians and patients search the Internet together for relevant information during office visits. During a recent appointment, my physical therapist popped quickly online to search for a particular style of walker, and then printed the Web page for me to take home for future reference. Some clinicians fear that consulting the Internet during office visits will reveal knowledge gaps, risking their position of professional authority. More likely, however, "wired patients will lose confidence in physicians if they fail to demonstrate real-time competence in using the resources of the information revolution. In the future, physicians must demonstrate that they are expert at marshalling . . . new information technologies for their patients' benefit—that they are as good at surfing the Web as listening to lungs or performing an appendectomy" (Blumenthal, 2002, p. 539).

Although Lester Goodall uses the Internet primarily to search for standard medical knowledge, the Web offers a trove of information about topics beyond these medical boundaries, such as computer technologies and related adaptive equipment; accessible technologies for self-care, such as home glucose monitoring and blood pressure cuffs; home modifications and furnishings to improve accessibility; devices and utensils to ease routine daily tasks; adapted cars, vans, and public and private transportation services; and all varieties of assistive technologies. Even clinicians experienced in caring for persons with disabilities cannot possibly know the full range of products available today to meet varying needs. Relatively few shops carry complete inventories of different products, and conducting Internet searches from home or local community centers offers tremendous ease and convenience. Internet searches are thus invaluable—even if only to research options.

Nonetheless, as elsewhere on the Web, consumers should scrutinize potential purchases carefully. Although searching online for function-related items and services offers obvious benefits, such virtual shopping carries ironic implications for persons with disabilities. Most assistive technology products have explicitly physical functions and attributes. Furthermore, these physical characteristics must fit a customer's specific needs, for example, by compensating for some functional impairment. Making purchases online is often a leap of faith—you don't always know exactly what you'll get until the box arrives.

Standard warnings to consumers therefore apply to Internet purchases. Getting professional advice could help, for example, by visiting a Web site during an appointment with a physical or occupational therapist to seek their advice about specific products. Asking persons with similar disabilities (e.g., by visiting chat rooms or sending questions over listservs) about experiences with various products could prove useful. Consumers should always understand a vendor's return policy in case a purchase fails to meet their expectations.

Healthy and Accessible Communities

Anything that separates and negates those with a chronic condition will ultimately invalidate not only them but everyone else.

—Irving K. Zola

As I planned to visit Atlanta a few months ago to give a seminar, one instruction from my host puzzled me. "We'll meet you in the hotel lobby at 8:00 a.m.," her message read, "and walk you across the street to our office building." Why, I wondered, did I need an escort simply to cross the street? When I arrived and saw the lay of the land, the answer became clear. The area appeared recently built: a sloping sweep of four-lane road with a luxuriantly planted median divider; office and apartment complexes set back from the street and screened by trees and tasteful landscaping. There were no sidewalks, pedestrian crosswalks, stop signs, or traffic signals to arrest the constant flow of vehicles. Rolling out on the active roadway in my scooter, below eye level of most drivers or hidden by foliage, would be foolhardy and dangerous. I gratefully accepted the escort of my walking host, who had worn a bright red sweater, joking that might help her to stop traffic. She, too, was nervous crossing the street.

Daily, this situation reprises itself countless times, as people venture out cocooned in cars, rarely on foot, bicycles, or wheels like mine or walking with a white cane like Bonnie. Sociological and literary critiques of early twenty-first century America lament our car-centric lifestyle, the isolation of urban sprawl, and built environments that impede communal life. Public health practitioners decry the negative consequences for population health and physical and emotional well-being. Is it a coincidence that the growing dependence on cars—even for taking children to school bus stops a block or two from home—closely tracks the alarming rise in obesity rates among both parents and progeny?

As discussed in previous chapters, the built environment significantly affects the daily lives, and even access to health care, of persons with disabilities. All too often, people with disabilities face barriers to navigating their communities, which can lead to isolation, inactivity, stress, and other negative consequences. Furthermore, because of low income, the need for ready access to public transportation,[1] and other considerations, persons with disabilities may have few choices about where they can live. These complex factors certainly compromise quality of life and could perhaps lead to further functional declines and worsening of overall health. In contrast, accessible neighborhoods and community facilities enable persons with disabilities to leave home and enjoy outside activities, enhancing opportunities to maximize overall emotional and physical wellness.

In this last chapter, we therefore adopt a public health perspective, arguing that efforts to improve the health and wellness of persons with disabilities cannot stop at the clinic door. For centuries, public health practitioners have linked population health to the environments in which persons live and work—especially those environments built by human beings.

> The built environment includes our homes, schools, workplaces, parks/recreation areas, business areas, and roads. It extends overhead in the form of electric transmission lines, underground in the form of waste disposal sites and subway trains, and across the country in the form of highways. The built environment encompasses all buildings, spaces, and products that are created or modified by people. It impacts indoor and outdoor physical environments (e.g., climatic conditions and indoor/outdoor air quality), as well as social environments (e.g., civic participation, community capacity and investment) and subsequently our health and quality of life. (Srinivasan, O'Fallon, and Dearry, 2003, p. 1446)

Numerous aspects of the built environment thus contribute to population health. In addition, how individuals interact daily with the built environment can affect population health, with so-called "lifestyle" factors now accounting for the preponderance of deaths in the United States. Tobacco use tops the list, but poor diet and physical inactivity also contribute to excess deaths among U.S. residents. Characteristics of the built environment strongly influence population lifestyle. For instance, urban sprawl appears linked to obesity (Lopez, 2004), and some poorer neighborhoods have fewer stores stocking healthy foods, such as fresh fruits and green vegetables, than nearby wealthier neighborhoods (Horowitz, 2004).

Numerous initiatives now aim to improve population health in cities and communities worldwide (see appendix 1). The Healthy Cities movement within the World Health Organization supports efforts around the globe, each addressing pressing local issues such as poverty, homelessness, environmental pollution, basic education, and classic public health (e.g., infectious disease prevention or eradication). To tackle local needs, initiatives typically bring together representatives from diverse sectors within the community, such as advocacy groups, business leaders, and health and ed-ucation professionals. In the United States, diverse programs have created community partnerships to improve population health, addressing a wide variety of concerns. In these initiatives, health care professionals and local medical institutions often serve as partners, under the presumption that "car-ing for the community" is part of their social contract with their neighbors (Omenn, 1999, p. 782). Community-based partnerships to improve popula-tion health have targeted such public health concerns as infant mortality, adolescent pregnancy, tobacco use, alcohol and substance abuse, immu-nizations, crime and violence, lead poisoning, HIV, cardiovascular diseases, and nutrition.

To focus our discussion here, we reach back to the independent living movement of the 1960s, which aimed to achieve full participation in com-munity life for persons with disabilities (see chapter 10). To attain that goal, an essential first step was building physical communities that persons with disabilities could access and navigate with safety and maximum independ-ence.[2] Building safe and accessible built environments figures prominently in today's efforts to create healthy communities for everyone.

The built environment affects the ability of people with and without dis-abilities to exercise, adopt healthy lifestyles, and spend enjoyable leisure time with family and friends—activities to maximize both physical and emotional health. A "reduction in the population-level prevalence of obesity requires changes in the environmental conditions (i.e., . . . opportunities for activity such as walking trails and bike routes) that support widespread changes in . . . activity habits" (Roussos and Fawcett, 2000, p. 375). Accessible exercise and recreation facilities convey advantages to everyone. For instance, paved bicycle trails offer safe exercise venues not only to bike riders but also to pedestrians, including Bonnie and her husband, who both walk with white canes. Paved bicycle trails allow my husband and me to take long walks together—he walks, I roll—cherished mental health breaks![3] Given looming epidemiologic trends, however, another compelling argument for environ-ments that encourage healthy lifestyles is the possibility of preventing or minimizing new disability relating to obesity and physical inactivity among otherwise fit individuals.[4]

Demographic Imperatives for Accessible Built Environments

By 2030, 20 percent of the U.S. population will be age sixty-five or older, just as the tail of the "baby boomer" generation—the 77 million persons born from 1946 through 1964—passes beyond that age milestone. The grandpar-ents and parents of these baby boomers enjoy better health and more robust functioning than have prior generations, although substantial numbers of elderly persons do report some debility (see table 1.1). Will their children share similar trends, with improved functional abilities into very old age?

Prognosticating future population health must concede numerous caveats, especially about potential benefits from as-yet unanticipated medical breakthroughs. Nevertheless, current numbers give pause.

Obesity among adult Americans is increasing, from 12 percent in 1991 to 20.9 percent (44.3 million adults) in 2001 (Mokdad et al., 2003, p. 77). On average, American adult men and women in 2002 weighed twenty-four pounds more than their 1960 counterparts, although they were only roughly an inch taller (Ogden et al., 2004, p. 2). More troubling, children are growing heavier. In 1999–2002, 31.0 percent of children age six through nineteen were either overweight or at risk for overweight, and 16.0 percent were actually overweight (Hedley et al., 2004, p. 2849). The precise contribution of obesity to excess deaths remains controversial (Flegal et al., 2005; Mark, 2005). Nonetheless, disability rates—specifically, limitations in activities of daily living—rise twofold with moderate obesity and fourfold with severe obesity in adults (Sturm, Ringel, and Andreyeva, 2004). Thus, if current trends continue, rising rates of obesity could substantially increase the numbers of persons with disabilities. Of particular concern, disability rates among younger persons are rising steeply, increasing 50 percent among persons age thirty to thirty-nine between 1984 and 1996 (Lakdawalla, Bhattacharya, and Goldman, 2004, p. 170).

Beyond its own disabling effects, obesity causes or contributes to other debilitating conditions, such as arthritis (especially degenerative joint disease), diabetes, and cardiovascular conditions. Arthritis or chronic joint symptoms— the leading cause of disability among adults—affected 70 million adults in 2001, including 60 percent of persons age sixty-five and older. If current arthritis rates persist, the number of persons over age sixty-five with arthritis will double by 2030 (to 41.1 million persons; Centers for Disease Control, 2003d, p. 489). In 2002, arthritis affected roughly 37 percent and 12 percent, respectively, of persons age forty-five through sixty-four and eighteen through forty-four (Centers for Disease Control, 2004b).[5] With rising obesity among youths, weight-related arthritis could similarly increase at younger ages.

Diabetes is closely associated both with obesity and disability. In 1999–2000, 14.4 percent (29 million) of Americans more than twenty years old had diagnosed diabetes, undiagnosed diabetes, or impaired fasting glucose levels (Centers for Disease Control, 2003b). Rates of diagnosed diabetes rise with age, from 1.4 percent for ages twenty through thirty-nine to 15.2 percent for sixty-five and older.[6] Annual surveys from 1980 through 2002 find substantial increases in rates of self-reported diabetes over time (Centers for Disease Control, 2004a). Most persons with diagnosed diabetes are heavy: 85.2 percent are overweight or obese, and 54.8 percent are obese (Centers for Disease Control, 2004c, p. 1066). Obesity exacerbates other chronic conditions among persons with diabetes, such as hypertension and high cholesterol levels, although precise relationships among overweight and various cardiovascular disease risk factors may be changing over time (e.g., because of new medications, lifestyle changes; Gregg et al., 2005).

In addition, diabetes is associated with relatively high levels of visual impairment. Among persons age fifty and older with diabetes, 10.2 percent have diabetic retinopathy (Centers for Disease Control, 2004d, p. 1069). In this age group, persons with diabetes have higher rates of other eye diseases than their non-diabetic counterparts: for cataracts, 31.8 percent and 21.2 percent, respectively; and for glaucoma, 8.0 percent and 4.3 percent.

Although increased physical activity confers numerous benefits, such as reducing obesity, diabetes, and premature mortality, fewer than half of adult Americans (45.4 percent) in 2001 regularly exercised at levels that could improve their health (Centers for Disease Control, 2003c).[7] Twenty-six percent of adults were physically inactive. Thus, huge gaps loom between exercise levels that could improve health, fitness, and overall well-being and the daily activities of U.S. adults.

These epidemiological trends carry consequences beyond health and disability: they also cost money. Annual U.S. medical expenditures attributable to overweight and obesity total $92.6 billion in 2002 dollars (9.1 percent of aggregate medical spending), rivaling costs related to smoking (Finkelstein, Fiebelkorn, and Wang, 2003). Obesity boosts annual medical spending per adult by 37.4 percent; Medicaid programs incur substantially higher obesity-related costs than do other insurers. In 1997, arthritis (and other rheumatic conditions) cost the United States $51.1 billion in direct costs, as well as $35.1 billion in indirect costs—the value of time lost from work (Centers for Disease Control, 2004f). In 1997, total economic costs of diabetes reached $98.2 billion, including $44.1 billion in direct medical costs (Centers for Disease Control, 2004e). Other societal costs could also increase. For instance, with growing numbers of persons with worsening vision or physical impairments making them unable to drive, cities and suburbs may need to build more accessible public transportation systems.

Thus, as the prevalence of lifestyle-related disabling conditions grows, so too will their costs, both to persons and to society. These costs unfurl against entrenched inequities in our health care system, especially the politically intransigent problem of uninsured persons (see chapter 3). By 2015, lack of health insurance may contribute to more than 30,000 excess deaths annually among people age fifty-five to sixty-four—greater than the number of deaths caused by stroke, diabetes, and lung disease in this age group (McWilliams et al., 2004, p. 229). Even among insured persons, health insurance rarely pays for programs to encourage healthy behaviors, such as exercise interventions and nutrition counseling.

Building Person-Centered and Healthy Communities

Impending demographic trends therefore compel efforts to build communities that encourage healthy lifestyles. "We now realize that how we design the built environment may hold tremendous potential for addressing many of the nation's greatest current public health concerns, including obesity, cardiovascular disease, diabetes, asthma, injury, depression, violence, and social inequities" (Jackson, 2003, p. 1382). These notions are not new—just the context and health targets have changed.

Direct connections between the built environment and public health became obvious during the nineteenth century, as the Industrial Revolution drove thousands of rural dwellers into cramped and filthy cities. Installing sewage systems, cleaning drinking water, and moving housing away from noxious industrial plants significantly reduced epidemic deaths and improved population health. Florence Nightingale, in 1860s England, observed that even hospitals located away from urban congestion, removed from raw sewage, with better sanitation, and less crowded wards had lower death rates. Nightingale's theory about miasmas—noxious vapors spreading disease—led her to introduce fresh air, light, and ample space into wards, thereby substantially reducing hospital deaths (Nightingale, 1863).

Health catastrophes produced by nineteenth-century industrial filth cemented the public's belief that close proximity between residences and business is inevitably unhealthy.

> This view was reflected in the esthetics of the City Beautiful movement as well as in the social agenda of many in the early 20th-century housing-reform movement. It is also reflected in the zoning ordinances that took hold in the 1920s. These ordinances separated neighborhoods for residential, business, and industrial uses. . . . They were consistently justified because population deconcentration and separation of uses improved "public health, safety, morals, [and] general welfare." (Perdue, Stone, and Gostin, 2003, p. 1390)

The 1926 U.S. Supreme Court case *Village of Euclid Ohio v. Ambler Realty Co.* set the precedent for exclusionary zoning. Before 1926, land use in the United States often intermixed residential and business properties, whereas afterward, "euclidean," or homogeneous use zoning, became dominant and persists today.

By the mid-twentieth century, zoning ordinances segregating commercial from residential properties had become less a matter of public health than aesthetics and economics. Suburbs physically isolated homes from the businesses essential to daily life, such as grocery stores, pharmacies, retailers, and workplaces. As distances grew between homes and job sites, shops, and services, so too did paradoxical implications for public health. In prior centuries, acute infectious diseases whipping through congested cities posed the greatest threat; however, in the late twentieth century, public health attention shifted largely to chronic conditions.[8] "Indeed, deconcentration of populations and the separation between residential and business areas, measures urged a hundred years ago to improve health, may contribute to chronic health problems" (Perdue, Stone, and Gostin, 2003, p. 1390). Distance encourages dependence on cars, sedentary lifestyles, weight gain, and even air pollution.[9] Failures of public transportation to effectively serve sprawling suburbs exacerbate the problem.[10]

In densely populated urban areas, poverty, which occurs at roughly twice the rates as in suburbs (16.4 percent versus 8.0 percent in 1999; Corburn, 2004, p. 543), compounds the ills of unhealthy built environments. Vacant lots might provide the only open spaces, even if covered with garbage and crawling with vermin. Without safe playgrounds, children must play in streets, if they exercise at all. People can perhaps buy groceries by walking to corner convenience stores. But typically these stores sell only expensive canned, processed, and packaged foods with low nutritional value, rather than the fresh fruits and vegetables plentiful at suburban markets. Crime and violence scare residents off the streets, making them unwilling to walk out for essential errands let alone exercise (Glass and Balfour, 2003, p. 318). Homelessness represents perhaps the ultimate failure of the built environment, albeit precipitated by complex economic, social, and political forces. In New York City, 85 percent of the 38,200 homeless residents represent families, including 17,000 children (Northridge, Sclar, and Biswas, 2003, p. 561).

Having access to the natural environment—everything not built by humans—is also essential to population health. "A theoretical basis for the notion that contact with nature is beneficial comes from E. O. Wilson, who introduced the term *Biophilia* almost 20 years ago, defined as the innately emotional affiliation of human beings to other living organisms" (Institute of Medicine, Roundtable, 2001, p. 12). Without green spaces, communities suffer. Parks and public gardens, even when small, encourage a sense of community, offering places for people to meet, interact, and relax. Exposure to natural areas extends longevity, reduces crime, lowers aggression and violence, and improves civility and neighborliness (Kaplan and Kaplan, 2003). Parks and public green spaces provide opportunities for walking, bicycling, sports, and other outdoor activities. The public strongly values open natural spaces, as suggested by generally successful local ballot initiatives to preserve nearby forests and farmlands, even if doing so requires higher taxes (e.g., to purchase property, maintain land).

Thus, urban blight, absent shared green spaces, and urban sprawl with dispersed and isolated residences bode ill for future population health—especially when compounded by constricted leisure time and poor health behavior choices. Several statistics highlight today's concerns.

- While the U.S. population has increased only 37 percent since 1970, the distance traveled by all cars, motorcycles, sport-utility vehicles, and small trucks rose 143 percent (Jackson, 2003, p. 1383).
- Twenty-eight percent of car trips in 2001 traveled less than one mile. Americans drive vehicles for 66 percent of all trips up to one

mile long and 89 percent of trips between one and two miles (Pucher and Dijkstra, 2003, p. 1509).

- In 1960, 10.3 percent of Americans walked to work, compared with 2.9 percent in 2000 (Pucher and Dijkstra, 2003, p. 1510).
- Today, only 10 percent of children walk or bicycle to school—a 40-percent decrease over the past two decades (Srinivasan, O'Fallon, and Dearry, 2003, p. 1447).

Although building and restructuring environments to promote healthy behaviors has garnered considerable attention in recent years, substantial barriers bar the way. Take, for example, efforts to increase walking and bicycling. Major obstacles include the mythic role of cars (and now sport-utility vehicles and light trucks) in American culture and fierce resistance to any initiatives that seemingly restrict choice or limit use of motor vehicles. Very real concerns include higher fatality and injury rates per mile and per trip for walking and cycling compared with car travel, as well as the absence of safe and convenient pedestrian walkways (e.g., sidewalks, bridges over major intersections) and cycling lanes.

Without careful thought and planning, efforts to improve safety may paradoxically yield unanticipated dangers. One study found that older pedestrians face a 2.1-fold greater risk of collisions with vehicles at locations marked with crosswalks only compared to those without crosswalks (Koepsell et al., 2002, p. 2141). One potential explanation is that marked crosswalks alone provide a false sense of security to older pedestrians, who erroneously believe that drivers will notice and defer to them as they cross streets.[11] Slower walking speeds also likely heighten risks for older pedestrians. Adding stop signs or traffic signals adjacent to crosswalks can reduce these risks, presumably by halting traffic flow. Audible cues, such as beeps, timed with automated walk signals inform persons with low vision when traffic signals have stopped vehicular traffic, presumably allowing them to safely cross streets.

Important lessons for environments that encourage safe physical activity come from abroad. An excellent example involves walking and bicycling experiences in the Netherlands and Germany compared with the United States (Pucher and Dijkstra, 2003). Differences are striking, especially among elderly persons.

> Walking increases with age in both [t]he Netherlands and Germany, while cycling falls off only slightly. Indeed, the Dutch and Germans who are 75 and older make roughly half their trips by foot or bike, compared with only 6% of Americans aged 65 and older. While cycling is almost nonexistent among the American elderly, it accounts for a fourth of all trips made by the Dutch elderly and for 7% of trips made by the German elderly. Equally stunning, walking accounts for 48% of trips by Germans aged 75 and older and 24% of

trips by Dutch aged 75 and older. This not only provides them with valuable physical exercise but also ensures them a level of mobility and independence that greatly enhances their quality of life. (Pucher and Dijkstra, 2003, p. 1510)

Many factors explain the differences between U.S. and European experiences. Land use patterns are more compact in Europe: trip lengths are roughly half those in U.S. cities. Americans pay less for car ownership, gasoline, parking, roadway tolls, and licensing fees than do Europeans. On a darker note, "Per kilometer and per trip walked, American pedestrians are roughly 3 times more likely to get killed than German pedestrians and over 6 times more likely than Dutch pedestrians. Per kilometer and per trip cycled, American bicyclists are twice as likely to get killed as German cyclists and over 3 times more likely as Dutch cyclists" (Pucher and Dijkstra, 2003, p. 1511). American pedestrians and bicyclists also are injured much more often than their European counterparts.

These excellent results from Germany and the Netherlands are no accident. Both countries have made extensive changes explicitly to increase the ease, safety, and convenience of walking and cycling. Between 1975 and 2001, total pedestrian fatalities dropped 82 percent in Germany and 73 percent in the Netherlands; during those years, cyclist fatalities fell by 64 percent in Germany and by 57 percent in the Netherlands (Pucher and Dijkstra, 2003, p. 1512). In Germany, this time period witnessed a cycling boom, with a 50-percent rise in the number of trips by bicycle, making the declining death rates doubly impressive. To achieve these gains, Germany and the Netherlands implemented wide-ranging interventions, including the following:

- Creating better facilities for walking and cycling, such as increasing auto-free zones often covering much of city centers; building wide, well-lit sidewalks on both sides of every street; installing pedestrian-activated crossing signals at intersections and midblock crosswalks; expanding bike paths and roadway bicycle lanes; designating "bicycle streets," which permit cars but give cyclists strict right-of-way; and installing traffic signals and advance turn lights just for cyclists.
- So-called "traffic calming" of residential neighborhoods, including reducing driving speeds (e.g., to 30 kilometers or 19 miles per hour); installing physical barriers, such as speed bumps, artificial dead-end road blocks, raised intersections and crosswalks, zigzag streets, and traffic circles; and extending traffic-calming techniques throughout entire neighborhoods, not just isolated streets.
- Designing urban environments for people, not cars, including locating shops, cultural activities, and services near residential areas, easily reached by foot or bicycle; adding safe and attractive pedestrian and bicycle lanes to all bridges built across waterways or

roads; and locating parking lots behind buildings so that front entrances offer easy access to walkers and cyclists.

- Restricting motor vehicle use, such as by prohibiting truck traffic in residential neighborhoods, lowering speed limits generally within cities, raising parking fees, and forbidding right turns on red traffic lights.
- Conducting extensive driver education, specifically teaching about avoiding collisions with pedestrians and bicyclists even when they disobey laws (e.g., by jaywalking or cycling in the wrong direction), as well as educating children on safe walking and cycling practices.
- Promulgating rigorous traffic regulations and enforcement that favor pedestrians and cyclists, including strict ticketing of motorists, pedestrians, and cyclists who violate traffic regulations; installing cameras at intersections to automatically photograph vehicles breaking traffic laws; and increasing the severity of punishment for violating traffic regulations.

Implementing such comprehensive reforms in the United States would likely prove challenging for many reasons, ranging from the larger expanses of most American towns and cities compared with those in Europe, to stiff cultural resistance to the economic and political clout of reluctant automotive and related industries. Numerous initiatives are introducing health concerns into designs of the U.S. built environment, but most have yet to make the measurable impact of the German and Dutch interventions. For instance, the federal Centers for Disease Control and Prevention sponsor the Active Community Environments (ACE) program to promote walking and bicycling through urban design, land use decisions, and transportation policies. ACE forges links with state and local governments and nonprofit organizations to pursue these goals within communities nationwide. The Robert Wood Johnson Foundation, a large health philanthropy, spends considerable resources on an "active living" initiative to promote physical activity through changes in the built environment. Its Active Living by Design program has funded twenty-five community partnerships, bringing together public health, city planning, architecture, transportation, crime prevention, safety, education, and other experts within communities to create and implement environmental strategies for increasing physical activity.[12]

The U.S. Department of Transportation, Federal Highway Administration, and state and local authorities have explored methods for "traffic calming" in American cities and neighborhoods, defined as "the combination of mainly physical measures that reduce the negative effects of motor vehicle use, alter driver behavior, and improve conditions for non-motorized street users" (Ewing, 1999, p. 2).[13] Traffic calming can offer secondary benefits beyond enhancing safety for non-vehicular users of roadways. For example,

limiting access to streets, installing speed bumps, and community beautifi-
cation efforts contributed to a 50-percent decline in violent crime and a
24-percent drop in nonviolent crime within a neighborhood of Dayton, Ohio
(Ewing, 1999, p. 113). In West Palm Beach, Florida, traffic calming was central to urban redevelopment efforts. Beyond the benefits of improved safety,
traffic calming helped foster neighborhood pride, attract private investment,
bolster downtown businesses, support home ownership, and advance his-
toric preservation. In Boulder, Colorado, installation of traffic circles significantly reduced vehicular noise: traffic circles slow cars (a relatively quiet
process), while STOP signs bring vehicles to a complete halt followed by
noisy acceleration (Ewing, 1999, p. 116).

Public health advocates acknowledge that more research must determine
the most effective and economical strategies for using built environment design to improve public health in the United States. Even basic issues, such
as optimal ways to encourage walking or cycling rather than driving for
short trips, remain poorly understood (Dannenberg et al., 2003). However,
as noted earlier, impending demographic shifts and the population burden
of chronic conditions provide a powerful impetus for finding answers.

Circling back to Disability

The precepts followed in building healthy communities should presumably
accommodate persons with disabilities. After all, constructing passageways
friendly to cyclists must contain curb cuts! But before making this assumption, designers must be sure. Fast-moving cyclists are scary for those less
adept at split-second directional shifts, especially when bike riders twist and
turn amongst other passersby. "Communities that are adequately designed
for a young adult with fast reflexes can be unnavigable for an elderly person" or someone with a disability (Jackson, 2003, p. 1383).

In 1972, the late sociologist Irving K. Zola spent a week at the Dutch community Het Dorp, constructed specifically to maximize independent
community-based living with dignity for persons with substantial physical
disabilities. Zola, who had had polio and typically used leg braces and
crutches to get around, moved with trepidation into a wheelchair for that
week, and he recorded not only his observations of Het Dorp residents but
also his growing understanding of his own disability. Het Dorp explicitly
segregated its residents within their own barrier-free environment. Nonetheless, on first encountering the community, Zola's initial impression involved
the uplifting independence offered by Het Dorp's design:

> Were it only the tilting of a finger, the raising of a palm, the moving
> of one's head, the controlling of one's breath—with this and the lat-
> est electronic ingenuity, the residents *themselves* could get into their

wheelchairs and propel themselves around *their* Village. What an enormous difference this made to the viewer, if not the viewed! They moved and *no one* pushed them, a small but important step to independence and dignity. (Zola, 1982, p. 33)

Today, opportunities for independence and dignity extend well beyond specialized settings like Het Dorp. Segregating persons with disabilities in such isolated enclaves defies the reality that, through the fullness of time, almost everyone will spend some months or years with disability. Designing built environments to facilitate access throughout the lifespan—from early years spent in strollers to later times with disability—allows everyone to retain those human connections so central to our sense of worth, dignity, and humanity.

Today's designers of healthy communities should think about creating built environments to *prevent* disability. More importantly, however, they must also explicitly design communities to welcome persons of varying abilities. Certainly, building communities that are safe and have clean air, well-lit and maintained sidewalks, audible and visual traffic controls at crosswalks, and good physical accessibility will encourage persons with disabilities who can exercise to do so, just as for other people. Additional goals for persons with disabilities include preventing injuries by minimizing risks of falls, reducing depression by luring people from homebound isolation, and maximizing independence within homes, workplaces, and neighborhoods.

As described in chapter 11, resources within communities provide important supports for self-management of chronic conditions. The built environment can facilitate or hinder certain self-management programs, notably exercise activities, weight reduction, stress management, and efforts to alleviate depression and anxiety. Planners of healthy communities should therefore remember to integrate self-management resources into their overall designs.

At the end of the day, people with disabilities want the same things from their communities as do others—safety, comfort, opportunities, freedom, choices, and independence. Today's assistive technologies allow persons with even substantial functional impairments to move freely and at will through the built environment, provided that designers think about their needs. Brianna, who is tetraplegic, navigates the world in her power wheelchair. She lives in a neighborhood of narrow, tree-shaded streets and century-old, bow-fronted, brick townhouses with steep granite steps. Her more modern apartment building, admittedly less charming, is completely accessible to her power chair. Brianna loves rolling along, going where she pleases. Most sidewalks have curb cuts, although—as often happens on congested Boston streets—drivers can block curb cuts with their parked cars. Brianna therefore sometimes must follow circuitous routes, backtracking and weaving to find accessible paths. But she knows how to get where she's going.

Brianna feels that she belongs to her community. Despite remaining barriers, she is not isolated or segregated from her neighbors.

> Some days, if I don't want to catch the bus, I'll ride my wheelchair downtown. I'll just go on my own. I used to work downtown. And if the weather was really nice, if it's not too hot, after work, I'd ride my wheelchair home, taking my time. Just browse, stop in a store. Don't have no money, but there's many places to go.

Getting to those places safely and independently immeasurably enriches Brianna's life and, through her, the community as a whole.

Appendix 1

Internet Resources Addressing
General Disability and Health Care Topics

This appendix lists Internet resources offering general information relating to disability, health care professionals, and topics addressed in this book, such as universal design, self-management, and building healthy and safe communities. We focus on governmental or nonprofit sites, acknowledging that this list is not exhaustive. The Internet contact information is current as of December 2004. Other useful web sites and links emerge continually, especially through condition-specific organizations (see appendix 2). Inclusion in this list does not imply our endorsement of specific organizations.

Federal Agencies and Departments

Simply typing "www.disability.gov" or "DisabilityInfo.gov" brings Internet surfers to the U.S. government's "gateway" to all federal resources relating to disability. The main menu offers links to the following topic areas: employment, education, housing, transportation, health, income, technology, independent living, civil rights, and accessibility. Each menu choice links users to more detailed menus and options for accessing the specific information sought. The Web site uses large print and is available with full, low, or no graphics and with high contrast.

Within the U.S. Department of Health and Human Services, two Web sites offer extensive information about health, health care, and persons with disabilities.

Medline Plus: Disabilities
National Library of Medicine and the National Institutes of Health
www.nlm.nih.gov/medlineplus/disabilities.html
This Web site provides links to current information about treatments
and research relating to specific disabling conditions, as well as information about assistive technologies, social and family issues,
consumer and provider organizations, special concerns relating to
children, law and policy, and many other disability-related topics.

Women with Disabilities
National Women's Health Information Center
Office on Women's Health
www.4women.gov/wwd/index.htm
This Web site, which specifically addresses women, contains extensive information on wide-ranging concerns, including access to
health care, aging with disability, reproductive health and sexuality, parenting, breast health, financial assistance, substance abuse,
laws and regulations, and information relating to specific types of
disabilities.

General Disability Advocacy and Information Organizations

American Association of People with Disabilities
Washington, DC
www.aapd-dc.org

American Association on Health and Disability
Rockville, MD
www.aahd.us

Consortium for Citizens with Disabilities
Washington, DC
www.c-c-d.org

Disability Rights Education & Defense Fund
Berkeley, CA
www.dredf.org

National Center on Physical Activity and Disability
Chicago, IL
www.ncpad.org

National Council on Disability
Washington, DC
www.ncd.gov

National Council on Independent Living
Arlington, VA
www.ncil.org

National Organization on Disability
Washington, DC
www.nod.org

North Carolina Office on Disability and Health
The Frank Porter Graham Child Development Institute at the
  University of North Carolina
Chapel Hill, NC
www.fpg.unc.edu/~ncodh

World Institute on Disability
Oakland, CA
www.wid.org

Health Care Professionals and Other Providers

Alliance for Technology Access
San Rafael, CA
www.ataccess.org

American Academy of Physical Medicine and Rehabilitation
Chicago, IL
www.aapmr.org

American Medical Rehabilitation Providers Association
Washington, DC
www.amrpa.org

American Occupational Therapy Association
Bethesda, MD
www.aota.org

American Physical Therapy Association
Alexandria, VA
www.apta.org

Association of Medical Professionals with Hearing Losses
Miamisburg, OH
www.amphl.org

Center for Disability Issues & the Health
  Professions—Western University
Pomona, CA
www.westernu.edu/xp/edu/cdihp/home.xml

Center for Personal Assistance Services, University of California
San Francisco, CA
www.pascenter.org/home/index.php

National Coalition for Assistive and Rehab Technology
Washington, DC
www.ncartcoalition.org

Registry of Interpreters for the Deaf, Inc.
Alexandria, VA
www.rid.org

Rehabilitation Engineering and Assistive Technology Society of
   North America (RESNA)
RESNA Technical Assistance Project
Arlington, VA
www.resna.org

Universal Design

Adaptive Environments
Boston, MA
www.adaptenv.org

Center for Universal Design, North Carolina State University
Raleigh, NC
www.design.ncsu.edu/cud/

Centre for Accessible Environments
London, England
www.cae.org.uk

Design for Ageing Network
London, England
www.hhrc.rca.ac.uk/programmes/designage/DAN/

European Design for All e-Accessibility: EDeAN
Hoensbroek, Netherlands
www.e-accessibility.org

European Institute for Design and Disability
Oliveto Lario, Italy
www.design-for-all.org

Building Healthy Communities

Active Community Environments Initiative: ACES
Atlanta, GA
www.cdc.gov/nccdphp/dnpa/aces.htm

ACES is sponsored by the Physical Activity and Health Branch, National Center for Chronic Disease Prevention and Health Promotion, Centers for Disease Control and Prevention

Active Living by Design
Chapel Hill, NC
www.activelivingbydesign.org
A national program of The Robert Wood Johnson Foundation administered by the University of North Carolina School of Public Health

National Center for Bicycling and Walking
Washington, DC
www.bikewalk.org

National Coalition for Promoting Physical Activity
Washington, DC
www.ncppa.org

World Health Organization Healthy Cities
Geneva, Switzerland
www.who.dk/healthy-cities

Appendix 2

Internet Resources Addressing Specific
Disabilities, Diseases, and Disorders

This appendix lists selected Internet resources to assist persons with managing their health and health conditions and learning more about specific disabilities, diseases, or disorders. Some sites provide primarily educational material about the target condition, while others list assistive technologies and links to various products that could help persons with daily activities, including self-management. This list is not exhaustive, and the Internet contact information is current as of December 2004. We concentrate on nonprofit organizations, although some Web sites contain links to commercial vendors of various products and services. Inclusion in this list does not imply an endorsement of specific organizations, the credibility of their information, or the utility and safety of specific products. Caveat emptor—"buyer beware"—remains a sensible principle for persons seeking information via the Internet about managing their health or health care. Ideally, when crafting self-management plans, persons should work collaboratively with informed clinicians or, at a minimum, review self-management plans with a knowledgeable health professional.

Blind and Low Vision

American Council of the Blind (ACB)
Washington, DC
www.acb.org
The ACB is a consumer organization of blind individuals with affiliates in all fifty states and with twenty special interest affiliates. The ACB focuses primarily on educational activities to improve economic and social opportunities for blind persons.

American Foundation for the Blind (AFB)
New York, NY
www.afb.org
The AFB Web site contains information on such topics as living with
   vision loss, education, employment, various assistive technologies,
   and braille. Some information addresses the families and friends of
   persons who are blind, seniors, children, and professionals.

Lighthouse International
New York, NY
www.lighthouse.org
Lighthouse International provides information and identifies resources addressing vision impairment, eye conditions, vision rehabilitation, and low vision services throughout the United States.

The Macula Foundation
New York, NY
www.macula.org
Along with the Association for Macular Diseases and the LuEsther
   T. Mertz Retinal Research Center, the Macula Foundation Web site
   gives information about macular conditions, aiming to help "people with macular diseases to lead independent lives." The other
   two organizations focus primarily on research.

Macular Degeneration Foundation, Inc.
Henderson, NV
www.eyesight.org
The Macular Degeneration Web site provides information for consumers about juvenile and adult macular degeneration, eye tests,
   and research.

National Federation of the Blind (NFB)
Baltimore, MD
www.nfb.org
The NFB is a membership organization of blind persons. Its Web site
   provides extensive information about aids and appliances to assist
   blind persons, employment, childhood education, braille, specific
   resources relating blindness to diabetes and to aging, and extensive other resources for blind individuals.

Deaf and Blind

American Association of the Deaf-Blind (AADB)
Silver Spring, MD
www.aadb.org
The AADB strives to enable deaf-blind persons to achieve their max-
    imum independence and productivity, through educational and
    mentoring programs and other activities.

Helen Keller National Center for Deaf-Blind Youths and Adults
    (HKNC)
Sands Point, NY
www.hknc.org
The HKNC provides family support and training, rehabilitation, and
    other educational services to deaf-blind children and adults
    following PATH principles—Person-centered Approach Toward
    Habilitation.

Deaf and Hard of Hearing

American Tinnitus Association (ATA)
Portland, OR
www.ata.org
The ATA provides information and support to persons with tinnitus,
    including suggestions for its prevention and treatment.

Association of Late Deafened Adults (ALDA)
Oak Park, IL
www.alda.org
ALDA is a membership organization of persons who became deaf af-
    ter the onset of speech or language. Its Web site offers links to
    products related to hearing loss, hosts chat rooms, and organizes
    gatherings and self-help support groups.

Gallaudet University Technology Access Program
Washington, DC
tap.gallaudet.edu
The Technology Access Program, based at Gallaudet University, con-
    ducts research in such areas as universal design in telecommunica-
    tions, video telecommunications, teletypewriters (TTY), relay serv-
    ices, captioning, wireless and paging technologies, telephone
    menus and voice mail, and equipment accessibility.

National Association of the Deaf (NAD)
Silver Spring, MD
www.nad.org
The NAD focuses on advocacy and legal assistance, expanding captioning, certification of American Sign Language interpreters,
deafness-related information and publications, public awareness,
and youth leadership development.

Self Help for Hard of Hearing People (SHHH)
Bethesda, MD
www.shhh.org
SHHH is an advocacy and support organization for persons with
hearing loss. Its Web site offers links to products related to hearing loss, as well as information about hearing-related assistive
technologies, cochlear implants, and tips for communicating with
family and friends.

Vestibular Disorders Association (VEDA)
Portland, OR
www.vestibular.org
VEDA provides information to the public and health care professionals about inner ear disorders, describing the range of vestibular
disorders and providing educational materials about addressing
and living with these conditions.

Diseases and Physical Disorders and Disabilities

Arthritis and Physical Disabilities, in General

Arthritis Foundation
Atlanta, GA
www.arthritis.org
The Arthritis Foundation Web site contains extensive information on
arthritis treatments, supplements and alternative therapies, assistive technologies and other useful products, and tips about living
with arthritis.

National Rehabilitation Hospital (NRH)
Center for Disability Issues and the Health Professions (CDIHP)
www.project-shield.org
This Web site contains the "Resource Kit for People with Physical
Disabilities," created by nearly 40 persons with physical disabilities along with researchers at NRH and CDIHP. The kit contains
information on staying healthy with a disability and specific tools
for identifying and minimizing risks to health.

Diabetes

American Diabetes Association (ADA)
Alexandria, VA
www.diabetes.org
The ADA Web site offers wide-ranging information about different types of diabetes, diabetes epidemiology, symptoms and complications, risks for heart disease and stroke, genetics of diabetes, treatments, research, and other topics.

Juvenile Diabetes Foundation (JDF)
New York, NY
www.jdf.org
The JDF aims to cure diabetes, but its Web site offers information on living with the disease, such as self-monitoring blood sugar, achieving good blood sugar control, diet and exercise, and nutrition for adults and children.

Heart, Vascular, and Lung Diseases

American Heart Association (AHA)
Dallas, TX
www.americanheart.org
The AHA Web site addresses healthy lifestyles as well as specific conditions, including heart attack, arrhythmias, congestive heart failure, cholesterol, high blood pressure, diabetes, and peripheral artery disease.

American Lung Association (ALA)
New York, NY
www.lungusa.org
Among extensive information about various lung diseases (e.g., asthma, chronic bronchitis, respiratory allergies), the ALA Web site offers an interactive decision support tool, the "Asthma Profiler," which aims to assist person with asthma and their physicians in making evidence-based decisions about treatments. Users must register an e-mail address with a confidential password.

American Stroke Association (ASA)
Dallas, TX
www.strokeassociation.org
The ASA, a division of the AHA, focuses on reducing death and disability from stroke through education, prevention, research, and advocacy.

National Stroke Association (NSA)
Englewood, CO
www.stroke.org
The NSA's major focus is preventing stroke, emphasizing implementation of clinical practice guidelines for stroke prevention and efforts to empower people to "ask your doctor" about their stroke risks.

Neurological Diseases and Selected Congenital Conditions

American Parkinson's Disease Association (APDA)
Staten Island, NY
www.apdaparkinson.org
The APDA offers extensive services aimed at patient support, education, and referrals to support groups nationwide.

Muscular Dystrophy Association (MDA)
Tucson, AZ
www.mdausa.org
The MDA offers a wide range of services and supports to individuals and families confronting not only the various forms of muscular dystrophy but also such disorders as amyotrophic lateral sclerosis (Lou Gehrig's disease), motor neuron disease, and myasthenia gravis.

National Multiple Sclerosis Society (NMSS)
New York, NY
www.nmss.org
The NMSS Web site contains extensive information about MS treatments and various issues confronted in daily life with MS, including suggestions for dealing with such concerns as difficulty walking, bladder and bowel dysfunction, cognitive function, dizziness and vertigo, emotional problems, fatigue, numbness, pain, sexual dysfunction, and vision problems.

Parkinson's Disease Foundation (PDF)
New York, NY
www.pdf.org
The PDF provides education and advocacy for persons with Parkinson's disease, as well as offering referrals to support groups around the country.

Spina Bifida Association of America (SBAA)
Washington, DC
www.sbaa.org
The SBAA provides support and resources to assist those living with
spina bifida and their families, as well as information about its potential prevention.

United Cerebral Palsy (UCP)
Washington, DC
www.ucp.org
The UCP provides advocacy and information to persons with cerebral palsy and their families, with extensive supports around ac-
quisition and payment policies regarding assistive technologies
(e.g., augmentive and alternative communication devices, wheeled
mobility aids).

Obesity

American Obesity Association (AOA)
Washington, DC
www.obesity.org
The AOA address a range of issues including prevention, treatment,
research, consumer protection, and employment and other discrimination relating to obesity.

Overeaters Anonymous (OA)
Rio Rancho, NM
www.overeatersanonymous.org
OA is not primarily about weight loss but instead "it addresses
physical, emotional, and spiritual well-being." OA provides a
twelve-step program for recovering from compulsive overeating;
persons can access meeting information through the OA Web site.

Spinal Cord Injury

American Spinal Injury Association (ASIA)
Atlanta, GA
www.asia-spinalinjury.org
The ASIA aims to educate persons with spinal cord injury, their families, and health care professionals about the treatment and prevention of these injuries, aiming to maximize activities of daily life
for persons with SCI.

National Spinal Cord Injury Association (NSCIA)
Bethesda, MD
www.spinalcord.org
The NSCIA provides information and referrals to individuals with
new and existing SCI, including peer support linking persons with
SCI with each other.

Paralyzed Veterans of America (PVA)
Washington, DC
www.pva.org
The PVA provides strong advocacy and support for veterans paralyzed during military service, as well as with certain disorders
connected with military services (e.g., multiple sclerosis). The PVA
also convenes clinical experts to issue practice guidelines around
various health conditions and complications of paralysis.

Appendix 3

Suggestions for Improving
Accessibility of Health Care Services

Meeting standards of the Americans with Disabilities Act (ADA) provides only a starting point for ensuring accessibility of health care services. Many physical settings and practices that comply with ADA regulations are nevertheless difficult and uncomfortable for certain persons with disabilities. In addition, the ADA does not address the interpersonal interactions that form the heart of many health care encounters. The persons we interviewed offered many suggestions for making health care services more accessible and improving patient-clinician communication. This appendix lists various recommendations from the interviewees, organized into broad categories. Clinicians and health care managers could consider implementing these ideas within their own health care delivery settings. Persons with disabilities could use these recommendations to help identify clinicians and health care providers that might be more "user friendly" and accessible. Administrators and policy-makers could use these recommendations to guide evaluations of whether health care settings are not only accessible but also comfortable and welcoming places for persons with disabilities. This list, however, is not exhaustive, and implementing some suggestions may prove infeasible in certain settings.

In many ways, these recommendations distill down to three overarching messages:

1. Never make any assumptions about the abilities, preferences, expectations, or desires of persons with disabilities.
2. Instead, just ask them—for example, about how clinic staff can best assist them and about what they prefer and expect.
3. Then, to the extent possible, respect and comply with their expressed preferences.

Following these three precepts is a clear road map toward achieving accessible and patient-centered care. Optimally, as clinicians and health care providers develop new facilities and practice environments, they should involve persons with disabilities from their communities. Designers should consider the universe of individuals—with and without disabilities, young and old—who might someday use their settings and services.

Basic Training and Organizational Policies

- Train all office staff, including clinicians, about professional, ethical, and legal obligations relating to disability. Repeat this training periodically.
- Emphasize the need to ensure effective communication during all interactions with all patients.
- Make clear that the call for treating persons with disabilities equally, with respect and dignity, comes from top leadership of the organization. Leadership should systematically assess physical and communication access within their health care delivery setting to identify needs for new equipment, renovations, staff training, and other changes. They should strive to implement required modifications, monitoring progress toward these goals.
- Identify an individual to oversee the full range of disability-related issues, not only for patients but also for employees.
- Establish procedures for registering complaints that maximize privacy for all parties but are expeditious and result in practical and productive solutions to identified problems.
- Develop and practice procedures for evacuating the facility in the case of emergency, specifically considering needs of persons with disabilities. Consider purchasing equipment to assist evacuations, such as lightweight frames for carrying wheelchair users safely down stairs.
- Train staff and administrators about the illegality of charging patients for specific accommodations, such as fees for sign language interpreters. Investigate potential federal tax credits and deductions for providing disability-related accommodations.
- Establish procedures for basic administrative functions. For example, determine who will work with patients to complete required paperwork and identify private settings for these interactions. Specify procedures for when and how to request sign language interpreters, as well as other specific communication or physical access accommodations.
- Specify policies relating to e-mail and other electronic communication with patients (e.g., access to test results, online medical records). Ensure that secure Internet portals are used to maximize confidentiality and that all Web site designs meet accessibility standards.

- Survey patients, including persons with disabilities (using accessible survey formats), about their experiences with care, and modify practices and procedures to rectify problems.

Communicating with Patients

- Always introduce yourself to persons when entering rooms. During encounters, introduce all other persons who newly enter the room.
- Look at persons when speaking to them. Communicate directly with patients, not family members, friends, or assistants who might accompany them.
- When using a sign language interpreter to facilitate communication, look at and speak to the patient, not the interpreter.
- Always speak clearly, at usual volume and a reasonable speed.
- Ask patients how best to communicate with them. After checking that patients agree, inform all clinicians and staff who interact with patients of these preferences through prominently placed information in medical charts and/or other procedures.
- Make appropriate efforts to comply with patients' preferred communication approach.
- Periodically check with patients to see if communication preferences have changed.
- Ask patients how best to attract their attention or assist them with movement or positioning during examinations and with moving in and around the office. Inform all clinicians and staff who interact with patients of their preferences.
- For established patients, plan ahead to ensure required communication accommodation (e.g., sign language interpreter). Stay on schedule, so interpreters do not leave before visit finishes.
- Ensure that office staff communicates discreetly with patients in public settings (e.g., do not raise voice).
- In waiting rooms, come up to patients who are deaf or hard of hearing to notify them when their appointment time comes.
- Describe all planned physical maneuvers, and inform patients immediately prior to touching.
- Periodically ask patients about effectiveness of communication; request suggestions to rectify unsatisfactory situations.
- Periodically ask patients to summarize their understanding of what has been said, particularly when conveying important technical information, to identify and correct miscommunications.

Accessible Information and Communication Methods

- Prepare easy-to-read written instructions, including in large-print and braille formats, about what to do before clinician arrives in examining room (e.g., which clothes to remove and why).
- Prepare easy-to-read written instructions, including in large-print and braille formats, about examining room or testing procedures. Whenever possible, use pictures or diagrams.
- Consider purchasing assistive listening devices to accommodate communication with persons who are hard of hearing (especially in practices with large numbers of elderly patients).
- Acquire and learn how to use a teletypewriter (TTY). Become familiar with telephone relay services.
- Place public TTY pay phones near specific locations (e.g., hospital waiting rooms, recovery rooms, emergency rooms, information desks) where public pay phones are available.
- Provide easy access to a chair for TTY use, so that persons do not need to bend over while typing on the TTY.
- Install knock sensors (small battery-powered units that attach to the inside of doors and flash a light when someone knocks— roughly $35) to examination and other room doors to alert patients who are deaf or hard of hearing when persons are outside and about to enter.
- Review automated telephone menu systems, considering alternatives for persons with sensory disabilities (e.g., e-mail, facsimile). Ensure that callers have a ready option to speak directly to a person, such as by dialing zero.
- In radiology units, install colored lights to signal when patients must take certain actions, such as holding their breath or resuming normal breathing.
- In waiting rooms, use vibrating pagers or other non-visual, non-auditory means to inform patients when their appointment time comes.
- Ensure that videos or DVDs containing educational material are captioned for persons with hearing impairments and audio-described for persons who cannot see the images.
- Consider communicating appointment times, reminders, and certain clinical information by e-mail through a secure Internet portal to patients who indicate they have access to the Internet.

Clinical and Technical Communication

- Focus first on the patient's chief complaint, not on their sensory or physical impairment.

- Assume that patients have detailed knowledge of their sensory or physical impairment. Sometimes this knowledge is highly technical. At a minimum, most persons know intimately the implications of their impairments for daily bodily functioning. Therefore, ask patients relevant questions and listen to and respect their responses (e.g., about pain, risks of certain physical maneuvers).
- Remain vigilant for risks of medical errors or iatrogenic injuries resulting from inadequate communication or inaccessible information (e.g., medication vials with labels patients cannot read, instructions given in inaccessible formats). Attempt to anticipate and prevent such situations.
- Prepare pictures or diagrams depicting tests or procedures; have books with relevant pictures available for more detailed discussions (e.g., concerning surgery).
- Provide brief, easy-to-read, written instructions, including in braille and large-print formats, about what to do after visits or procedures.
- Consider making a tape recorder and cassettes available so that persons who have difficulty reading can record verbal instructions.
- Work collaboratively and respectfully with patients, as partners to their care. Develop plans of care and self-management that take into consideration the person's disability, preferences, values, and lifestyle.
- Address patients' interests in screening, wellness, lifestyle modification, and other services oriented toward maximizing overall health and quality of life.
- Consider offering lists of appropriate Web sites that provide information about self-management, improving overall health, and specific diseases, disorders, and disabilities.

Physical Environment, Resources, and Equipment

Specific attributes and access issues vary widely depending on the nature of the health care facility. Many of the suggestions below might apply to most settings, although small private physicians' offices obviously differ in terms of their size and resources from large, multispecialty practices in academic centers.

Cross-Cutting Issues

- Physical environment meets basic safety standards (e.g., visual and auditory signals for fire emergency).

- Lighting is non-glare, uses warm tones when possible.
- Provide bright task lighting for areas where patients complete forms or read documents.
- Avoid backlighting in examination rooms or settings where clinicians communicate extensively with persons who are deaf or hard of hearing.
- Minimize background noise, such as canned music.
- Use baffling materials on walls to absorb ambient noise.
- Flooring should minimize glare and attenuate sounds, in addition to being durable, easy to clean, and reducing risks of slips and falls. Vinyl flooring is generally preferable to ceramic tiles because it is softer and has higher friction ratings.
- Carpeting is unpadded and has a short pile height, thus minimizing the force required to propel wheelchairs.
- Fix any loose seams and curled edges of carpeting, vinyl tiles, linoleum, or other flooring.
- Avoid flooring with broad stripes, large geometric designs, or wavy patterns.
- Label all doorways and passages using clearly visible and easily understood signage, including in raised print and braille.

Entryways

- Accessible parking near entrance, including wide spaces to allow vans with automatic lifts or ramps on their sides to unload wheelchair users.
- Recognize problems posed by densely built urban locations that have little exterior space close by for accessible parking. May need to create alternatives, such as complementary valet parking for persons with disabilities.
- If parking is in a multistory garage nearby, access to the health care facility should be through covered spaces with elevators kept in good order and automatic openers on all doors.
- Smooth transitions from the loading areas and parking lot surface to sidewalks and other walkways, with detectable warnings (e.g., changes in pavement surface to cue persons with visual disabilities) at curbless crosswalks that cross vehicular traffic.
- Covered entryways to protect persons from inclement weather.
- Smooth, level entry into building, without steps or steep ramps.
- Automatic door opener located so the door does not swing into persons immediately after they push the opener. When automatic revolving doors are present, they should have an easily accessible button to slow down their speed. A regular door, preferably with

automatic opener, should be available for persons who cannot use revolving doors.

- Lever handles for doors requiring manual entry.

Waiting Rooms

- Understand purpose of waiting room, patient volumes, and visit lengths. For instance, in busy emergency rooms, persons without immediately life-threatening conditions could wait for hours; they may nevertheless feel ill, need spaces to consult triage staff privately and expeditiously, and require places for anxious relatives or friends. Waiting areas outside of surgical suites, where visitors await news about loved ones, may demand quieter, contemplative settings, with private areas for conversations with clinicians and telephone calls with family members. Outpatient primary care practices may strive for short waits for patients who are generally not acutely ill but may need privacy to complete routine paperwork.
- Automatic opener for door, positioned so that the door will not open into persons who just pressed the button.
- Doors should have glass windows or sidelights to see persons approaching from opposite side; lever handles.
- Rods or hooks for hanging coats at both standing height and wheelchair height.
- Reception area desks at standing and sitting heights; sitting height desk has knee space to accommodate wheelchair users. Freestanding chairs available for persons who cannot stand long enough to transact business but do not use wheelchairs.
- Private spaces nearby for office staff to assist patients confidentially with required paperwork.
- Chairs at different heights, including for children as appropriate; some chairs with armrests and some without.
- Open spaces dispersed through waiting room but next to seating so wheelchair users can sit with other people but outside foot traffic. Passageways within seating area wide enough to accommodate wheelchairs; these open spaces and wide passages will also accommodate baby strollers and carriages.
- Dual-height water fountains for standing and seated users; refreshment counters accessible to wheelchair users, with knee space under table.
- Adequate lighting for reading.
- Racks with informational brochures, magazines, and other reading materials within easy reach; offer materials in large-print format.

- Television controls, if any, easily reachable, with closed captioning; television volume not too loud.

Restrooms

- Doors with lever handles and glass sidelights; automatic door opener optimal.
- Minimize height of threshold; having no threshold is best.
- If there is a second door immediately beyond outside door (e.g., to protect privacy), ensure wheelchair users have enough room to maneuver and to open inner door. If automatic door opener is installed (optimal), it should open both doors.
- Nonslip flooring; if ceramic tiles, use small-sized tiles to minimize likelihood of slipping.
- Wheelchair-accessible toilet door should open out, with handle and lock devices that are easy to grasp and operate.
- Grab bars on either side of toilet, with adequate turning space within toilet stall.
- Toilet should be slightly higher than standard height, making it easier for persons who use their legs to stand but still allowing easy transfer from wheelchair. Installing lifts to position persons with very limited mobility is optimal but requires larger space and careful planning.
- Position toilet tissue and bins for sanitary product disposal within easy reach of person seated on toilet.
- Tilt mirror over sink slightly forward to reflect wheelchair users.
- Sink basin should come to edge of counter. Use lever rather than turn faucet handles. If water flow is operated by an electronic sensor device, make sure persons in wheelchairs can easily trigger sensor.
- Soap dispenser and paper towels easily accessible to persons in wheelchairs.
- Avoid having hot air blower as the only way to dry hands. Some people may find it difficult to stand in front of the blower long enough to dry hands; furthermore, this device can pose problems for some walker and cane users.

Examination Rooms

See relevant suggestions above.

- Automatically adjustable examination table with ample space for wheelchair maneuverability; if not, have appropriate lift devices, with trained staff to operate them.
- Wheelchair-accessible scale readily available within clinic.

Specialized Facilities and Services

See relevant suggestions above.

- Surgery units, recovery rooms, labor and delivery suites, emergency departments, radiology suites, and other specialized units should establish specific protocols for effective communication during all phases of care.
- When purchasing new equipment, search for models that are accessible, maximizing independence for patients and minimizing injury risks to staff (e.g., from transferring patients).
- Review policies about removing and returning hearing aids to maximize patients(safety and comfort; discuss policies and safeguards with patient before procedures.
- Consider using colored lights to signal when patients must take certain actions during radiology studies (see above).

Transportation Awareness

- Have listing of accessible bus and transportation routes that serve facility.
- Ensure that office staff can give accurate directions using nonvisual cues from the bus or subway stop to the health care facility.
- Be aware if patients are using paratransit services; ensure they are finished with their visit by the paratransit pick-up time.

Other Recommendations

- Become familiar with various clinical disciplines, such as physiatry (physicians who specialize in physical medicine and rehabilitation) and physical and occupational therapy, that provide care to persons with certain disabilities. Learn about when to refer patients to these other specialists.
- Become familiar with broad classes of assistive technologies used by persons with disabilities, and learn about where to refer patients to obtain more specific information and, when relevant, about writing prescriptions for this equipment. Learn more about preparing effective "medical necessity" documentation justifying health insurance purchases of necessary assistive technologies.
- Become aware of devices that aid persons with physical and sensory disabilities with self-management tasks, such as "talking" glucose monitoring equipment and thermometers and adapted pill

minders. Know where to refer patients to get more information.

- Learn about local resources, such as sign language interpreters specifically trained for medical encounters, telephone and video relay services, and pharmacies that provide large-print and/or braille labeling and instructions for medications.
- Identify local consumer groups of persons with disabilities that might offer peer support and consider referring certain patients to these groups.
- Keep fresh hearing aid batteries in stock. These batteries come in a few standard sizes and will keep for several years. If patients with hearing aids lose battery power unexpectedly, providing them with a new battery can help restore their ability to communicate.
- If state telephone carrier has a program for providing free or discounted TTY equipment, amplified telephones, alerting devices, or other equipment to qualified residents, health care office could display leaflets for the program and keep application forms and contact information to distribute to appropriate patients.

Appendix 4

Identifying Disability Using National Survey Data

Tables A.1, A.2, and A.3 present the question wording and responses used to define disability categories with the Medical Expenditure Panel Survey (MEPS), Medicare Current Beneficiary Survey (MCBS), and National Health Interview Survey (NHIS) disability supplements, respectively. Within disability groups (i.e., vision, hearing, lower extremity, upper extremity, and hand difficulties), we assigned individuals to the most severe level suggested by their responses. Some questions in the surveys fail to yield completely accurate impressions of certain disabilities. For instance, MEPS Question HE30 (table A.1) asks if a respondent can "not see anything at all, that is, is—blind?" However, many persons who qualify as blind still retain some vision, such as the ability to see light, broad shapes, or colors or vision in a specific region of the visual field. The perception conveyed by the wording of the question (that only persons who cannot see anything at all are blind) is inaccurate.

Table A.1. Questions and Responses from the Medical Expenditure Panel Survey (MEPS) Used to Define Disability

Disability	Questions and Responses from the MEPS
Vision	HE26. "Does ___ wear eyeglasses or contact lenses?" (yes, no)
	HE28. "Does ___ have any difficulty seeing [with glasses or contacts if they use them]?" (yes, no)
	HE30. "Can ___ not see anything at all, that is, is ___ blind?" (yes, no)
	HE31. "[With glasses or contacts], can ___ see well enough to read ordinary newspaper print, even if ___ cannot read?" (yes, no)
	HE32. "[With glasses or contacts], can ___ see well enough to recognize familiar people if they are two or three feet away?" (yes, no)
Blind or major difficulty	"Blind" on HE30 OR "no" on HE31 OR "no" on HE32
Some difficulty	"Yes" on HE28
Hearing	HE33. "Does ___ use a hearing aid?" (yes, no)
	HE35. "Does ___ have any difficulty hearing [even with a hearing aid, if they use one]?" (yes, no)
	HE37. "Can ___ not hear any speech at all, that is, is ___ deaf?" (yes, no)
	HE38. "[With a hearing aid], can ___ hear *most* of the things people say?" (yes, no)
	HE39. "[With a hearing aid], can ___ hear *some* of the things people say?" (yes, no)
Deaf or major difficulty	"Deaf" on HE37 OR "no" on HE38 OR "no" on HE39
Some difficulty	"Yes" on HE35
Lower extremity mobility difficulty	HE12. "How much difficulty does ___ have walking up 10 steps without resting?" (no difficulty, some difficulty, a lot of difficulty, completely unable to do it, completely unable to walk)
	HE13. "How much difficulty does ___ have walking 3 city blocks or about a quarter of a mile?" (no difficulty, some difficulty, a lot of difficulty, completely unable to do it)
	HE15. "How much difficulty does ___ have standing for about 20 minutes?" (no difficulty, some difficulty, a lot of difficulty, completely unable to do it)

(continued)

Table A.1. (continued)

Disability	Questions and Responses from the MEPS
Major difficulty Moderate difficulty Minor difficulty	"Completely unable" on HE12 OR HE13 OR HE15 "A lot of difficulty" on HE12 OR HE13 OR HE15 "Some difficulty" on HE12 OR HE13 OR HE15
Upper extremity mobility difficulty Major difficulty Some difficulty	HE17. "How much difficulty does ___ have reaching overhead, for example to remove something from a shelf?" (no difficulty, some difficulty, a lot of difficulty, unable to do it) "Unable" OR "a lot of difficulty" on HE17 "Some difficulty" on HE17
Difficulty using hands Major difficulty Some difficulty	HE18. "How much difficulty does ___ have using fingers to grasp or handle something, such as picking up a glass from a table or using a pen to write?" (no difficulty, some difficulty, a lot of difficulty, un- able to do) "Unable" OR "a lot of difficulty" on HE18 "Some difficulty" on HE18

Table A.2. Questions and Responses from the Medicare Current Beneficiary Survey (MCBS) Used to Define Disability

Disability	Questions and Responses from the MCBS
Vision	"Do you wear eyeglasses or contact lenses?" (yes, no, blind)
	"Which statement best describes your vision?" (wearing glasses/contact lenses)
Blind	Blind on eyeglasses/contact lens question
Very low vision	"A lot of trouble" on vision question
Hearing	"Do you use a hearing aid?" (yes, no, deaf)
	"Which statement best describes your hearing (even with a hearing aid)?"
Deaf/very hard of hearing	Deaf on hearing aid question OR "a lot of trouble" on hearing question
Hard of hearing	Uses hearing aid or has "a little trouble" hearing
Walking	"How much difficulty do you have walking a quarter of a mile (two or three blocks)?"
	"Because of a health or physical problem, do you have any difficulty walking by yourself and without special equipment?"
Major difficulties	"Unable to walk two to three blocks" OR "Doesn't walk" by self without special equipment
Moderate difficulties	"A lot of difficulty" walking two to three blocks OR "difficulty" walking by self without equipment
Reaching overhead	"How much difficulty do you have reaching or extending your arms above shoulder level?"
Major difficulties	Reports being "unable to do" or having "a lot" of difficulty reaching
Moderate difficulties	Reports "some" difficulty reaching
Grasping and writing	"How much difficulty do you have either writing or handling and grasping small objects?"
Major difficulties	Reports being "unable to do" or having "a lot" of difficulty with hands
Moderate difficulties	Reports "some" difficulty with hands

Table A.3. Questions and Responses from the National Health Interview Survey Disability (NHIS-D) Supplement Used to Define Disability

Disability	Questions and Responses from the NHIS-D
Blind or seriously impaired vision	Reports being "legally blind" OR having "SERIOUS difficulty seeing, even when wearing glasses or contact lenses?" that will last for ≥12 months
Deaf or seriously hard of hearing	Reports using a hearing aid OR having "trouble hearing what is said in normal conversation (even when wearing a hearing aid)" that will last for ≥12 months
Lower extremity mobility difficulty	"Has ___ used or is ___ expected to use" various mobility aids "for 12 months or longer?" "Does ___ have any difficulty walking up 10 steps without resting?" "Does ___ have any difficulty walking a quarter of a mile—about three city blocks?" "Does ___ have any difficulty standing for about 20 minutes?"
Major, long-term difficulty	Uses manual or electric wheelchair or scooter OR reports being "completely unable" to climb steps, walk, or stand, lasting for ≥12 months
Some difficulty	Uses cane, crutches, or walker OR reports "some" or "a lot" of difficulty climbing stairs, walking, or standing
Upper extremity mobility difficulty	"Does ___ have any difficulty reaching up over the head or reaching out as if to shake someone's hand?"
Major difficulty	Reports being "completely unable" or having "a lot" of difficulty reaching
Some difficulty	Reports "some" difficulty reaching
Difficulty using hands	"Does ___ have any difficulty using fingers to grasp or handle something such as picking up a glass from a table?" "Does ___ have any difficulty holding a pen or pencil?"
Major difficulty	Reports being "completely unable" or having "a lot" of difficulty with hands
Some difficulty	Reports "some" difficulty with hands

Notes

Chapter 1

1. The numbers in table 1.1 derive from civilian non-institutionalized individuals. The long form of the 2000 Census questionnaire asked two questions relating to disability (items 16 and 17, U.S. Census Bureau, 2003b). Item 16, asked of a sample of respondents age five and older, contained two parts inquiring about long-lasting conditions as follows: "(a) blindness, deafness, or a severe vision or hearing impairment (sensory disability); and (b) a condition that substantially limits one or more basic physical activities such as walking, climbing stairs, reaching, lifting, or carrying (physical disability)." Item 17 had four parts and asked if the respondent had a physical, mental, or emotional condition lasting at least six months that made it difficult to perform specified tasks. The four activity categories were "(a) learning, remembering, or concentrating (mental disability); (b) dressing, bathing, or getting around inside the home (self-care disability); (c) going outside the home alone to shop or visit a doctor's office (going outside the home disability); and (d) working at a job or business (employment disability)." A sample of respondents age five and older was asked activity categories 17a and 17b, while a sample age 16 and over was asked categories 17c and 17d.

2. Life expectancies also differ importantly by race. White males born in 2002 can expect to live 75.1 years, compared with 68.8 years for black males (Arias, 2004, p. 3). White females born in 2002 have average life expectancies of 80.3 years, compared with 75.6 years for black women.

3. Life expectancies for persons with spinal cord injury decline with increasing level of the injury (i.e., injuries at higher segments of the spinal cord have worse prognoses than do lower-level injuries). However, even persons with high tetraplegia (injuries at C1–C4 of the cervical spinal cord), injured at age forty and surviving for a year, have life expectancies of twenty-one years, while those who require a ventilator to breathe will live another fourteen years (National Spinal Cord Injury Statistical Center, 2001).

4. A study of 7,258 Medicare beneficiaries older than age sixty-four who died between 1993 and 1998 found the following distribution across the four functional decline trajectories: 7 percent had sudden death; 22 percent had terminal illnesses; 16 percent had organ system failures; and 47 percent met frailty definitions (Lun-

ney, Lynn, and Hogan, 2002, p. 1110). Fewer than 8 percent fell into an "other" category.

5. As indicated in footnotes to table 1.2 and subsequent tables throughout the book using MEPS 2001 data, we sometimes used direct standardization methods to account for age category and sex distributions before calculating population percentages. Age categories generally used seven groupings (ages 18–44, 45–64, 65–69, 70–74, 75–79, 80–84, and 85+ years); analyses split by older and younger ages (age 16–64 years and age 65+) used only age categories in appropriate ranges. We performed this standardization to account for the differences in disability distributions by age and sex and their possible implications for the topic of specific analyses (e.g., regarding education levels, poverty income, and employment).

6. As noted in preface note 6, in some instances relative standard errors for given analyses exceeded 30, the threshold at which figures begin becoming unreliable. In these instances, we collapsed disability levels together to bolster the number of cases within each disability type. We originally separated "other race" into "Asian" and "other," but this split also yielded unreliable estimates so we grouped these categories together (table 1.3). Thus, "other" race respondents contain distinct subpopulations; Asians, who generally report low disability rates; and such populations as Native Americans and Asian and Pacific Islanders, who report very high rates.

Chapter 2

1. We use the lowercase "d" to refer to the sensory condition of deafness and the uppercase "D" to identify Deaf culture or Deaf community.

2. In England from the sixteenth through nineteenth centuries, reports circulated of vagrants self-mutilating and feigning impairments (Stone, 1984). In France, some beggars allegedly learned medicine to make their duplicitous ailments more realistic. Local leaders may have fabricated these reports to solidify their political control by stoking public fears of vagrants. For centuries, officials viewed vagrants, including those with disabilities, as dishonest and dangerous.

3. Studies performed in 1924 and 1925 using the audiometer suggested that children who were born deaf or became deaf very early in life (prelingually) and who had minimal if any residual hearing were less likely than other deaf children to learn to speak proficiently or to benefit from oral educational programs (Burch, 2001, p. 226). The data bolstered the position of the Deaf community that purely oral educational methods would fail for an important subset of deaf children. Oralists, however, refused to accept the pedagogical implications of these findings.

4. The American Occupational Therapy Association and American Physical Therapy Association were established in 1917 and 1921, respectively, while the American Congress of Rehabilitation Medicine was founded only in 1933 and the Physical Medicine and Rehabilitation Academy in 1938 (Institute of Medicine, Committee on Assessing, 1997, p. 31).

5. Goffman viewed many other characteristics beyond disability as potentially stigmatizing, including virtually any attribute that makes an individual different or unusual within specific contexts and is putatively associated with weakness, inferiority, or other undesirable traits. In certain contexts, minority race and ethnicity could be stigmatizing, as could specific religions, poverty, illiteracy, and many other factors.

6. Franklin Delano Roosevelt, who had contracted polio in 1921, mastered this craft. Although Roosevelt never truly walked again, he also rarely complained or talked about his impairment to family or friends. To achieve his political goals, he created a fiction. After arduous practice, Roosevelt learned to swing his legs sequentially forward while being carried by his elbows, thus appearing to walk. Endeavoring to avoid crutches, Roosevelt strove to "stand easily enough in front of people so that they'll forget I'm a cripple" (Gallagher, 1994, p. 63). With the press guarding this deception, the public largely remained unaware that Roosevelt used a wheelchair.

7. Critics argue that the ICF fails to distinguish clearly between activities and participation, making the classification difficult to apply reliably. Concerns about these potentially overlapping concepts almost derailed final agreements on the ICF's classification scheme. WHO staff and member organizations plan to characterize these concepts more explicitly in future versions of the ICF.

8. Persons receive cash benefits five months after qualifying for SSDI. Two years later, they get Medicare coverage. In 2001, Social Security waived the two-year waiting period for Medicare coverage for persons with amyotrophic lateral sclerosis. This generally rapidly progressive, debilitating, neurological illness often kills persons within three years of diagnosis, so the two-year wait was unreasonable. Persons disabled by other life threatening conditions, like cancer, still have to wait for two years to receive Medicare coverage.

9. Social Security Act amendments of 1956 introduced cash benefits for disabled workers between fifty and sixty-five years old; 1958 amendments granted cash benefits to children and dependent spouses of disability recipients; 1960 amendments extended benefits to workers under age fifty; and 1965 amendments changed the definition of "permanent disability" to one "expected to continue for at least 12 months" (Stone, 1984, p. 78). SSI passed in 1972 and extended coverage to persons disabled before age twenty-two who had never worked. The Institute of Medicine (Committee to Review, 2002) offers a comprehensive account of the complicated history of disability programs and policies overseen by the Social Security Administration.

10. This dichotomous judgment diverges from the tactic taken by other Western nations. In the late 1800s, Germany, for example, stipulated that injured workers perform other suitable labor rather than quit entirely. From its inception, German pension policy "anchored disability to the inability to earn a certain amount, rather than to a total incapacity to earn" (Stone, 1984, p. 66). When persons could no longer perform their former jobs, the question became what alternative work should be expected or required.

11. The SSA created the List to streamline decision-making in the face of its burgeoning work load: between 1960 and 1965, SSDI applications had increased

26.4 percent, from 418,600 to 529,300 (Institute of Medicine, Committee to Review, 2002, p. 36).

12. State DDSs evaluate persons with impairments that are severe but not included in the List for their "residual functional capacity"—what persons can still do in their prior work setting despite their present physical or mental impairments. In 2002, roughly 60 percent of disability decisions were based on the List, without conducting complete functional and vocational assessments (Institute of Medicine, Committee to Review, 2002, p. 124).

13. State vocational rehabilitation agencies supposedly must routinely evaluate Social Security recipients to evaluate their job potential and need for training and assistive technologies, but this process is haphazard at best. Over the years, Congress has periodically passed initiatives to encourage return to work, some of which include provisions to support assistive devices, workplace accommodations, and retention of health insurance coverage. One such initiative is the Ticket to Work and Work Incentives Improvement Act of 1999 (P.L. 106-170). Evaluations of the effectiveness of the Ticket to Work program continue.

14. Title I ADA employment provisions apply only to employers with "15 or more employees in each working day in each of 20 or more calendar weeks in the current or preceding calendar year" or organizations meeting other specified criteria [Sec. 101(5)].

15. According to the Code of Federal Regulations (CFR), the ADA did use different language to define its target population than had the Rehabilitation Act and Section 504, although the ADA's intentions are virtually identical:

> The use of the term "disability" instead of "handicap" . . . represents an effort by the Congress to make use of up-to-date, currently accepted terminology. The terminology applied to individuals with disabilities is a very significant and sensitive issue. As with racial and ethnic terms, the choice of words to describe a person with a disability is overlaid with stereotypes, patronizing attitudes, and other emotional connotations. (28 CFR Part 36, Sec. 36.104)

16. On May 29, 2001, the Supreme Court ruled seven to two that walking five miles or so around a golf course is not fundamental to the game and therefore Martin (given his serious physical impairment) merits that accommodation. In his dissent, Justice Antonin Scalia called the majority's opinion a misguided intrusion of compassion into the rule of law (and the rules of golf) rather than as a matter of justice.

17. Many other important Supreme Court cases have addressed additional provisions of the ADA. Two particularly critical rulings preclude persons from suing states for monetary damages under Title I of the ADA. In *Board of Trustees of the University of Alabama et al. v. Garrett et al.*, decided five to four on February 21, 2001, two employees of Alabama sued the State under Title I. Patricia Garrett, a registered nurse, had been a director of nursing at the University of Alabama in Birmingham Hospital when she developed breast cancer. During her cancer treatment, she took extensive leave from work, and when she returned, Garrett had lost her nursing director position and was demoted to nurse manager, a lower-

paying job. Milton Ash, who filed a separate suit, had worked as a security officer for the Alabama Department of Youth Services. Because of asthma and at his physician's recommendation, Ash requested that his employer limit his exposure to cigarette smoke and carbon monoxide; Ash later developed sleep apnea and requested reassignment to daytime shifts. His employer denied Ash's requests. The Supreme Court ruled that individuals cannot bring lawsuits for monetary damages against states under the ADA. Writing for the majority, Chief Justice William H. Rehnquist asserted that, in passing the ADA, Congress had failed to show a convincing pattern of discrimination by states against people with disabilities, as would be required for these persons to meet the "equal protection" assurances of the Fourteenth Amendment. Rehnquist continued, "Thus, the Fourteenth Amendment does not require States to make special accommodations for the disabled, so long as their actions toward such individuals are rational. They could quite hardheadedly—and perhaps hardheartedly—hold to job-qualification requirements which do not make allowance for the disabled." Writing for the four dissenting justices, Justice Stephen G. Breyer rejected Rehnquist's assertion that states did not demonstrate a pattern of discrimination against people with disabilities: "The powerful evidence of discriminatory treatment throughout society in general, including discrimination by private persons and local governments, implicates state governments as well, for state agencies form part of that larger society."

18. Chapter 2 of the Body Functions section relates to "seeing and related functions" (codes b210–b229) while chapter 3 addresses "hearing and vestibular functions" (codes b230–b249) (WHO, 2001, p. 33). Chapter 7 addresses "neuromusculoskeletal and movement-related functions" in three parts: "functions of the joints and bones" (codes b710–b729); "muscle functions" (codes 730–b749); and "movement functions" (codes b750–b789) (WHO 2001, pp. 35–36).

Chapter 3

1. Legislative reports and statements during congressional deliberations guide interpretation of the ADA (Feldblum, 1991, p. 101). This record contains four relevant points. First, employers may not refuse to hire persons because they will generate higher insurance or health care costs. Second, employers and health insurers may keep "preexisting condition clauses" in their health plans, even if such provisions deny benefits for specified periods to persons with disabilities (e.g., a health plan could exclude diabetes care for some period for workers with preexisting diabetes). Third, employers and health insurers may limit coverage for specified procedures or treatments. Finally, employers may not allow health plans to deny coverage completely based on a person's diagnoses. Even if plans exclude payments for preexisting conditions or specified therapies, they must cover other health problems, procedures, or treatments. Title V of the ADA [Sec. 501(c)] addresses aspects of the insurance issue.

2. We focus here on Medicare and Medicaid because these are the largest public insurers of individuals with disabilities. However, other federal health care programs—the Veterans Health Administration and CHAMPUS (the Civilian

Health and Medical Program of the Uniformed Services)/TRICARE (a medical program for active duty members, qualified family members, and specified other individuals)—cover substantial numbers of individuals with disabilities. Especially when disabilities relate to their military service, both veterans and active-duty military personnel often have more generous benefit options around rehabilitation services and assistive technologies, such as sophisticated prosthetic devices, than in other public and private programs. Specific benefit packages vary depending on various factors, including an individual's military status and the nature of his or her health conditions.

3. Other reasons for failing to comply with medication regimens include forgetfulness, 47.4 percent; side effects, 24.5 percent; perceived lack of need, 22.0 percent; and inability to pick up or obtain medications from the pharmacy, 3.3 percent (Kennedy and Erb, 2002, p. 1121).

4. The 1972 legislation made persons with end-stage renal disease (ESRD) eligible for Medicare after waiting for three months. Although ESRD can be profoundly disabling, the ESRD Medicare benefit represents its own special entitlement separate from Social Security policies.

5. The Consolidated Omnibus Budget Reconciliation Act of 1985 makes employer-sponsored health insurance available for eighteen months after persons leave jobs, with monthly premiums set at 102 percent of employers' costs (Dale and Verdier, 2003, p. 7). Persons with disabilities can receive eleven additional months of coverage at 150 percent of employers' costs.

6. Even persons with sufficiently low incomes and assets to meet Medicaid's financial requirements can face administrative barriers to enrolling in the program (Dale and Verdier, 2003, p. 4). Sometimes states pose more stringent disability determinations than those of Social Security. Typical income limits range from 74 percent to 100 percent of poverty levels, with assets limited to $2,000 for individuals and $3,000 for couples.

7. Riley (2004) estimated costs of eliminating the twenty-four month waiting period at $5.3 billion in 2000 dollars, lower than the $8.7 billion in 2002 dollars estimated by Dale and Verdier (2003). The latter estimate, however, includes disabled adult children and widow(er)s instead of only the disabled workers considered by Riley.

8. We do not address the thorny topic of what happens to Medicare coverage if SSDI recipients become able to return to work. Loss of Medicare (and Medicaid) coverage poses a huge hurdle to moving persons who could return to work off the SSDI rolls. The Ticket to Work and Work Incentive Improvement Act of 1999 makes it easier for SSDI recipients to retain Medicare when returning to work and to remove limits on Medicaid buy-in programs for disabled workers. Anecdotal evidence suggests that the Ticket to Work program has yet to yield its anticipated widespread benefits.

9. Although President Franklin D. Roosevelt wanted to add health insurance to his 1935 Social Security bill, he did not, concerned that opponents, such as organized medicine, would derail his entire Social Security plan. Decades later, Johnson administration officials underscored Medicare's focus on acute care in short-stay hospitals to gain congressional support. Policy-makers feared that adding chronic

care would exacerbate concerns about uncontrollable costs and block political approval (Fox, 1993, p. 75).

10. Although the major political impetus behind the Medicare Prescription Drug, Improvement, and Modernization Act (MMA) was providing drug benefits to elderly individuals, disabled beneficiaries actually use more prescription medications than persons age sixty-five and older: in 1998, disabled and elderly beneficiaries filled an average of thirty-four and twenty-five drug prescriptions, respectively; and annual drug spending totalled $1,284 versus $841 for disabled versus elderly beneficiaries (Briesacher et al., 2002, p. 6). However, political debates about prescription drug benefits largely disregarded disabled beneficiaries. Section 721 of the MMA directly targets potentially disabled individuals by calling for fee-for-service beneficiaries to voluntarily participate in chronic care improvement programs, including disease management programs (see chapter 11). The program initially targets persons with diabetes, congestive heart failure, and chronic obstructive pulmonary disease.

11. Prohibitions against covering exercise programs might change for obese Medicare beneficiaries: in July 2004, the Secretary of Health and Human Services, Tommy G. Thompson, announced that Medicare would henceforth consider obesity to be a disease and thus be eligible for treatment under the Medicare statute. Over the next years, CMS will determine which obesity-related services Medicare will cover.

12. As of 1982, Medicare added health maintenance organizations (HMOs) to traditional indemnity coverage. Many of these plans provided prescription drugs and other benefits not covered by traditional Medicare, but they also tended to recruit healthier Medicare beneficiaries than average. The Balanced Budget Act of 1997 and the Balanced Budget Refinement Act of 1999 introduced new types of health plans—managed care organizations (MCOs)—and reimbursement policies (risk adjustment and new ways of setting local payment rates). Many MCOs revised their benefits packages, with some eliminating the additional services and others dropping Medicare enrollees.

13. Although Medicare is a federal program, specific coverage decisions for certain items and services can sometimes vary depending on the geographic region and local Medicare carrier policies and procedures. While some Medicaid programs closely follow Medicare's definition of medical necessity, others promulgate their own standards, which can differ widely.

14. The 1997 Balanced Budget Act also changed the way that Medicare pays SNFs for rehabilitation therapies. Under the new payment methodology, SNFs receive fairly generous reimbursement for providing moderate to high amounts of rehabilitation, but once therapy minutes exceed 720 per week, SNFs get no additional payments. "The average SNF rehabilitation charge per hospital stay dropped by 44.6 percent after the new [payment system] was phased in, from $421 in 1997 to $233 in 2000" (White, 2003, p. 219).

15. The home health agency discharge after the football game was actually the second time that home care had ousted David Jayne for breaking Medicare's homebound rule. The first instance occurred one year earlier when he attended the funeral of a friend who had died from ALS. That time, Jayne worked with a disability advocacy organization to restore his home care (Byzek, 2003).

Chapter 4

1. According to the 2000 MEPS, only 0.2 percent of the 53.3 percent of persons with any disability who used a private clinician's office as their usual source of care saw a nurse practitioner and 0.1 percent saw another nonphysician—all others visited physicians (see also table 8.2 using MEPS 2001 data looking at specialty of usual source of care). However, 46.7 percent of persons with any disability used a clinic rather than a private office as their usual source of care. Nonphysicians and physicians practice in teams at many clinics.

2. These estimates come from the 2000 MEPS survey cycle so represent different respondents than those in table 4.1. Among persons age eighteen to sixty-four, 32.1 percent said they did not have a usual source of health care because they are seldom sick, while 9.4 percent were new to their area. The numbers of individual respondents to the 2000 MEPS age sixty-five and older who did not have a usual source of care were too small to produce rigorous estimates about why elderly persons did not have usual care sources.

3. The percentages come from the 2000 MEPS and are adjusted by age category and sex. Among persons with any major disability, 19.8 percent of those with Medicare coverage only reported not having a usual source of care, as did 6.9 percent with Medicaid only and 3.1 percent with Medicare and Medicaid.

4. The 1990 and 1991 National Health Interview Survey Hearing Supplement asked detailed questions about hearing, including timing of onset, whether respondents had bilateral hearing deficits, and extent of hearing difficulties (using two scales, the self-rated scale and Gallaudet Hearing Scale). This permitted researchers to separate prelingually from postlingually deafened individuals and to determine fairly precisely the extent of hearing loss. Using these data, Barnett and Franks (2002) found that, even adjusting for age, health status, income, education, and other demographic characteristics, prelingually deafened adults were much less likely than postlingually deafened and hearing persons to have seen a physician in the prior two years.

5. Private insurance paid for 58.8 percent of office visits in 2001, of which Medicare reimbursed 21.8 percent and Medicaid or the state children's health insurance program paid 7.2 percent. Patients themselves paid for 4.0 percent of visits.

6. In 2001, the median length of an office visit across physician specialties was 14.7 minutes (Cherry, Burt, and Woodwell, 2003, p. 35). Median visit lengths by specialty were 14.6 minutes for internal medicine, general and family practice, and ophthalmology; 14.5 minutes for otolaryngology; 14.2 minutes for orthopedic surgery; and 19.3 minutes for neurology.

7. Because of spending patterns in the early 2000s, by statute Medicare had to cut fees for physicians. The pressing question became whether continued cuts would prompt physicians to withdraw from Medicare, making it harder for beneficiaries like Joe Alto to find routine care. According to the Medicare Payment Advisory Commission (MedPAC, 2003b, p. 157), 70.1 percent of physicians accepted new Medicare fee-for-service beneficiaries in 2002, down from 76.4 percent in 1999. MedPAC warned that physicians might stop accepting new Medicare pa-

tients because of falling fees. The Medicare Prescription Drug, Improvement, and Modernization Act of 2003 (MMA) raises fees to certain physicians in specified years (MedPAC, 2004a, p. 106).

8. One focus group participant asked Judi Pitt why she did not get traditional Medicare and purchase a Medigap policy to cover prescription drugs. Judi responded that she couldn't pay the Medigap premium and that state Medicaid programs, which purchase Medigap policies for poor Medicare beneficiaries, would not apply to her since she is under sixty-five years old. "In fact, very few states offer guaranteed access to Medigap plans for the under-65 Medicare population with disabilities" while poor elderly individuals can get this benefit (Blanchard and Hosek, 2003, pp. 14–15). It is unclear how the prescription drug benefit in the MMA, scheduled to take effect in 2006, would affect Judi Pitt.

9. Facial expressions, such as raised eyebrows, are often part of ASL vocabulary. However, persons unfamiliar with ASL can misinterpret such facial expressions, viewing them as indicating emotion or as nonverbal aspects of spoken English (Barnett, 2002b). Sometimes the ASL-associated body movements and facial expressions can lead clinicians to misdiagnose expressive Deaf persons as having inappropriate affect, personality or mood disorders, or tics.

10. One study involving focus group interviews of persons age fifty-five and older who had become deaf before age ten found that participants never actually asked their physicians for sign language interpreters, even if they desired that communication accommodation. Complex reasons underlay reluctance to make this request, including fear of physicians' refusals, reluctance to upset the physician or patient-physician relationship, concerns about hiring an inadequate interpreter, and expectations that the physician would deny payment for the interpreter (Witte and Kuzel, 2000).

11. Quadriplegia and tetraplegia are synonyms, each meaning paralysis involving all four limbs. Especially for international usage, some now prefer the term "tetraplegia." The American Spinal Injury Association (www.asia-spinalinjury.org) maintains the *International Standards for Neurological Classification of SCI* (spinal cord injury), revised in 2002, aiming to improve the consistency of measurement of spinal cord injury across practitioners and researchers. Spinal cord injuries, even at the same vertebral level, have diverse manifestations.

12. Autonomic dysreflexia can be life-threatening and requires emergency treatment. In persons with cervical or high thoracic spinal cord injuries, autonomic dysreflexia presents as hypertensive crisis, with blood pressures exceeding 200/100 mm Hg. Painful, irritating, or uncomfortable stimuli below the level of the spinal cord injury generally precipitate these episodes; such stimuli include certain bladder and bowel conditions, urinary catheterization or bowel evacuation programs, injuries, pressure ulcers, and labor and delivery.

13. According to the Spina Bifida Association of America (2003), spina bifida is the most common permanently disabling birth defect, occurring in 1 in 1,000 live births in the United States. One of three types of neural tube defects (the others are anencephaly and encephalocele), the lesion causing spina bifida occurs in the first month of pregnancy. In severe cases, the spinal cord protrudes through the gap in the bony neural tube, requiring surgery within twenty-four hours of birth.

Most children born with spina bifida now live into adulthood because of sophisticated medical interventions.

14. According to MEPS 2001 data, 92.4 percent of persons with any impairment drive or are driven to their usual health care provider, while 5.3 percent take public transportation or taxis and 2.4 percent walk. Comparable figures for persons without any impairment are 95.1 percent, 3.0 percent, and 1.9 percent—not substantially different. Persons with hand difficulties demonstrate the least reliance on private cars: 88.5 percent of them drive or are driven, while 9.1 percent take public transportation or taxis and 2.4 percent walk.

15. In 2001, about 62 percent of hospital emergency departments (ED) were located in metropolitan statistical areas (MSA, major urban centers), and they saw 82.4 percent of the ED visits (McCraig and Burt, 2003, p. 4). The number of ED visits per 100 persons per year was 39.5 in MSAs and 33.7 in non-MSAs, not a statistically significant difference (12).

Chapter 5

1. All statements quoted in this chapter date from 2000 or later. Sometimes interviewees, like Todd Paulson, describe experiences that happened years earlier but explicitly note this timing. We did not include any examples that appear (from the context of the person's comments) to have happened long ago if the interviewee did not clearly specify the timing. Therefore, unless otherwise noted, all incidents described here occurred well after implementation of the ADA.

2. A Web site maintained by the U.S. Department of Justice (www.usdoj.gov/crt/ada/qasrvc.htm, accessed October 28, 2004) addresses common questions about service animals, starting by emphasizing that these animals are not pets. The site states, "Any service animal that displays vicious behavior towards other guests or customers may be excluded. You may not make assumptions, however, about how a particular animal is likely to behave based on your past experience with other animals."

3. The figures in table 5.1 come from the 1994 NHIS-D and Healthy People 2000 supplements, which queried people who had had a routine health care visit in the last three years about services recommended by the U.S. Preventive Services Task Force (Iezzoni et al., 2000a). For example, the surveys asked women over age forty-nine if they had had mammograms in the prior two years and asked women age eighteen through seventy-five who had not had a hysterectomy if they had had a Pap smear in the last three years. After adjusting for age category, race, Hispanic ethnicity, education, income, health insurance, and having a usual source of care, women with major mobility difficulties were 40 percent less likely than women without any mobility problems to have had Pap smears and 30 percent less likely to have had mammograms. We also examined relative use of preventive services for women who have vision or hearing impairments but found few differences with rates for women without disabilities (Iezzoni et al., 2001).

4. Data from 2001 MEPS suggest that these patterns may have changed somewhat from 1994–1995, the dates represented in table 5.1. Although women with

major lower extremity mobility difficulties still have lower rates of Pap smears and mammograms than women without any impairments, the differences are modest: 4.5 percentage points for Pap smears and 2.1 percentage points for mammograms. However, gaps have widened for other groups. For instance, only 68.1 percent of women with major hand difficulties received Pap smears compared with 84.4 percent of women without any impairments; 58.4 percent of women who are deaf or have major hearing impairments obtained mammograms, compared with 75.0 percent of women without any impairments.

5. In the study funded by AHRQ, we had initially planned to conduct systematic interviews of physicians and visits to practice sites—not to conduct formal accessibility evaluations but to make descriptive observations and talk with office staff about their experiences with patients with disabilities. However, these plans generated considerable resistance. We heard informally that physicians worried that we planned to conduct ADA audits and that our findings could potentially result in legal actions for ADA noncompliance. Several practices allowed us to visit and speak with roughly twenty physicians, nurses, and office staff. Their observations are not generalizable. Nonetheless, because what we learned is completely consistent with interviewees' reports and more general observations about the health care system, we feel comfortable presenting this information here.

6. Beginning November 1, 2002, the National Institute for Disability and Rehabilitation Research in the federal Department of Education funded the Rehabilitation Engineering Research Center on Accessible Medical Instrumentation at Marquette University, Milwaukee, Wisconsin. Among various activities, this five-year project aims to analyze the accessibility of medical diagnostic and therapeutic equipment, develop guidelines for improving accessibility, and educate health care professionals about this issue.

7. The Television Decoder Circuitry Act of 1990 (P.L. 101-431) amended Section 303 of the Communications Act of 1934 (47 U.S.C. 303) to require all televisions with picture screens thirteen inches large or greater manufactured or imported for use in the United States after July 1, 1993, to have built-in decoder circuitry designed to display closed-captioned television transmissions. In passing the act, Congress noted that closed-captioned television would assist not only persons who are deaf or hard of hearing but also immigrant populations trying to learn English as a second language.

8. In filing his lawsuit, John Lonberg, the Kaiser Permanente member, reported that he had not been weighed in the eighteen years since his spinal cord injury. As Sid Wolinsky, the attorney who filed the lawsuit, noted, "When it comes to recording the weight of disabled people, doctors just take their word for it, which is incredible . . . changes in weight tell a great deal about the progress of an illness (Glionna, 2000, p. 3).

9. Some fraction of persons report disability because of serious systemic illness, such as cancer, heart disease, or emphysema. Those persons cannot exercise, and they are often underweight because of tissue wasting caused by their diseases. The NHIS-D found that 5.2 percent of persons without disability were underweight (<18.5 kg/m^2), as were 5.6 percent of blind/low vision; 5.5 percent of deaf/hard of hearing; 12.6 percent with severe lower extremity mobility difficulties; 8.9 per-

cent with severe upper extremity mobility difficulties; and 10.9 percent with severe manual dexterity problems (Weil et al., 2002, p. 1267).

Chapter 6

1. Schmittdiel and colleagues (2000, p. 761) surveyed 10,205 patients age thirty-five to eighty-five, grouping them for analysis into four dyads: female patients of female physicians; male patients of female physicians; female patients of male physicians; and male patients of male physicians. Among patients who chose their physicians, women who chose female physicians were generally the least satisfied with their care, while men who chose female physicians were the most satisfied.

2. This study analyzed audiotapes of 537 office visits in eleven sites (including clinics and private and group practices) across the United States and Canada (Roter et al., 1997). However, the visits occurred in 1985 and 1986. Changes in attitudes and goals of patients as health care consumers since then may make findings from this unique study somewhat out of date.

3. Several factors could explain lesser participation in their health care among persons who self-identify as "sick." One cause could relate to becoming a "'sick person,' which relieves him or her of some or all of the ordinary obligations, depending on the severity of the illness" (Murphy, 1990, p. 19). We do not discuss the "sick role" concept, advanced by mid-twentieth century sociologist Talcott Parsons and much studied by others. When people become newly disabled, aspects of the sick role may affect their behaviors and expectations at various points.

4. In this study, Murray-García and colleagues (2000, p. 301) received responses from 11,494 persons enrolled in a large California health plan (71.4 percent response rate). The percentage responding that they "worry about my health more than other people my age" varied by race and ethnicity: 17 percent of white, 33 of black, 38 percent of Latino, and 55 percent of Asian respondents (p. 305). Feeling that their physician is "courteous, respectful, sensitive, friendly" was rated as "more important than anything else" by only 15 percent of whites but by 27 percent of blacks, 24 percent of Latinos, and 22 percent of Asians. Having their physician show "concern for emotional and physical well-being" was viewed as "more important than anything else" by 17 percent of whites compared with 27 percent of blacks, 25 percent of Latinos, and 22 percent of Asians (p. 304).

5. Regardless of health status, people should document their preferences for specific clinical interventions if they become unable to make or articulate decisions. Explicit advance care planning involves specific legal documents meeting standards set by each state. A "living will" documents an individual's instructions for treatment should a person become unable to express his or her preferences. A "health care proxy" is someone assigned the legal authority to make medical decisions when individuals no longer can; the "durable power of attorney" is a written form used to appoint a health care proxy (Lynn and Harrold, 1999, p. 121).

6. Inevitably, disagreements can arise between clinicians and patients (or their proxies), particularly around appropriate interventions at the very end of life. Although technological interventions can now temporarily maintain certain core

physiologic functions, such as machine-assisted ventilation to oxygenate blood and powerful drugs to elevate falling blood pressures, at some point preserving these functions becomes futile. The question then becomes what to do when the inevitable catastrophic event occurs (e.g., when the heart stops beating). Should physicians intervene to "resuscitate" the patient and reinstitute "life support"? In good medical practice, this question is discussed between clinicians and patients well before patients lose their abilities to articulate their preferences. Following patients' wishes, physicians can write "do not resuscitate" orders, meaning that clinicians would not intervene after catastrophic events. Sometimes, patients and/or family members have unrealistic expectations about the ability of technological interventions to restore or preserve basic physiologic functioning. In these instances, physicians can ethically withhold resuscitation because it is physiologically futile (Waisel and Truog, 1995).

7. Some deaf interviewees noted that hearing people learn routine health facts and preventive practices from public service announcements on television and radio (as "background noise") and in print media that deaf persons rarely access: for instance, a primary ASL speaker, for whom English is a second language, may not pick up newspapers or magazines prepared for general audiences. Sometimes, special health education programs prepared specifically for the Deaf community provide people's first knowledge of such topics as HIV infection and prevention. Limited amounts of health information are available in ASL or by TTY on public Internet sites, such as video clips or TTY connections at the HIV "frequently asked questions" Web site sponsored by the Centers for Disease Control and Prevention (www.ashastd.org/nah/tty/ttyfaq.html, accessed December 17, 2004).

8. Gallaudet University, founded in 1864, is dedicated to higher education of persons who are deaf or hard of hearing. The March 1988 uprising of students demanding appointment of a deaf president—all prior leaders had been hearing—catapulted Gallaudet to national prominence and helped spur the disability rights movement. The protests succeeded when Gallaudet appointed I. King Jordan as its first deaf president (Fleischer and Zames, 2001, p. 28).

9. The physician's office staff did not have legal authority to force Brad Pepperill to have a urine test to check for traces of cocaine. However, because Brad did not know what was going on—and because events apparently happened so rapidly—he had limited ability to protest. Without an ASL interpreter present, the physician and office staff could have easily misinterpreted Brad's vigorous protestations (most likely conveyed with rapid hand gestures, bodily movements, and pointed facial expressions) as threatening, even manifestations of active cocaine use. The situation could have rapidly escalated out of control.

10. To some people, the attitudes and actions of the actor and later activist Christopher Reeve, who died in 2004, personified the conflict between reality and irrational hope. Reeve became tetraplegic after falling from his horse in 1995. Immediately following his spinal cord injury, Reeve heard uniformly gloomy predictions from his clinicians about his prognosis—no one with such a massive injury had ever recovered his or her ability to walk. Within the year, however, Reeve turned with energy and hope to medical science. "I've always been a practical person, not one to waste time in the pursuit of unrealistic goals or dreams," Reeve

wrote in his autobiography *Still Me* (1998, p. 133). "By the end of 1995 I was firmly convinced that the push for a cure was based on reality and not on unfounded optimism." Reeve (p. 135) began his advocacy with an address to an American Paralysis Association fundraiser, proposing to challenge medical researchers to find this cure just as President John F. Kennedy had proposed landing a man on the moon decades earlier: "This time the mission would be the conquest of *inner* space, the brain and central nervous system. . . . To create a sense of urgency, and to give the quest a human face, I declared my intention to walk by my fiftieth birthday, only seven years away." Reeve's advocacy did motivate massive spending increases on spinal cord injury and other medical research. However, some people worried that the cure Reeve sought was many years away and that his fame and single-minded focus diverted scarce resources away from other, perhaps more achievable lines of scientific inquiry. Some felt that Reeve's example might give other persons with spinal cord injury a false sense of hope, delaying the "acceptance" of disability and postponing their willingness to move on and live their lives as they now are.

11. Of course, things are never simple. Later in the interview, Vic admitted to another reality that derails even the most thoughtful mobility plan: "I can't use my wheelchair because I don't have accessible housing. The places where I go are not accessible. So if I was to use the wheelchair, I'd have a really hard time. What am I going to do? Stay in my house all day?"

12. The 1994 National Health Interview Survey Healthy People 2000 supplement asked questions about reproductive health issues only of respondents under age fifty. However, sexuality also concerns many elderly persons. Physical conditions often associated with aging, such as diabetes, cardiopulmonary diseases, and various medications for common chronic conditions can compromise sexual functioning, as can many other factors (Sipski, Alexander, and Sherman, 2005, p. 1584). Therefore, clinicians should broach sexuality with older patients and follow patients' wishes about additional discussions.

13. We used separate multivariable logistic regression models to examine the association between each provider query and each disabling condition, adjusting for age, race, ethnicity, family income (<$15,000, $15,000– ≤$30,00, $30,000– ≤$50,000, >$50,000), and education (≤high school, college, >college). After adjusting for these factors, women in several disability categories reported significantly fewer contraception queries than other women: adjusted odds ratio = 0.3 (95 percent confidence interval = 0.1, 0.8; p = 0.02) for major lower extremity mobility difficulties; 0.6 (0.5, 0.8; p = 0.002) for some lower extremity mobility difficulties; 0.5 (0.3, 0.9; p = 0.02) for some upper extremity mobility difficulties; and 0.4 (0.2, 0.7; p = 0.002) for some hand difficulties. For men, no differences in contraception queries were statistically significant. No comparisons of sexually transmitted disease queries were significant for either men or women.

14. When discussing sexuality among women with disabilities, a troubling historical backdrop involves the forced sterilization of disabled women (especially those with developmental disabilities) living in institutions, aiming to prevent them from having children (Asch and Fine, 1988). According to a 1999 Committee Opinion of the American College of Obstetricians and Gynecologists, involuntary sterilization should be viewed as "ethically not acceptable because of the violation

of privacy, bodily integrity, and reproductive rights" (Quint, 2004, p. 267). Connie Wilder, in her late thirties with muscular dystrophy (generally an inherited condition, although it can occur through spontaneous genetic mutations), offered hints that vestiges of such views persist. "I was taught early on in life that I should go on birth control because, God, they would not want me to get pregnant." Connie's gynecologist repeatedly underscored this point, making her feel devalued and uncomfortable. "They didn't want me to have babies like me."

15. Intracavernosal injection of various medications can treat most forms of erectile dysfunction by relaxing the sinusoidal smooth muscle and enhancing corporeal filling (Sipski, Alexander, and Sherman, 2005, p. 1598). These injections are less useful in men with impaired arterial blood flow. The procedure can cause various complications, including penile pain during injections and prolonged erections.

16. Cognitive dysfunction (e.g., in brain injury or certain diseases) can complicate assessment of mental health (Rohe, 2005). Various questionnaire and testing instruments can help skilled clinicians disentangle cognitive and emotional functioning.

17. After getting an affirmative answer to any of the mental health questions, NHIS-D interviewers asked, "During the past 12 months, did any of these problems SERIOUSLY interfere with [your] ability to work or attend school or manage [your] day-to-day activities?" The percentages responding "yes" to this question for being frequently depressed or anxious were as follows: 0.9 percent, no disability; 10.9 percent, blind or low vision; 6.8 percent, deaf or hard of hearing; 20.4 percent, major lower extremity mobility difficulty; 18.5 percent, major upper extremity mobility difficulty; and 19.5 percent, major hand dexterity difficulty.

18. Figures from the 2001 MEPS suggest that smoking rates may have fallen since 1994, the date of the NHIS-D (table 6.4). According to the 2001 MEPS, the following percentages of individuals currently smoke or use other tobacco products (figures account for age category and sex): 21.7 percent, no impairment; 30.5 percent, blind or very low vision; 32.0 percent, deaf or very hard of hearing; 34.9 percent, moderate lower extremity mobility difficulty and 42.9 percent for major difficulty; 32.2 percent, some upper extremity mobility difficulty and 38.3 percent for major difficulty; and 35.4 percent for some hand difficulty and 39.5 percent for major difficulty.

19. As for the modeling described earlier in note 13, we conducted multivariable logistic regression analyses predicting physician queries about substance use. Differences in queries across the impairment categories did not reach statistical significance except for tobacco queries for persons with major lower extremity mobility difficulties: adjusted odds ratio = 0.7 (0.6, 0.9; p = 0.05).

Chapter 7

1. The HIPAA Privacy Rule, implemented April 14, 2003, primarily addresses access to medical records, limits use of private health information, and prohibits marketing activities using private health data. In addition, the Privacy Rule re-

quires health care providers to "permit individuals to request an alternative means or location for receiving communications of protected health information by means other than those" typically employed (U.S. Department of Health and Human Services, 2003, p. 13). Health care providers must train their workforces on policies and procedures for protecting private health information and must sanction employees who fail to comply.

2. These figures come from the 2001 MEPS and are not adjusted for age category and sex. The impairment associated with the longest waits is major upper extremity mobility difficulties: 16.3 percent of these individuals report waiting thirty-one to fifty-nine minutes, and 10.5 percent waited an hour or more.

3. Many women with limited hip range of motion, postmenopausal vaginal atrophy, women who have not had children, and those who are not sexually active may find insertion of the speculum especially uncomfortable (Welner et al., 1999). A speculum with narrower blades can minimize discomfort in these situations. Women with neurologic conditions that relax their pelvic structures can require a larger speculum to compensate for this anatomic laxity.

4. Questions arise about whether "chaperones" should be present during physical examinations. In the past, standard practice held that male physicians needed chaperones while examining female patients, but this simple rule fails to recognize other gender-related complexities (Gabbard and Nadelson, 1995). No systematic guidelines exist today about the need for chaperones during physical examinations. However, chaperones are strongly recommended in certain situations, including exams of patients with histories of sexual or physical abuse, extreme anxiety or psychiatric conditions, and litigious tendencies.

5. In the study by Young and colleagues (1997), roughly 62 percent of women with and without disabilities reported physical, sexual, or emotional abuse at some point during their lives. About 4 percent of women reported emotional abuse by attendants, with 4.6 percent reporting emotional abuse by health care providers.

6. Among Medicare beneficiaries with very low vision, 17.0 percent and 8.6 percent (for those younger than and older than age sixty-five years, respectively) report dissatisfaction with telephone access (Iezzoni et al., 2002, p. 375). For Medicare beneficiaries who are deaf or hard of hearing in these two age groups, 17.2 percent and 8.7 percent express dissatisfaction with telephone access.

7. Since Sylvie Park survived four days without long-term consequences, obviously the medication side effect was not serious. However, this after-the-fact judgment misses the point. Anti-seizure medications are powerful drugs and require careful monitoring when patients switch regimens. Sylvie could have had a dangerous reaction to her new medication. Her nurse should have responded quickly to Sylvie's telephone call.

Chapter 8

1. Relying heavily on communication between patients and clinicians for making diagnoses and managing care is inappropriate in certain contexts. Neonatal

care is one obvious example, as is intensive care of patients who are not fully conscious or able to speak. In both instances, evaluation of physiological parameters (e.g., heart and respiratory rates, serum chemistry and hematology studies, arterial oxygenation), as well as physical examinations, drive clinical assessments and therapeutic decision-making. In pediatrics, clinicians rely heavily upon reports from parents about very young children.

2. These words appeared in a letter, enclosed in the book, dated February 9, 1982, from the president of the Harvard Medical Alumni Association to members of the Harvard Medical School Class of 1984.

3. According to Shattuck, "Success in the practice of medicine lies in a happy marriage between science and art." He viewed the seven elements of success as (a) knowing clinical science; (b) thoroughness; (c) common sense; (d) character, including high ideals; (e) enthusiasm and love for the profession; (f) sympathy, empathy, and cheerfulness; and (g) honesty of mind.

4. Clinical interviews also provide opportunities to observe patients' functioning, such as breathing rates and patterns; skin color, moistness, and tone; coherence and pace of speech; eye, hand, limb, and other movements; and appearance of pain, energy, and alertness. These observations guide clinicians' subsequent questioning and physical examinations.

5. These numbers come from 876 women age sixty-five and older who participated in the second interviews of the Women's Health and Aging Study, a longitudinal, population-based study of the one third of women in this age group who live with at least mild disabilities in communities (Leveille, Fried, and Guralnik, 2002). The study started in 1992 and sampled women living in the city and county of Baltimore, Maryland. Complete details about the Women's Health and Aging Study are available on the National Institute on Aging Web site at www.nia.nih.gov/health/pubs/whasbook/title.htm, accessed April 6, 2004.

6. These numbers also come from the Women's Health and Aging Study (see note 5), from the baseline assessment of 1,002 women in this longitudinal study (Leveille et al., 2001). Among these women—all with at least some mild disability—24 percent reported widespread musculoskeletal pain.

7. "C-5 quad" indicates that Mrs. Patrick's spinal cord injury occurred at the level of her fifth cervical vertebra. In situations that cause pain, persons with high-level spinal cord injuries are susceptible to autonomic dysreflexia (see note 12, chapter 4). Tylenol might help assuage Mrs. Patrick's pain from her hemorrhoidectomy. But different types of pain control (i.e. techniques that block pain sensations from reaching the spinal cord, such as epidural anesthetics) are needed to prevent autonomic dysreflexia. When Mrs. Patrick delivered her son, she received epidural anesthesia to reduce her risks of autonomic dysreflexia. For women with high spinal cord injuries, anesthesiologists may insert epidural catheters not necessarily for pain control during labor and delivery but for blocking the sensory input to the spinal cord that could precipitate autonomic dysreflexia.

8. Today, most blind and low-vision children attend public schools rather than special schools for blind students, and the percentage of school-aged children who use braille as their primary reading medium has dropped from 50 percent in the 1960s to just over 10 percent today. New computer tools, such as screen readers,

and audio recordings lessen the impetus for children with vision deficits to learn braille. Some believe that these technologies allow students to attain sufficient literacy levels, although this position is controversial. More information about teaching braille to children and legal, policy, and practical issues raised by braille usage is available at the Web site of the National Federation of the Blind at: www.nfb.org/brailco.htm, accessed December 21, 2004.

9. A closed-circuit television (CCTV), or video magnifier, uses video cameras, either handheld or stand-mounted, to project a magnified image onto a video or computer monitor or a television screen. Cameras with zoom lenses provide variable levels of magnification. More information about CCTV and video magnifier technologies is available in the "Browse Products" section of the American Foundation for the Blind Web site at www.afb.org/ProdBrowseCatResults.asp?CatID=53, accessed April 4, 2004.

Chapter 9

1. The Program of All-Inclusive Care for the Elderly (PACE) patterned itself after a model program called On Lok, a senior day health care center started in San Francisco's Chinatown neighborhood in 1971. In 1979, On Lok obtained Medicare funding to demonstrate its comprehensive program of interdisciplinary care involving physicians, nurses, physical and occupational therapists, social workers, dieticians, health workers, and drivers. In 1986, newly named PACE programs began disseminating elsewhere, and the Balanced Budget Act of 1997 certified PACE as a specific Medicare provider type. More information about On Lok, which continues today, is available at www.onlok.org and information about PACE is posted by the National PACE Association at www.npaonline.org

2. Many factors have slowed the spread of PACE programs, including difficulties competing for participants with other providers, unwillingness of potential enrollees to transfer all their care to PACE physicians, high start-up costs, and logistical and financial challenges of maintaining staffing and comprehensive services (Gross et al., 2004).

3. Medicare covers eyeglasses under narrow circumstances but virtually never reimburses hearing aids, although some private insurers do. Medicare pays for cochlear implant surgery if persons meet five guidelines: (a) diagnosis of bilateral severe-to-profound sensorineural hearing impairment with limited benefit from appropriate hearing aid; (b) cognitive ability to use auditory cues and willingness to receive extensive rehabilitation; (c) middle ear and relevant neurologic functioning conducive to implant; (d) no contraindications to surgery; and (e) use meets requirements of Food and Drug Administration (American Medical Association, 2003, p. 192). Medicare covers augmentative and alternative communication devices or communicators for persons with severe speech impairments but only when the device's sole purpose is generating speech: personal computers that do other tasks (such as word processing), as well as performing speech synthesis functions, do not qualify.

4. The name "Quickie" is a lighthearted, double entendre, mocking the assumption that sex life ends when legs stop working.

5. Anecdotally, these situations reflect calculations that are cynical at best. Insurers anticipate that once the enrollee enters the nursing home, they can transfer coverage to another insurer, most likely Medicaid. Thus, they would no longer bear responsibility for repairing or replacing an expensive power wheelchair.

6. Total Medicare reimbursements for power wheelchairs grew from $289 million in 1999 to more than $845 million in 2002 and are projected at $1.2 billion in 2003 (CMS, 2003b). In 1999, just over 55,000 Medicare beneficiaries had at least one claim for a motorized wheelchair, compared with almost 159,000 in 2002—a 189 percent increase. By contrast, total Medicare costs rose only 11 percent during that time period, and the overall Medicare population grew only 1 percent per year. An investigation by the Office of the Inspector General in the Department of Health and Human Services uncovered frequent fraudulent billings and documentation, as well as charges for equipment never delivered, especially in certain regions (Harris County, Texas, was a particular hot spot, with Medicare reimbursing 31,000 power wheelchairs in 2002, compared to just over 3,000 in 2001). In 2003, Medicare initiated "Operation Wheeler Dealer" to expose vendors exploiting Medicare. The Medicare agency is currently considering a policy change that would greatly restrict coverage of all mobility aids.

7. The Cash and Counseling Demonstration and Evaluation Project, co-funded by The Robert Wood Johnson Foundation and the U.S. Department of Health and Human Services, is exploring the feasibility and outcomes of directly paying cash benefits to Medicaid recipients in several states who, in turn, arrange their own PAS (Mahoney et al., 2004). Current law prohibits states from giving federal funds in cash directly to Medicaid recipients. This demonstration will assess whether changing that prohibition for PAS is warranted.

8. The MiCASSA legislation includes a provision for quality assurance programs to promote consumer control and satisfaction with their community attendant services.

9. Often collaborating with senior citizen's organizations, disability advocates have filed lawsuits against local transportation authorities nationwide, asserting the right to accessible public transportation under Section 504 of the 1973 Rehabilitation Act (see chapter 2). Many transit agencies fought back, citing the prohibitive costs of making local buses and subway systems accessible. In some jurisdictions, years of litigation and vocal protests ensued (Fleischer and Zames, 2001).

10. The Bay Area Rapid Transit (BART) system, built in the 1960s, became an exemplar of barrier-free mass transit design, motivated largely by the tireless actions of Harold Willson, the senior economic analyst of the Kaiser Medical Care Program and a wheelchair user (Fleischer and Zames, 2001, p. 63). Using designs and specifications from the American National Standards Institute, Willson demonstrated how designs to improve physical access to buildings could transfer to subway design. He and other advocates lobbied the California legislature for additional funding to construct elevators and make BART widely accessible.

11. If patients are not ready when The RIDE van arrives, it may leave without them to pick up other scheduled passengers. Because The RIDE is often heavily booked, drivers may not return to retrieve a late passenger.

12. These numbers come from Phase II of the 1994–1995 NHIS-D. Among persons with major difficulty walking, 39 percent live in houses with more than one level, 32 percent have difficulty reaching or opening cabinets, and 16 percent have difficulty opening or closing doors at home.

13. These injury figures come from a 1997 nationwide survey conducted by the National Center for Health Statistics. Setting of injuries differs by sex: among men, 17.6 percent of injuries occurred within homes, while 32.0 percent of injuries among women happened within homes (Warner, Barnes, and Fingerhut, 2000, p. 23). Across sexes, 17.8 percent of injuries occurred at home but outdoors; 17.4 and 18.2 percent of injuries among men and women, respectively, had this location.

14. Housing discrimination prohibitions of the Civil Rights Act of 1968 (Title VIII, also known as the Fair Housing Act) did not apply to persons with disabilities.

Chapter 10

1. After graduating with a master's degree in political science from the University of California at Berkeley in 1966, Roberts (1939–1995) became a world leader in the disability rights movement, founding important organizations (such as the Center for Independent Living in the Bay Area in 1972 and the World Institute on Disability in 1983, along with Judith Heumann and Joan Leon) and leading the California Department of Vocational Rehabilitation from 1975 to 1983 (Pelka, 1997, pp. 266–267).

2. Other relevant federal statutes include the Individuals with Disabilities Education Act of 1975, the Fair Housing Amendments Act of 1988, and Section 508 of the Rehabilitation Act Amendments of 1998. By 1973, forty-nine states had enacted their own accessibility legislation, although some of the standards were voluntary and thus not enforceable.

3. In the early 1970s, Mace (1941–1998) left the practice of conventional architecture and began designing the first building codes for accessibility in the United States. North Carolina mandated this code in 1973; the code became a model for other states. In 1989, Mace founded the Center for Universal Design at the School of Design at North Carolina State University, which became a leader in universal design innovation and teaching (www.design.ncsu.edu/cud/center/history/ronmace.htm, accessed June 8, 2004). Recent cuts in federal funding for universal design activities have put the future of this center at risk.

Chapter 11

1. One complication of diabetes is decreased sensations in the toes, feet, and lower limb. Thus, patients may not detect injuries in these areas, increasing the risks of wounds that fail to heal and develop gangrene. Sighted persons could simply visually inspect their feet periodically, but someone who is blind cannot. Standard prac-

tice guidelines for persons with diabetes, regardless of their visual acuity, stipulate annual visits to podiatrists for professional assessments of foot health.

2. Marcia McDonough had a sufficiently low spinal cord injury that autonomic dysreflexia was unlikely. Persons with higher thoracic and cervical spinal cord injuries face the greatest risks of this dangerous complication (see note 9 of chapter 4 and note 7 of chapter 8).

3. Although patients legally have the right to obtain and read their medical records, historically physicians and other health care providers have honored this right reluctantly. As one rationale, health care professionals often cite concerns that patients might be troubled by what appears in their records. This, in turn, may cause clinicians to limit or skew what they write in medical records. With new electronic medical records potentially offering easier access to patients, some health care providers are revisiting their resistance, considering not only allowing open availability to patients but also letting patients make additions and corrections to their medical records (Slack, 2004).

4. Persons with neurologic bladder problems face increased risks of urinary tract stones, which are the leading cause of kidney failure in this population. Calcium loss from bones following spinal cord injury, paralysis, or body immobilization is well recognized but difficult to control. Reducing dietary intake of calcium (to 400 to 500 mg/day) can lower risks of stones for some patients. Other dietary modifications, as well as medications, can also reduce stone formation. Increasing fluid intake, to dilute the urine and decrease mineral crystallization, is also important but may present difficulties for persons who must catheterize themselves to empty their bladders (Williams and Hopkins, 2005, p. 1284).

5. Evidence suggests that being obese or overweight reduces the development of osteoporosis in older women. Multiple factors likely contribute to this finding, such as mechanical forces and higher hormone levels associated with elevated weight (including estrogen synthesis in adipose tissues). However, the myriad negative consequences of excess weight, especially for a manual wheelchair user like Candy Bonner, far outpace any potential benefits from lower bone loss. Furthermore, little evidence about the protective effects of added weight derives from persons with physical disabilities.

6. Our description draws primarily from the perspectives of Stanford University's Chronic Disease Self-Management Study (Lorig et al., 2000) and the Chronic Care Model developed at the MacColl Institute for Healthcare Innovation, Group Health Cooperative of Puget Sound (Bodenheimer, Wagner, and Grumbach, 2002). Funded largely by The Robert Wood Johnson Foundation, both programs have undergone extensive research and are described in numerous publications and on Web sites: for example, patienteducation.stanford.edu and www.improvingchroniccare.org for the MacColl Institute. Various self-management initiatives and chronic care proposals share the goal of maximizing patients' goals and preferences. Details of specific approaches vary across programs. In particular, because of important differences in their health care systems, European perspectives on chronic care and self-management diverge somewhat from U.S.-derived models.

7. The critical concept underlying the self-management approach is "self-efficacy"—patients' confidence that they can perform an action necessary to

achieve a desired goal (Bodenheimer et al., 2002, p. 2472). The psychologist Albert Bandura first described self-efficacy in the late 1970s, drawing upon personality and social cognitive theory. Self-efficacy serves as the key element in motivating behavior change, and self-efficacy beliefs predict persons' abilities to achieve good treatment outcomes in certain disorders (Miller and Rollnick, 1991, p. 60).

8. The reviewed studies varied in terms of the nature of the self-management intervention, experimental design, patient populations, and specific outcomes of interest. These differences impeded direct comparisons of results (Bodenheimer et al., 2002). Research on self-management has important limitations, notably the reliance on volunteers rather than randomly selected participants. Volunteers would likely have greater motivation to achieve benefits and comply with self-management precepts than persons recruited randomly from the community. In addition, studies typically do not follow participants across years; effects of self-management may fade over time.

9. Section 721 of the Medicare Prescription Drug, Improvement, and Modernization Act of 2003 calls for voluntary chronic care improvement programs, including self-management training, for fee-for-service beneficiaries, starting in certain regions of the country (MedPAC, 2004b, p. 35). If the initial projects go well, CMS would disseminate the program elsewhere. The program targets persons with diabetes, congestive heart failure, and chronic obstructive pulmonary disease.

10. Two organizations at the forefront of developing shared decision-making tools are the Center for Shared Decision Making associated with Dartmouth Medical School and Dartmouth-Hitchcock Medical Center in Hanover, New Hampshire (www.hitchcock.org); and the Foundation for Informed Medical Decision Making in Boston (www.fimdm.org/shared_decision_making.php).

Chapter 12

1. The researchers surveyed 233 emergency providers at three Level I trauma centers in metropolitan Denver (including emergency medical technicians, emergency nurses, emergency medicine residents, and attending physicians), achieving a 63 percent response rate. Different professionals responded differently to key questions. When asked if they would want everything possible done to ensure survival if they themselves arrived with a high cervical spinal cord injury (therefore with obvious tetraplegia), only 14 percent of nurses agreed, compared with 29 percent of emergency medical technicians and 37 percent of physicians (Gerhart et al., 1994, p. 809).

2. According to the Curriculum Directory maintained by the American Association of Medical Colleges, none of the 125 U.S. or 16 Canadian medical schools in the database offer formal courses on disability. A search of courses using "disability" as the keyword found no listings: services.aamc.org/currdir/section4/start.cfm, accessed November 12, 2004.

3. We interviewed fourteen students during their final year at medical school (Iezzoni, Ramanan, and Drews, 2005). By this time, students have had considerable clinical experience and their styles for interacting with patients have matured.

To recruit students, we approached the three Boston medical schools—Boston University, Harvard, and Tufts—for permission to recruit their students. Two schools gave permission and provided e-mail lists of their final-year students. We wrote a solicitation e-mail describing our project about how students are taught about communicating with patients with sensory and physical disabilities. We invited all students who responded affirmatively to this e-mail to participate in one of two focus groups conducted in February 2002.

4. Levodopa is a synthetic compound of L-dopa used to treat Parkinson's disease. Shortly after ingesting the drug, patients who previously appeared frozen in place can once more initiate movement. The drug can also precipitate unintentional body movements that are difficult to control.

5. Scoliosis involves curvature of the spine. In this instance, the student is likely describing "kyphosis," where the spine curves forward as vertebrae collapse and persons increasingly appear bent over.

6. Techniques for so-called "motivational interviewing" originated in efforts by therapists to motivate behavior change among persons addicted to alcohol and illicit drugs. It builds upon precepts of Carl Rogers, who asserted that client-centered interpersonal relationships between therapists and clients could encourage behavior change when therapists offer three critical conditions: "accurate empathy, nonpossessive warmth, and genuineness" (Miller and Rollnick, 1991, p. 5).

7. Inquiring about a patient's typical day takes six to eight minutes on average, which may be too long in busy practices. However, as Rollnick, Mason, and Butler (1999, p. 110) note, it could replace up to twenty questions clinicians might ask about a patient's situation and furthermore "helps to cement rapport between the parties."

8. Each medical school is responsible for determining "essential functions" or "technical standards" (i.e., "essential eligibility" requirements) for its own program (Cohen, 2004). What might constitute "reasonable accommodations" using the ADA framework (see chapter 2) ties directly to these essential functions: if students ask for accommodations that fundamentally differ from standard training program requirements or that pose excessive burdens on the school, institutions could claim that the request does not meet the "reasonableness" test. Medical schools differ widely in how they establish these criteria.

9. The Association of Medical Professionals with Hearing Loss (AMPHL), founded in 2000, targets physicians, veterinarians, dentists, nurses, physician's assistants, therapists, and other health care professionals, including trainees. AMPHL aims to disseminate information about useful technologies and services, including amplified, electronic, and visual stethoscopes; see-through surgical masks; and sign language interpreters, Communication Access Realtime Translation (CART), and assistive listening devices (www.amphl.org/htmlindex.html, accessed May 24, 2004).

Chapter 13

1. Title III of the ADA covers private health care providers. The Department of Justice issued regulations concerning the obligations of private organizations at 28

CFR Part 36 (the Department's analysis of this regulation is at 56 *Federal Register* 35544-35691, 26 July 1991). Title II of the ADA covers health care facilities operated by state and local governments. Title II and III regulations concerning communication access are similar.

2. Sometimes the goals of Deaf persons who communicate in ASL diverge from this overarching goal of avoiding segregation of persons with disabilities. These individuals do not view deafness as a disability (see chapter 2), instead seeing themselves as a linguistic and cultural minority. Some Deaf persons advocate for services that are separate but equal to those provided hearing persons, rather than receiving services integrated with the majority community. Differing perspectives on advocacy goals and disability can cause friction between Deaf ASL speakers and other disability advocates, as well as with health care providers. Communication barriers can impede efforts to resolve such differences.

3. In discussing the ADA requirements for interpreter services, the National Association of the Deaf Law Center (2004) underscores the inadequacy of lip reading and note writing during critical medical discussions. On average, the best lip readers accurately understand only 25 percent of spoken words, and this comprehension level falls with unfamiliar medical terms. Note writing is especially problematic for ASL users who have limited English facility. Furthermore, note writing is slow and cumbersome, likely limiting clinicians' discourse with patients (chapters 6 and 7).

4. Definitions of what poses "undue burden" vary depending on the financial resources of organizations (and "parent" organizations, as appropriate), number of persons employed, and legitimate safety requirements (28 CFR, Sec. 36.104).

5. Tax credits are deducted from an organization's tax liability after it calculates its taxes. In contrast, tax deductions are subtracted from an organization's total income before taxes, thus setting its "taxable income." To gain tax relief, all accommodations cited as expenses must meet ADA regulatory standards. "Tax Incentives Packet on the Americans with Disabilities Act," a 2001 document from the Department of Justice, is available at www.usdoj.gov/crt/ada/taxpack.htm, accessed May 30, 2004.

6. The American Foundation for the Blind Web site has a Technology section that includes excellent descriptions of various information, computer, and communication technologies. Much of the discussion in this chapter derives from that Web site at www.afb.org/Section.asp?SectionID=4, accessed June 9, 2004. The National Federation of the Blind Web site (www.nfb.org) offers information about numerous "Aids & Appliances," which visitors can purchase online.

7. Video Relay Services (VRS) differ importantly from Video Relay Interpreting (VRI), described later in chapter 13. In VRI, both the deaf and hearing communication partners are in the same room, but the sign language interpreter is in a remote location. With VRS, the deaf and hearing persons are in different locations, and they are linked through a communications assistant sign language interpreter through the telecommunications relay service.

8. The University of Rochester Medical Center in Rochester, New York, conducted these tests of sign language interpretation, and video clips of the results are available at: www.urmc.rochester.edu/strongconnections/videohtml, accessed December 17, 2004. ISDN stands for Integrated Services Digital Network and rep-

resents the system of digital telephone connections that allows voice and data to be transmitted simultaneously. The University of Rochester experiment compared one line ISDN (128 kbs or 1,000 bits per second) versus three line ISDN (384 kbs).

9. The Registry of Interpreters for the Deaf had, at one time, offered twenty different types of certificates, but RID now sponsors only a few specific certificates (www.rid.org/expl.html, accessed May 19, 2004). Different certificates address various skills, including ASL, transliteration between English-based sign language and spoken English, and silent oral techniques and natural gestures. One certificate specifically applies to interpretation in legal settings. No certificate explicitly addresses medical encounters.

10. "Clear" surgical face masks are basically standard masks with a window cut into them around the mouth area and covered with transparent material. Given hopes that these clear face masks would facilitate lip reading, their tendency to "fog up" as the wearer's breathe condenses posed an initial problem. The patent holder on these masks has worked largely successfully to eliminate fogging (Carroll, 2002).

11. Infrared systems transmit sounds by invisible light beam; therefore, they do not work outdoors or near bright incandescent lights. Receivers (in lavaliere or headset styles) must fall directly in line with the infrared light beam that transmits the sound. Infrared systems work well for television viewing and small group meetings. FM systems transmit sound using radio waves, which can penetrate walls and ceilings. Speakers wear a compact transmitter and microphone, while listeners use a portable receiver with headphones or earphones. FM systems work well in groups, both indoors and outdoors. Loop systems, based on electromagnetic principles, assist persons with hearing aids with a telecoil circuit. This ALD involves placing a loop wire around a listening area; the primary speaker then uses a special amplifier and microphone. The loop wire amplifies and circulates speech signals, while telecoil-equipped hearing aids pick up the signal. Persons without these hearing aids can access this magnetic signal using special receivers with earphones. Loop technologies work particularly well in automobiles and classrooms. When installing these technologies in medical settings, users must consider whether the infrared beam, radio waves, or electromagnetic fields would interfere with medical equipment. Prices for ALD technologies vary from less than $200 to around $1,800.

12. When printing texts of conversations, typical TTYs automatically use all capital letters for one party and lower case letters for the other, so that readers can easily differentiate who was speaking. When typing on TTYs, ASL users do not follow any specific conventions about using capital letters. Capital letters are not part of ASL since ASL does not spell using an alphabet. It relies instead upon hand movements and other gestures and facial expressions to convey complete concepts.

Chapter 14

1. This statement pertains to building or renovation projects involving private properties. When constructing or adapting public-sector properties, attention to accessibility standards is typically strict. State or local governmental programs gen-

erally cannot lease space that fails accessibility standards, and they cannot contract with any entity that does not comply with access requirements (Duprey, 2004, p. 21).

2. Beyond ADA and comparable Section 504 regulations, various state and local laws and federal and state building codes address physical accessibility (Carpman and Grant, 1993, pp. 218–219). The American National Standards Institute (ANSI) developed the first accessibility standard in 1961. ANSI has renewed and revised this standard, known as ANSI A117.1, over the years, and many states use it as their code. Federal building codes include the Minimum Guidelines of the Architectural and Transportation Barriers Compliance Board (an independent federal agency) and the Uniform Federal Accessibility Standard (UFAS). Conflicts among technical specifications of some building codes and the way they are applied have generated considerable controversy. Efforts are under way to resolve differences among various building codes and standards.

3. Title III regulations contain ADA construction guidelines, which apply to private entities; the Architectural and Transportation Barriers Compliance Board develops these guidelines. Title II entities (state or local government providers) can either follow the ADA guidelines or the UFAS standard mentioned in note 2, this chapter (Duprey, 2004).

4. Connecticut Senator Lowell Weicker introduced the first draft of the ADA as S. 2345 on April 28, 1988 (Young, 1997, p. 207). When Joseph Lieberman defeated Weicker, the ADA lost a powerful advocate and sponsor in the Senate. Iowa Senator Tom Harkin and Representative Tony Coelho assumed leadership on the legislation, jointly reintroducing the ADA as S. 933 and H.R. 2273 on May 9, 1989.

5. For instance, when renovating a "primary function area" (e.g., lobby, waiting room), an accessible path of travel to that area is required; furthermore, the restrooms, telephones, and water fountains serving that area must also be accessible. These accessibility requirements are waived if the additional costs are "disproportionate," defined as exceeding 20 percent of the costs of the original alteration (Duprey, 2004, p. 22).

6. Various governmental agencies enforce other statutes that grant civil rights to persons with disabilities. For instance, the U.S. Department of Housing and Urban Development oversees provisions of the Fair Housing Act of 1988, and the U.S. Department of Transportation enforces the Air Carrier Access Act of 1986.

7. On January 13, 2004, the U.S. Supreme Court heard arguments in *Tennessee v. Lane*, where the main issue revolved around Section 502 of the ADA: "A State shall not be immune under the eleventh amendment to the Constitution of the United States from an action in Federal or State court . . . for a violation of the Act." Congress added this section based on their findings of systematic discrimination by states in the past against persons with disabilities.

8. Beverly Jones, who is paraplegic and works as a certified court reporter, joined George Lane in the lawsuit. Jones alleged that, unable to enter several Tennessee county courthouses, she had lost employment and income and been unable to participate fully in the judicial process.

9. In his dissent to *Tennessee v. Lane*, joined by Associate Justices Anthony Kennedy and Clarence Thomas, Chief Justice Rehnquist wrote, "We have never

held that a person has a *constitutional* right to make his way into a courtroom without any external assistance. Indeed, the fact that the State may need to assist an individual to attend a hearing has no bearing on whether the individual successfully exercises his due process right to be present at the proceeding. Nor does an 'inaccessible' courthouse violate the Equal Protection Clause, unless it is irrational for the State not to alter the courthouse to make it 'accessible.' But financial considerations almost always furnish a rational basis for a State to decline to make those alterations" (p. 10).

10. Title III of the ADA prohibits providers from segregating or isolating individuals with disabilities from other persons, unless doing so will ensure equal opportunity. For instance, health care providers cannot require persons with disabilities to use a side entrance or wait in private waiting rooms because their presence makes other people uncomfortable (Duprey, 2004).

11. The Department of Justice resolved all 114 cases either through lawsuits or alternative resolution approaches (Reis et al., 2004, p. 15). In addition to the access cases, other issues included sixty-five cases concerning effective communication for persons who are deaf or hard of hearing, including twenty-five in hospitals and thirty-four in offices; eight cases regarding HIV status; and one relating to intellectual disabilities.

12. The complete text of the March 2001 settlement of *Metzler v. Kaiser Foundation Health Plans, Inc.*, No. 829265-2 (California Superior Court, Alameda County) is available at: www.resna.org/taproject/policy/health/kaiser-s.doc, accessed July 20, 2004.

13. The 2001 JCAHO accreditation manual for hospitals contains more explicit language about communication access (Reis et al., 2004, p. 26). In particular, hospitals are to provide access to translation services when necessary; have TTY access through their switchboards; provide amplification devices for telephones in patients' rooms as appropriate; and supply patient information in braille or on audiocassette.

14. This discussion draws upon information from various sources: the Center for Universal Design at North Carolina State University's guide for removing barriers to health care (Mace, 1998; this guide can be downloaded as a PDF file at www.design.ncsu.edu/cud); Adaptive Environments, a nonprofit organization in Boston that specializes in human-centered design (www.adaptenv.org); IDEO, a company with offices worldwide (Palo Alto, San Francisco, Chicago, Boston, London, and Munich, www.ideo.com) that helps design health care settings, as well as diverse products and services; and books and pamphlets (Ferreyra and Hughes, 1984; Carpman and Grant, 1993; Welner, 1999; Duprey, 2004; Welner and Temple, 2004).

15. *Design That Cares* (Carpman and Grant, 1993) uses this sequential approach and offers detailed checklists for planning health care facilities that make patients and visitors feel welcome, safe, and confident. Other publications also provide space-by-space guidance for designing health care settings specifically for persons with disabilities (Mace, 1998; Welner and Temple 2004).

16. Information about independent living centers in various communities, updated weekly, is available through the Independent Living Research Utilization or-

ganization (www.ilru.org/jump1.htm, accessed November 14, 2004). Many local independent living centers maintain their own Web sites.

17. Many different technologies can assist with alerting persons about emergencies, but each has pros and cons and specific requirements. For instance, strobe lights should emit five or fewer flashes per second due to the risk of triggering seizures in some individuals. Details about different alerting devices and other assistive technologies for evacuation planning are available in Batiste and Loy (2004). The "Emergency Preparedness Initiative" of the National Organization on Disability, begun in response to the terrorist attacks of September 11, 2001, offers useful information for emergency managers, planners, and responders (www.nod.org).

18. In 2002, nursing aides and orderlies had the second highest number (79,000) of occupational injuries and illnesses involving days away from work following truck drivers (112,200); registered nurses experienced 21,900 such events (Bureau of Labor Statistics, 2004a). Across all occupations, the most common site of injuries is the trunk of the body (522,100 injuries), including 345,300 involving the back and 83,900 the shoulders (Bureau of Labor Statistics, 2004b). Contact with health care patients caused 70,000 illnesses or injuries in 2002, but the statistics do not indicate precisely how.

19. To determine weights, wheelchair users such as Gretchen (figure 14.5) ride onto the scale. Then the wheelchair's weight is measured without its occupant, perhaps when he or she is on the examining table. Subtracting the wheelchair's weight from the total weight yields the weight of the user. After weighing the wheelchair, staff could record its weight in the patient's medical record or affix a waterproof sticker with the weight onto the wheelchair's frame. That way, the wheelchair never needs to be weighed again without its user.

20. Carpman and Grant (1993, pp. 229–231) review research findings and recommendations about chairs, focusing particularly on needs of elderly persons. They recommend that seat angles not exceed 4 degrees and that chairs not have crossbars below the seat that prevent the user from tucking their legs under the front edge of the seat. Older persons typically position their heels under the front edge of the seat and grab onto arm rests to guide themselves as they sit down. When rising, they also use their heels, positioned under the front of the seat, to push themselves out and forward to standing positions. Nonabsorbent upholstery, such as vinyl, is uncomfortable, as are cushions that are exceedingly hard. These situations can contribute to skin ulcers for some persons who sit too long in these conditions.

Chapter 15

1. This number comes from telephone interviews conducted in late 2002 among a national sample of roughly 2,000 persons eighteen years of age and older. Since 2000, the Pew Internet & American Life Project has conducted this and other surveys aiming to explore how the Internet affects American society. Funded by The Pew Charitable Trusts, the project is part of the Pew Research Center for the Peo-

ple & the Press, based in Washington, DC. More information about this initiative and its multiple reports and tracking surveys is available at: www.pewinternet.org

2. Section 508 of the Rehabilitation Act Amendments of 1998 requires the Architectural and Transportation Barriers Compliance Board to publish standards for ensuring access for individuals with disabilities to electronic information produced by federal agencies, unless the agency would be unduly burdened by the requirements (36 CFR Part 1194). More information about these standards is available at www.access-board.gov/sec508/508standards.htm

3. According to a survey conducted by the Pew Internet & American Life Project in February 2004, the percentages of Americans who go online, by basic demographic characteristics, are as follows: women, 61 percent, men, 65 percent; age 18–29 years, 77 percent, 30–49 years, 74 percent; 50–64 years, 58 percent, 65+ years, 23 percent; white non-Hispanic, 64 percent, black non-Hispanic, 46 percent, Hispanic, 63 percent; urban, 65 percent, suburban, 67 percent, rural, 48 percent; household income less than $30,000 per year, 41 percent, $30,000–$50,000, 69 percent, $50,000–$75,000, 86 percent, more than $75,000, 89 percent; and less than high school education, 24 percent, high school, 54 percent, some college, 78 percent, and college+, 85 percent. These results are available at 207.21.232.103/trends/DemographicsofInternetUsers.jpg, accessed June 9, 2004.

4. These numbers and others that follow in this paragraph come from the 2002 survey described in note 1, this chapter.

5. Among Internet users, 85 percent of women seek health information compared with 75 percent of men; 87 percent of those with chronic health conditions search for health information online, as do 79 percent of those without chronic illness or disability.

6. Persons, largely middle-aged and female, seeking information for others often aim to assist family members or friends in making medical decisions (Fox and Fallows, 2003, pp. 20–23). The Internet facilitates immediate contact with their intended audience: for instance, a daughter can easily e-mail information to an ailing parent living in a distant state. Six million home caregivers go online, and they are more likely than other searchers to seek information about specific medical treatments, medications, experimental therapies, mental health care, and health insurance.

7. The Pew Internet & American Life Project conducted this survey between March 1 and May 19, 2002, with telephone surveys of 3,553 Americans nationwide (Horrigan et al., 2003). In-depth interviews with selected non-users and new Internet users, conducted in summer 2002, give additional insight into attitudes and experiences in these subgroups. Eighteen percent of the survey respondents reported having some disability—a fraction close to the nearly 20 percent identified by the U.S. Census. From published information, we cannot determine the nature of these disabling conditions (e.g., sensory or physical impairments). Persons also self-reported whether their disability impedes Internet use; non-users may have inadequate knowledge about the Internet to answer this question accurately.

8. This small study conducted by the Nielsen Norman Group involved twenty persons age sixty-five and older and twenty persons between ages twenty-one and fifty-five (Nielsen, 2002). Most older subjects were in their seventies, but the study did include some persons age eighty and older.

9. Comprehensive details about the Web Accessibility Initiative, as well as technical guidelines, checklists, and techniques to promote accessibility, appear at: www.w3.0rg/WAI/, accessed October 1, 2004.

10. The third component of e-health—after communication and decision support (i.e., electronic exchange of health information)—involves medical records (Bodenheimer and Grumbach, 2003). Although the transition to electronic medical records (EMR) is expensive (prohibitively so for some small medical offices), EMR technologies offer tremendous advantages, from guaranteeing legibility of medical records to rapid access of digital images (e.g., radiographs, electrocardiograms). EMR also provides the potential for monitoring health and health care experiences of patient populations and individual providers' panels (e.g., for quality improvement); identifying specific patients requiring particular services (e.g., screening tests); and enhancing medication safety (e.g., by tracking prescribed medications).

11. Lester Goodall's wry comment about Internet use at the office rings true. Persons with Internet and e-mail access in the workplace likely use these technologies mostly for work-related activities but might sneak in personal uses, although some employers monitor deviations from company policies. Most employees probably do not know that "employers own their e-mail systems and any messages sent or received over them. They have the right to review any e-mail message and may be subject to disclosing their contents in legal proceedings" (Spielberg, 1998, p. 1356).

12. This study, conducted by researchers at RAND in California, concentrated on health information relating to breast cancer, depression, obesity, and childhood asthma (Berland, et al., 2001). The first pages of links identified by search engines led to relevant information for only 20 percent of English and 12 percent of Spanish searches. On average, only 45 percent of English and 22 percent of Spanish language Web sites provided completely accurate and more than minimal information; 24 percent of English and 53 percent of Spanish language Web sites did not cover important clinical information.

Chapter 16

1. Access to public transportation, both fixed-route and paratransit systems, is particularly pressing for persons with visual disabilities who cannot drive. In sprawling suburbs, even simple errands, such as purchasing groceries or getting a hair cut, require driving. Persons with vision impairments who live alone or with others who do not drive may therefore need to find housing in urban settings or neighborhoods with good transportation access and nearby services.

2. The word "community" can have many different meanings. "Community is characterized by a sense of identification and emotional connection to other members, common symbol systems, shared values and norms, mutual—although not necessarily equal—influence, common interests, and commitment to meeting shared needs" (Israel et al., 1998, p. 178). Communities of identity (e.g., by race, ethnicity, religious faith) may live geographically dispersed rather than concentrated in specific locations. Given the fundamental importance to people with disabilities of physical accessibility within their neighborhoods and regions, we use "community" in its geographic sense.

3. The actual safety of paved bicycle trails to walkers and wheelchair users depends largely upon the behavior of the bicycle riders. Bonnie reports that cyclists largely respect and understand her white cane; I find congested urban bike trails more problematic than trails in less frequented parks (however, these are often more difficult to get to). A Web site linked to the nonprofit Rails-to-Trails Conservancy (www.railstrails.org) lists more than 1,200 paved bicycle trails built along abandoned railway corridors nationwide.

4. Historically, public health has had an uneasy relationship with some persons with disabilities. Since the mid-1800s, public health experts have focused on eliminating specific threats to population health, including infectious, environmental, occupational, nutritional, and other causes of disease or injury. "Public health messages have often depicted people with disabilities as the negative result of 'unhealthy' actions," and many people with disabilities have therefore "rejected public health as inimical to their very existence" (Lollar, 2001, p. 754). We acknowledge that our arguments here explicitly presume that, in most instances, persons would wish to avoid developing significant obesity, complicated diabetes, and debilitating arthritis. But we believe that the ability to prevent these conditions, which are admittedly sometimes unavoidable, resides not only with individual actions but also with the social and physical environments.

5. These percentages represent the median percentage reported within each of thirty states that asked questions about arthritis in their 2002 Behavioral Risk Factor Surveillance System survey (Centers for Disease Control, 2004b). For the three age groups studied (18–44, 45–64, and 65+), rates of reported arthritis and possible arthritis varied widely across states. For instance, rates of physician-diagnosed arthritis ranged from 17.8 percent in Hawaii to 35.8 percent in Alabama.

6. Rates of diagnosed diabetes are 5.8 percent for persons age forty through fifty-nine (Centers for Disease Control, 2003b). These figures, based on the National Health and Nutrition Examination Survey, failed to show rising rates of diabetes between 1988–1994 and 1999–2000, which the authors acknowledged as surprising, giving obesity trends. They suggest that additional research must hone these estimates and account for a 1997 change in the way physicians diagnosed diabetes (as recommended by an expert committee). Using the National Health Interview Survey, crude prevalence rates of self-reported diabetes have risen 89 percent from 1980 to 2002, but changes in the survey methodology in recent years could have artificially accentuated this trend (Centers for Disease Control, 2004a).

7. In 2001, for its annual Behavioral Risk Factor Surveillance System survey, the Centers for Disease Control and Prevention (2003c) broadened the list of what constitutes adequate exercise, including some physical activities that people routinely do throughout their day (so-called "lifestyle activity questions"), such as brisk walking, bicycling, vacuuming, gardening, or other actions that increase heart rate for at least ten minutes at a time. In addition, they collected more traditional measures of vigorous activity, such as running, calisthenics, golfing, jogging, and swimming. Because of the expanded definition, 45.4 percent of respondents in 2001 met criteria for adequate exercise, compared with 26.2 percent using the narrower 2000 definition.

8. With continually expanding populations infected with HIV and other localized infectious threats (e.g., drug-resistant tuberculosis, persistent polio in certain

locales), public health practitioners still closely monitor and address infectious diseases. But, especially in developed nations, chronic conditions now consume the majority of public health attention.

9. Car emissions contribute to air pollution, which exacerbates respiratory ailments among young and old and has long-term environmental consequences that could affect population health. Ample evidence makes the connection between density of cars and public health. For instance, when the Olympic games reduced vehicular traffic in Atlanta, peak ozone concentrations fell 27.9 percent, and the number of emergency asthma cases dropped 41.6 percent (Perdue, Stone, and Gostin, 2003, p. 1391). However, in this chapter, we focus primarily on the physical implications of the built environment, rather than the effects on air, water, and the natural environment. These less visible factors hold obvious implications, not only for the health of humans but also for the long-term well-being of all inhabitants of our planet and the Earth itself.

10. The inadequacies of public mass transportation for supporting healthy communities are legion. Not only would more effective mass transportation systems ameliorate vehicular congestion and pollution, but also they could encourage physical activity as persons walk to and from bus or subway stops.

11. Enforcing existing traffic safety laws could potentially reduce risks to pedestrians using crosswalks without traffic signals or stop signs. All states model their traffic laws upon the uniform vehicle code (11-502[a]), which reads, "when traffic control signals are not in place or not in operation, the driver of a vehicle shall yield the right of way . . . to a pedestrian crossing in the roadway within a crosswalk" (Runge and Cole, 2002, p. 2173). Unfortunately, traffic laws vary across states, and pedestrians and drivers may not know local rules. In addition, local police officers may not have adequate resources for comprehensive enforcement.

12. Much more information about various active living, as well as obesity programs, is available on The Robert Wood Johnson Foundation Web site at www.rwjf.org. The Active Living by Design program is run by the University of North Carolina at Chapel Hill School of Public Health; it offers grants to communities to design and implement activities (www.activelivingbydesign.org, accessed July 30, 2004). Research about the relationship of the built environment to physical activity receives funding through the Active Living Research Program, administered by San Diego State University (www.activelivingresearch.org/index.php, accessed July 30, 2004).

13. "Traffic calming" carries different names across the country. San Jose, California, officially calls it "neighborhood traffic management," while Boulder, Colorado, labels it "traffic mitigation" and Sarasota, Florida, refers to it as "traffic abatement." More information about this approach and examples of existing programs are available at www.trafficcalming.org

References

Accreditation Council for Graduate Medical Education. 1999. *General Competencies. Minimum Program Requirements Language,* approved by the ACGME September 28, 1999. www.acgme.org/outcome/comp/compMin.asp, accessed May 25, 2004.

Adaptive Environments. 2004. *Universal Design.* www.adaptenv.org, accessed June 4, 2004.

Albrecht, G. L., K. D. Seelman, and M. Bury, eds. 2001. *Handbook of Disability Studies.* Thousands Oaks, CA: SAGE Publications.

Allen, K., and J. Blascovich. 1996. The Value of Service Dogs for People with Severe Ambulatory Disabilities: A Randomized Controlled Trial. *Journal of the American Medical Association* 275(13):1001–1006.

American Medical Association. 2003. *Healthcare Common Procedure Coding System 2004. Medicare's National Level II Codes.* Chicago: AMA Press.

Andriacchi, R. 1997. Primary Care for Persons with Disabilities. The Internal Medicine Perspective. *American Journal of Physical Medicine and Rehabilitation* 76(3 Supplement):S17–S20.

Arias, E. 2004. United States Life Tables, 2002. *National Vital Statistics Reports* 53(6). Booklet. Hyattsville, MD: National Center for Health Statistics.

Asch, A., and M. Fine. 1988. Introduction: Beyond Pedestals. In *Women with Disabilities, Essays in Psychology, Culture, and Politics,* edited by M. Fine and A. Asch, 1–37. Philadelphia: Temple University Press.

Bakker, R. 1997. *Elder Design. Designing and Furnishing a Home for Your Later Years.* New York: Penguin Books.

Barnard, D. 1995. Chronic Illness and the Dynamics of Hoping. In *Chronic Illness. From Experience to Policy,* edited by S. K. Toombs, D. Barnard, and R. D. Carson, 38–57. Bloomington and Indianapolis: Indiana University Press.

Barnett, S. 2002a. Communication with Deaf and Hard-of-Hearing People: A Guide for Medical Education. *Academic Medicine* 77(7):694–700.

Barnett, S. 2002b. Cross-Cultural Communication with Patients Who Use American Sign Language. *Family Medicine* 34(5):376–382.

Barnett, S., and P. Franks. 1999. Smoking and Deaf Adults: Associations with Age at Onset of Deafness. *American Annals of the Deaf* 144(1):44–50.

Barnett, S., and P. Franks. 2002. Health Care Utilization and Adults Who Are Deaf: Relationship with Age at Onset of Deafness. *Health Services Research* 37(1):103–118.

Barry, M. J. 2002. Health Decision Aids to Facilitate Shared Decision Making in Office Practice. *Annals of Internal Medicine* 136(2):127–135.

Batavia, A. I. 2000. Ten Years Later. The ADA and the Future of Disability Policy. In *Americans with Disabilities: Exploring Implications of the Law for Individuals and Institutions,* edited by L. P. Francis and A. Silvers, 283–292. New York: Routledge.

Batiste, L. C., and B. Loy. 2004. *Employers' Guide to Including Employees with Disabilities in Emergency Evacuation Plans.* Job Accommodations Network. www.jan.wvu.edu/media/emergency.html, accessed July 9, 2004.

Beatty, P. W., and K. R. Dhont. 2001. Medicare Health Maintenance Organization and Traditional Coverage: Perceptions of Health Care among Beneficiaries with Disabilities. *Archives of Physical Medicine and Rehabilitation* 82(8):1009–1017.

Becker, H., A. Stuifbergen, and M. Tinkle. 1997. Reproductive Health Care Experiences of Women with Physical Disabilities: A Qualitative Study. *Archives of Physical Medicine and Rehabilitation* 78(12 Supplement 5):S26–S33.Beckman, H. B., and R. M. Frankel. 1984. The Effect of Physician Behavior on the Collection of Data. *Annals of Internal Medicine* 101(5):692–696.

Beckman, H. B., K. M. Markakis, A. L. Suchman, and R. M. Frankel. 1994. The Doctor-Patient Relationship and Malpractice. Lessons from Plaintiff Depositions. *Archives of Internal Medicine* 154(12):1365–1370.

Beckmann, C. R., M. Gittler, B. M. Barzansky, and C. A. Beckmann. 1989. Gynecologic Health Care of Women with Disabilities. *Obstetrics and Gynecology* 74(1):75–79.

Berkman, N. D., D. A. DeWalt, M. P. Pignone, S. L. Sheridan, K. N. Lohr, L. Lux, S. F. Sutton, T. Swinson, and A. J. Bonito. 2004. *Literacy and Health Outcomes. Summary, Evidence Report/Technology Assessment No. 87.* AHRQ Publication No. 04-E00701. Rockville, MD: Agency for Health Care Research and Quality, January.

Berland, G. K., M. N. Elliott, L. S. Morales, J. I. Algazy, R. L. Kravitz, M. S. Broder, D. E. Kanouse, J. A. Muñoz, J.-A. Puyol, M. Lara, K. E. Watkins, H. Yang, and E. A. McGlynn. 2001. Health Information on the Internet. Accessibility, Quality, and Readability in English and Spanish. *Journal of the American Medical Association* 285(20):2612–2621.

Betancourt, J. R., A. R. Green, and J. E. Carrillo. 2002. *Cultural Competence in Health Care: Emerging Framework and Practical Approaches.* New York: The Commonwealth Fund, October.

Blanchard, J., and S. Hosek. 2003. *Financing Health Care for Women with Disabilities.* RAND Health White Paper WP-139. Santa Monica, CA: RAND.

Blumenthal, D. 2002. Doctors in a Wired World: Can Professionalism Survive Connectivity? *Milbank Quarterly* 80(3):525–546.

Bodenheimer, T., and K. Grumbach. 2003. Electronic Technology. A Spark to Revitalize Primary Care? *Journal of the American Medical Association* 290(2):259–264.

Bodenheimer, T., K. Lorig, H. Holman, and K. Grumbach. 2002. Patient Self-Management of Chronic Disease in Primary Care. *Journal of the American Medical Association* 288(19):2469–2475.

Bodenheimer, T., E. H. Wagner, and K. Grumbach. 2002. Improving Primary Care for Patients with Chronic Illness. *Journal of the American Medical Association* 288(14):1775–1779.

Boult, C., M. Altmann, D. Gilbertson, C. Yu, and R. L. Kane. 1996. Decreasing Disability in the 21st Century: The Future Effect of Controlling Six Fatal and Nonfatal Conditions. *American Journal of the Public Health* 86(10):1388–1393.

Briesacher, B., B. Stuart, J. Doshi, S. Kamal-Bahl, and D. Shea. 2002. *Medicare's Disabled Beneficiaries: The Forgotten Population in the Debate over Drug Benefits.* New York: The Commonwealth Fund and Menlo Park, CA: Kaiser Family Foundation, September.

Burch, S. 2001. Reading between the Signs. Defending Deaf Culture in Early Twentieth-Century America. In *The New Disability History: American Perspectives,* edited by P. K. Longmore and L. Umansky, 214–235. New York: New York University.

Bureau of Labor Statistics, U.S. Department of Labor. 2004a. *Table 3. Number of nonfatal occupational injuries and illnesses involving days away from work by selected occupation and industry division, 2002.* www.bls.gov/news.release/osh2.t03.htm, accessed July 15, 2004.

Bureau of Labor Statistics, U.S. Department of Labor. 2004b. *Table 4. Number of nonfatal occupational injuries and illnesses involving days away from work by selected injury or illness characteristics and industry division, 2002.* www.bls.gov/news.release/osh2.t04.htm, accessed July 15, 2004.

Byrom, B. 2001. A Pupil and a Patient. Hospital-Schools in Progressive America. In *The New Disability History: American Perspectives,* edited by P. K. Longmore and L. Umansky, 133–156. New York: New York University.

Byzek, J. 2003. David Jayne: 2002 Person of the Year. *New Mobility* 14(112):32–38.

Calkins, D. R., R. B. Davis, P. Reiley, R. S. Phillips, K. L. Pineo, T. L. Delbanco, and L. I. Iezzoni. 1997. Patient-Physician Communication at Hospital Discharge and Patients' Understanding of the Postdischarge Treatment Plan. *Archives of Internal Medicine* 157(9):1026–1030.

Calkins, D. R., L. V. Rubenstein, P. D. Cleary, A. R. Davies, A. M. Jette, A. Fink, J. Kosecoff, R. T. Young, R. H. Brook, and T. L. Delbanco. 1991. Failure of Physicians to Recognize Functional Disability in Ambulatory Patients. *Annals of Internal Medicine* 114(6):451–454.

Calkins, D. R., L. V. Rubenstein, P. D. Cleary, A. R. Davies, A. M. Jette, A. Fink, J. Kosecoff, R. T. Young, R. H. Brook, and T. L. Delbanco. 1994. Functional Disability Screening of Ambulatory Patients: A Randomized Controlled Trial in a Hospital-Based Group Practice. *Journal of General Internal Medicine* 9(10):590–592.

Callahan, J. 1989. *Don't Worry, He Won't Get Far on Foot.* New York: Vintage Books.

Carpman, J. R., and M. A. Grant. 1993. *Design That Cares. Planning Health Facilities for Patients and Visitors. Second Edition.* San Francisco: Jossey-Bass.

Carroll, S. M. 2002. Progress with Clear Face Mask Project. *Journal of the Association of Medical Professionals with Hearing Losses.* www.amphl.org/jamphl/fal12002/cordwellcarroll.html, accessed December 17, 2004.

Cassell, E. J. 1985a. *Talking with Patients, Volume 1. The Theory of Doctor-Patient Communication.* Cambridge, MA: MIT Press.

Cassell, E. J. 1985b. *Talking with Patients, Volume 2. Clinical Technique.* Cambridge, MA: MIT Press.

Cassell, E. J. 1997. *Doctoring. The Nature of Primary Care Medicine.* New York: Oxford University Press.

Center for Health Policy Research. 1996. *Interdisciplinary Education and Training of Professionals Caring for Persons with Disabilities.* Washington, DC: George Washington University Medical Center, December.

Centers for Disease Control and Prevention. 2003a. Adults Who Have Never Seen a Health-Care Provider for Chronic Joint Symptoms—United States, 2001. *Morbidity and Mortality Weekly Report* 52(18):416–419.

Centers for Disease Control and Prevention. 2003b. Prevalence of Diabetes and Impaired Fasting Glucose in Adults—United States, 1999–2000. *Morbidity and Mortality Weekly Report* 52(35):833–837.

Centers for Disease Control and Prevention. 2003c. Prevalence of Physical Activity, Including Lifestyle Activities among Adults—United States, 2000–2001. *Morbidity and Mortality Weekly Report* 52(32):764–769.

Centers for Disease Control and Prevention. 2003d. Public Health and Aging: Projected Prevalence of Self-Reported Arthritis or Chronic Joint Symptoms among Persons Aged >65 Years—United States, 2005–2030. *Morbidity and Mortality Weekly Report* 52(21):489–491.

Centers for Disease Control and Prevention. 2004a. *Crude and Age-Adjusted Prevalence of Diagnosed Diabetes per 100 Population, United States, 1980–2002.* National Center for Chronic Disease Prevention and Health Promotion, Diabetes Surveillance System. www.cdc.gov/diabetes/statistics/prev/national/figage.htm, accessed July 26, 2004.

Centers for Disease Control and Prevention. 2004b. Prevalence of Doctor-Diagnosed Arthritis and Possible Arthritis—30 States, 2002. *Morbidity and Mortality Weekly Report* 53(18):383–386.

Centers for Disease Control and Prevention. 2004c. Prevalence of Overweight and Obesity among Adults with Diagnosed Diabetes—United States, 1988–1994 and 1999–2002. *Morbidity and Mortality Weekly Report* 53(45):1066–1068.

Centers for Disease Control and Prevention. 2004d. Prevalence of Visual Impairment and Selected Eye Diseases among Adults with and without Diabetes—United States, 2002. *Morbidity and Mortality Weekly Report* 53(45):1069–1071.

Centers for Disease Control and Prevention. 2004e. *Studies on the Cost of Diabetes.* National Center for Chronic Disease Prevention and Health Promotion, Division of Diabetes Translation. www.cdc.gov/diabetes/pubs/costs/intro.htm, accessed July 26, 2004.

Centers for Disease Control and Prevention. 2004f. Update: Direct and Indirect Costs of Arthritis and Other Rheumatic Conditions—United States, 1997. *Morbidity and Mortality Weekly Report* 53(18):388–389.

Centers for Medicare and Medicaid Services. 2002. *2002 CMS Statistics.* Office of Research, Development and Information. Baltimore, MD. CMS Pub No. 03437, April.

Centers for Medicare and Medicaid Services. 2003a. *Your Medicare Benefits.* Baltimore, MD: Centers for Medicare and Medicaid Services Pub. No. CMS-10116. April.

Centers for Medicare and Medicaid Services. 2003b. *New Efforts Aimed at Stopping Abuse of the Power Wheelchair Benefit in the Medicare Program.* Office of the Inspector General. Washington, DC: September 9.

Centers for Medicare and Medicaid Services. 2004. *2003 Data Compendium.* www.cms.hhs.gov/researchers/pubs/datacompendium/current/, accessed October 16, 2004.

Chan, S. 2003. Patients Allege Rights Violations, Inadequate Care. *Washington Post.* November 26:A8.

Charlton, J. I. 1998. *Nothing about Us without Us: Disability Oppression and Empowerment.* Berkeley: University of California Press.

Cherry, D. K., C. W. Burt, and D. A. Woodwell. 2003. National Ambulatory Medical Care Survey: 2001 Summary. *Advance Data from Vital and Health Statistics.* No. 337. Hyattsville, MD: National Center for Health Statistics, August 11.

Chow, A. W. 2002. Epidemiology, Pathogenesis, and Clinical Manifestations of Odontogenic Infections. *UpToDate Online 12.2.* March 21. www.uptodate.com, accessed August 9, 2004.

Cohen, J. J. 2004. A Word from the President. Reconsidering "Disabled" Applicants. *AAMC Reporter.* Washington, DC: American Association of Medical Colleges, June. www.aamc.org/newsroom/reporter/june04/word.htm, accessed June 14, 2004.

Cooper-Patrick, L., J. J. Gallo, J. J. Gonzales, H. T. Vu, N. R. Powe, C. Nelson, and D. E. Ford. 1999. Race, Gender, and Partnership in the Patient-Physician Relationship. *Journal of the American Medical Association* 282(6):583–589.

Corburn, J. 2004. Confronting the Challenges in Reconnecting Urban Planning and Public Health. *American Journal of Public Health* 94(4):541–546.

Crowley, J. S., and R. Elias. 2003. *Medicaid's Role for People with Disabilities.* Menlo Park, CA: Kaiser Commission on Medicaid and the Uninsured, August.

Dale, S. B., and J. M. Verdier. 2003. *Elimination of Medicare's Waiting Period for Seriously Disabled Adults: Impact on Coverage and Costs.* Publication No. 660. New York: Commonwealth Fund, July.

Daley, J. 1993. Overcoming the Barrier of Words. In *Through the Patient's Eyes,* edited by M. Gerteis, S. Edgman-Levitan, J. Daley, and T. L. Delbanco, 72–95. San Francisco: Jossey-Bass.

Dannenberg, A. L., R. J. Jackson, H. Frumkin, R. A. Schieber, M. Pratt, D. Kochtitzky, and H. H. Tilson. 2003. The Impact of Community Design and Land-Use Choices on Public Health: A Scientific Research Agenda. *American Journal of Public Health* 93(9):1500–1508.

Day, J. C. 1996. *Population Projections of the United States by Age, Sex, Race, and Hispanic Origin: 1995–2050.* Washington, DC: U.S. Bureau of the Census, Current Population Reports, P25-1130.

DeJong, G., S. E. Palsbo, P. W. Beatty, G. C. Jones, T. Kroll, and M. T. Neri. 2002. The Organization and Financing of Health Services for Persons with Disabilities. *Milbank Quarterly* 80(2):261–301.

Delichatsios, H., M. Callahan, and M. Charlson. 1998. Outcomes of Telephone Medical Care. *Journal of General Internal Medicine* 13(9):579–585.

DeNavas-Walt, C., B. D. Proctor, and R. J. Mills. 2004. *Income, Poverty, and Health Insurance Coverage in the United States: 2003.* U.S. Census Bureau, Current Population Reports, P60-226. Washington, DC: U.S. Government Printing Office, August.

Dolan, P. 1996. The Effect of Experience of Illness on Health State Valuations. *Journal of Clinical Epidemiology* 49(5):551–564.

Donabedian, A. 1980. *Explorations in Quality Assessment and Monitoring. Volume I. The Definition of Quality and Approaches to Its Assessment.* Ann Arbor, MI: Health Administration Press.

Drey, E. A., and P. D. Darney. 2004. Contraceptive Choices for Women with Disabilities. In *Welner's Guide to the Care of Women with Disabilities,* edited by S. L. Welner and F. Haseltine, 109–130. Philadelphia: Lippincott, Williams & Wilkins.

Duprey, M. 2004. Americans with Disabilities Act and the Women's Health Provider: What the Women's Health Provider Needs to Know about the ADA, Case Law Ramifications of Noncompliance, and the Like. In *Welner's Guide to the Care of Women with Disabilities,* edited by S. L. Welner and F. Haseltine, 17–24. Philadelphia: Lippincott, Williams & Wilkins.

Eichner, J., and D. Blumenthal, eds. 2003. *Medicare in the 21st Century: Building a Better Chronic Care System. Final Report of the Study Panel on Medicare and Chronic Care in the 21st Century.* Washington, DC: National Academy of Social Insurance, January.

Ewing, R. H. 1999. *Traffic Calming: State of the Practice.* Washington, DC: Institute of Transportation Engineers.

Feldblum, C. R. 1991. Employment Protections. In *The Americans with Disabilities Act. From Policy to Practice,* edited by J. West, 81–110. New York: Milbank Memorial Fund.

Ferreyra, S. and K. Hughes. 1984. *Table Manners. A Guide to the Pelvic Examination for Disabled Women and Health Care Providers.* San Francisco: Planned Parenthood Alameda/San Francisco.

Finkelstein, E. A., I. C. Fiebelkorn, and G. Wang. 2003. National Medical Spending Attributable to Overweight and Obesity. How Much, and Who's Paying? *Health Affairs Web Exclusive.* May 16. www.healthaffairs.org/WebExclusive/FinkelsteinWebExcl051403.htm, accessed May 14, 2003.

Flegal, K. M., B. I. Graubard, D. F. Williamson, and M. H. Gail. 2005. Excess Deaths Associated with Underweight, Overweight, and Obesity. *Journal of the American Medical Association* 293(15):1861–1867.

Fleischer, D. Z., and F. Zames. 2001. *The Disability Rights Movement. From Charity to Confrontation.* Philadelphia: Temple University Press.

Ford, J. A., M. K. Glenn, L. Li, and D. C. Moore. 2004. Substance Abuse and Women with Disabilities. In *Welner's Guide to the Care of Women with Disabilities,* edited by S. L. Welner and F. Haseltine, 315–331. Philadelphia: Lippincott, Williams & Wilkins.

Fox, D. M. 1993. *Power and Illness. The Failure and Future of American Health Policy.* Berkeley: University of California Press.

Fox, S. 2004. *Older Americans and the Internet. Just 22% go Online, but Their Enthusiasm for Email and Search May Inspire Their Peers to Take the Leap.* Washington, DC: Pew Internet & American Life Project, March 25.

Fox, S., and D. Fallows. 2003. *Internet Health Resources. Health Searches and Email Have Become More Commonplace, but There Is Room for Improvement in Searches and Overall Internet Access.* Washington, DC: Pew Internet & American Life Project, July 16.

Francis, L. P., and A. Silvers, eds. 2000. *Americans with Disabilities: Exploring Implications of the Law for Individuals and Institutions.* New York: Routledge.

Frankel, R., and H. Beckman. 1989. Evaluating the Patient's Primary Problem(s). In *Communicating with Medical Patients,* edited by M. Stewart and D. Roter, 86–98. Newbury Park, CA: Sage Publications.

Freedman, V. A, L. G. Martin, and R. F. Schoeni. 2002. Recent Trends in Disability and Functioning among Older Adults in the United States. A Systematic Review. *Journal of the American Medical Association* 288(24):3137–3146.

Friedman, R. H., J. E. Stollerman, D. M. Mahoney, and L. Rozenblyum. 1997. The Virtual Visit: Using Telecommunications Technology to Take Care to Patients. *Journal of the American Medical Informatics Association* 4(6):413–425.

Gabbard, G. O., and C. Nadelson. 1995. Professional Boundaries in the Physician-Patient Relationship. *Journal of the American Medical Association* 273(18):1445–1449.

Gallagher, H. G. 1994. *FDR's Splendid Deception.* Arlington, VA: Vandamere Press.

Gallagher, H. G. 1998. *Black Bird Fly Away. Disabled in an Able-Bodied World.* Arlington, VA: Vandamere Press.

Gandhi, T. K., S. N. Weingart, J. Borus, A. C. Seger, J. Peterson, E. Burdick, D. L. Seger, K. Shu, F. Frederico, L. L. Leape, and D. W. Bates. 2003. Adverse Drug Events in Ambulatory Care. *New England Journal of Medicine* 348(16):1556–1564.

Ganter, B. K., R. P. Erickson, M. A. Butters, J. H. Takata, and S. F. Noll. 2005. Clinical Evaluation. In *Physical Medicine and Rehabilitation: Principles and Practice,* edited by J. A. DeLisa, B. M. Gans, and N. E. Walsh, 1–48. Philadelphia: Lippincott-Raven Publishers.

Gerhart, K. A., J. Koziol-McLain, S. R. Lowenstein, and G. G. Whiteneck. 1994. Quality of Life following Spinal Cord Injury: Knowledge and Attitudes of Emergency Care Providers. *Annals of Emergency Medicine* 23(4):807–812.

Gerteis, M., S. Edgman-Levitan, J. Daley, and T. L. Delbanco, eds. 1993. *Through the Patient's Eyes.* San Francisco: Jossey-Bass.

Glass, T., A., and J. L. Balfour. 2003. Neighborhoods, Aging, and Functional Limitations. In *Neighborhoods and Health,* edited by I. Kawachi and L. F. Berkman, 303–334. New York: Oxford University Press.

Glionna, J. M. 2000. California and the West: Suit Faults Kaiser's Care for Disabled. *Los Angeles Times.* July 27:3.

Glionna, J. M. 2001. Kaiser Will Improve Treatment of Disabled. *Los Angeles Times.* April 13:A1.

Goffman, E. 1963. *Stigma. Notes on the Management of Spoiled Identity.* New York: Simon & Schuster.

Goldzweig, C. L., S. Rowe, N. S. Wenger, C. H. MacLean, and P. G. Shekelle. 2004. Preventing and Managing Visual Disability in Primary Care. Clinical Applications. *Journal of the American Medical Association* 291(12):1497–1502.

Green, A. R., J. R. Betancourt, and J. E. Carrillo. 2002. Integrating Social Factors into Cross-Cultural Medical Education. *Academic Medicine* 77(3):193–197.

Greenhouse, L. 1999. Justices Wrestle with the Definition of Disability: Is It Glasses? False Teeth? *New York Times*. April 28:A20.

Gregg, E. W., Y. J. Cheng, B. L. Cadwell, G. Imperatore, D. E. Williams, K. M. Flegal, K. M. Venkat Narayan, and D. F. Williamson. 2005. Secular Trends in Cardiovascular Disease Risk Factors According to Body Mass Index in US Adults. *Journal of the American Medical Association* 293(15):1868–1874.

Groce, N. E. 1985. *Everyone Here Spoke Sign Language. Hereditary Deafness on Martha's Vineyard.* Cambridge, MA: Harvard University Press.

Gross, D. L., H. Temkin-Greener, S. Kunitz, and D. B. Mukamel. 2004. The Growing Pains of Integrated Health Care for the Elderly: Lessons from the Expansion of PACE. *Milbank Quarterly* 82(2):257–282.

Hanson, K. W., P. Neuman, D. Dutwin, and J. D. Kasper. 2003. Uncovering the Health Challenges Facing People with Disabilities: The Role of Health Insurance. *Health Affairs Web Exclusive.* November 19:W3-552–565.

Harris Interactive, Inc. 2000. *2000 National Organization on Disability/Harris Survey of Americans with Disabilities.* Conducted for the National Organization on Disability. New York: Harris Interactive, Inc.

Harris Interactive, Inc. 2004. *2004 National Organization on Disability/Harris Survey of Americans with Disabilities.* Conducted for the National Organization on Disability. www.nod.org/content.cfm?id=1537, accessed December 21, 2004.

Hedley, A. A., C. L. Ogden, C. L. Johnson, M. D. Carroll, L. R. Curtin, and K. M. Flegal. 2004. Prevalence of Overweight and Obesity among U.S. Children, Adolescents, and Adults, 1999–2002. *Journal of the American Medical Association* 291(23):2847–2850.

Hockenberry, J. 1995. *Moving Violations: War Zones, Wheelchairs, and Declarations of Independence.* New York: Hyperion.

Hoenig, H. 1993. Educating Primary Care Physicians in Geriatric Rehabilitation. *Clinics in Geriatric Medicine* 9(4):883–893.

Horowitz, C. R. 2004. Barriers to Buying Healthy Foods for People with Diabetes: Evidence of Environmental Disparities. *American Journal of Public Health* 94(9):1549–1554.

Horrigan, J., L. Rainie, K. Allen, A. Boyce, M. Madden, and E. O'Grady. 2003. *The Ever-Shifting Internet Population. A new look at Internet access and the digital divide.* Washington, DC: Pew Internet & American Life Project, April 16.

Hurley, R. E., and S. A. Somers. 2003. Medicaid and Managed Care: A Lasting Relationship? *Health Affairs* 22(1):77–88.

Iezzoni, L. I. 1999. Boundaries. *Health Affairs* 18(6):171–176.

Iezzoni, L. I. 2003. *When Walking Fails. Mobility Problems of Adults with Chronic Conditions.* Berkeley: University of California Press.

Iezzoni, L. I., and B. L. O'Day. 2003. *Quality of Care and Service Use for Persons with Disabilities. Final Report.* R01 HS10223, Agency for Healthcare Research and Quality. Boston: Beth Israel Deaconess Medical Center, June 12.

Iezzoni, L. I., E. P. McCarthy, R. B. Davis, and H. Siebens. 2000a. Mobility Impairments and Use of Screening and Preventive Services. *American Journal of Public Health* 90(6):955–961.

Iezzoni, L. I., E. P. McCarthy, R. B. Davis, and H. Siebens. 2000b. Mobility Problems and Perceptions of Disability by Self-Respondents and Proxy-Respondents. *Medical Care* 38(10):1051–1057.

Iezzoni, L. I., E. P. McCarthy, R. B. Davis, L. Harris-David, and B. O'Day. 2001. Use of Screening and Preventive Services among Women with Disabilities. *American Journal of Medical Quality* 16(4):135–144.

Iezzoni, L. I., R. B. Davis, J. Soukup, and B. O'Day. 2002. Satisfaction with Quality and Access to Health Care among People with Disabling Conditions. *International Journal for Quality in Health Care* 14(5):369–381.

Iezzoni, L. I., R. B. Davis, J. Soukup, and B. O'Day. 2003. Quality Dimensions That Most Concern People with Physical and Sensory Disabilities? *Archives of Internal Medicine* 163(4):2085–2092.

Iezzoni, L. I., B. L. O'Day, M. Killeen, and H. Harker. 2004. Communicating about Health Care: Observations from Persons Who Are Deaf or Hard of Hearing. *Annals of Internal Medicine* 140(5):356–362.

Iezzoni, L. I., R. Ramanan, and R. E. Drews. 2005. Teaching Medical Students about Communicating with Patients Who Have Sensory or Physical Disabilities. *Disability Studies Quarterly* 25(1). Online at www.dsq-sds.org

Iglehart, J. K. 2003. The Dilemma of Medicaid. *New England Journal of Medicine* 348(21):2140–2148.

Illingworth, P., and W. E. Parmet. 2000. Positively Disabled. The Relationship between the Definition of Disability and Rights under the American Disability Act. In *Americans with Disabilities: Exploring Implications of the Law for Individuals and Institutions*, edited by L. P. Francis and A. Silvers, 3–17. New York: Routledge.

Institute of Medicine, Committee on Assessing Rehabilitation Science and Engineering. E. N. Brandt, Jr. and A. M. Pope, eds. 1997. *Enabling America: Assessing the Role of Rehabilitation Sciences and Engineering.* Washington, DC: National Academy Press.

Institute of Medicine, Committee on the Consequences of Uninsurance. 2001. *Coverage Matters. Insurance and Health Care.* Washington, DC: National Academy Press.

Institute of Medicine, Committee on the Consequences of Uninsurance. 2002a. *Care Without Coverage. Too Little, Too Late.* Washington, DC: National Academy Press.

Institute of Medicine, Committee on the Consequences of Uninsurance. 2002b. *Health Insurance Is a Family Matter.* Washington, DC: National Academy Press.

Institute of Medicine, Committee on the Consequences of Uninsurance. 2003a. *Hidden Costs, Value Lost. Uninsurance in America.* Washington, DC: National Academy Press.

Institute of Medicine, Committee on the Consequences of Uninsurance. 2003b. *A Shared Destiny. Community Effects of Uninsurance.* Washington, DC: National Academy Press.

Institute of Medicine, Committee on Health Literacy. L. Nielsen-Bohlman, A. M. Panzer, and D. A. Kindig, eds. 2004. *Health Literacy. A Prescription to End Confusion.* Washington, DC: National Academy Press.

Institute of Medicine, Committee on a National Agenda for the Prevention of Disabilities. A. M. Pope and A. R. Tarlov, eds. 1991. *Disability in America: Toward a National Agenda for Prevention.* Washington, DC: National Academy Press.

Institute of Medicine, Committee on Quality of Health Care in America. 1999. *To Err Is Human: Building a Safer Health System.* Washington, DC: National Academy Press.

Institute of Medicine, Committee on Quality of Health Care in America. 2001. *Crossing the Quality Chasm: A New Health System for the 21st Century.* Washington, DC: National Academy Press.

Institute of Medicine, Committee to Review the Social Security Administration's Disability Decision Process Research. National Research Council. Committee on National Statistics. G. S. Wunderlich, D. P. Rice, and N. L. Amado, eds. 2002. *The Dynamics of Disability. Measuring and Monitoring Disability for Social Security Programs.* Washington, DC: National Academy Press.

Institute of Medicine, Committee on Understanding and Eliminating Racial Disparities in Health Care. B. D. Smedley, A. Y. Stith, and A. R. Nelson, eds. 2002. *Unequal Treatment: Confronting Racial and Ethnic Disparities in Health Care.* Washington, DC: National Academy of Sciences.

Institute of Medicine, Roundtable on Environmental Health Sciences, Research, and Medicine. K. Hanna and C. Coussens. 2001. *Rebuilding the Unity of Health and the Environment. A New Vision for the 21st Century.* Washington, DC: National Academy Press.

Israel, B. A., A. J. Schulz, E. A. Parker, and A. B. Becker. 1998. Review of Community-Based Research: Assessing Partnership Approaches to Improve Public Health. *Annual Review of Public Health* 19:173–202.

Jackson, R. J. 2003. The Impact of the Built Environment on Health: An Emerging Field. *American Journal of Public Health* 93(9):1382–1384.

Janofsky, M. 2004. Costs and Savings in Medicare Change on Wheelchairs. *New York Times.* January 30:A10.

Johnson, R. L., S. Saha, J. J. Arbelaez, M. C. Beach, and L. A. Cooper. 2004. Racial and Ethnic Differences in Patient Perceptions of Bias and Cultural Competence in Health Care. *Journal of General Internal Medicine* 19(2):101–10.

Kahn, P. 2003. Teaching Tomorrow's Doctors. *New Mobility* 14(119):45–48.

Kaiser Family Foundation/Harvard School of Public Health. 2004. *Views of the New Medicare Drug Law: A Survey of People on Medicare. Opinions and Experiences of Non-Elderly People with Disabilities on Medicare. Supplemental Chartpack.* Menlo Park, CA, and Boston: Kaiser Family Foundation and Harvard School of Public Health, October.

Kane, B., and D. Z. Sands. 1998. Guidelines for the Clinical Use of Electronic Mail with Patients. *Journal of the American Medical Informatics Association* 5(1):104–111.

Kaplan, B., R. Farzanfar, and R. H. Friedman. 2003. Personal Relationships with an Intelligent Interactive Telephone Health Behavior Advisor System: A Multimethod Study Using Surveys and Ethnographic Interviews. *International Journal of Medical Informatics* 71(1):33–41.

Kaplan, S. and R. Kaplan. 2003. Health, Supportive Environments, and the Reasonable Person Model. *American Journal of Public Health* 93(9):1484–1489.

Kaplan, S. H., B. Gandek, S. Greenfield, W. Rogers, and J. E. Ware. 1995. Patient and Visit Characteristics Related to Physicians' Participatory Decision-Making Style. Results from the Medical Outcomes Study. *Medical Care* 33(12):1176–1187.

Karp, G. 1998. *Choosing a Wheelchair. A Guide for Optimal Independence.* Sebastopol, CA: O'Reilley & Associates.

Karp, G. 1999. *Life on Wheels. For the Active Wheelchair User.* Sebastopol, CA: O'Reilley & Associates.

Katz, S. J., and C. A. Moyer. 2004. The Emerging Role of Online Communication between Patients and Their Providers. *Journal of General Internal Medicine* 19(9):978–983.

Keating, N. L., D. C. Green, A. C. Kao, J. A. Gazmararian, V. Y. Wu, and P. D. Cleary. 2002. How Are Patients' Specific Ambulatory Care Experiences Related to Trust, Satisfaction, and Considering Changing Physicians? *Journal of General Internal Medicine* 17(1):29–39.

Kennedy, J., and C. Erb. 2002. Prescription Noncompliance Due to Cost among Adults with Disabilities in the United States. *American Journal of Public Health* 92(7):1120–1124.

Kirschner, K. L., C. J. Gill, J. P. Panko Reis, and C. Hammond. 2005. Health Issues for Women with Disabilities. In *Physical Medicine and Rehabilitation: Principles and Practice,* edited by J. A. DeLisa, B. M. Gans, and N. E. Walsh, 1561–1582. Philadelphia: Lippincott-Raven Publishers.

Kleinman, A. 1988. *The Illness Narratives.* New York: Basic Books.

Klopsteg, P. E., and P. D. Wilson. 1954. *Human Limbs and Their Substitutes.* Washington, DC: National Academy of Sciences.

Koepsell, T., L. McCloskey, M. Wolf, A. V. Moudon, D. Buchner, J. Kraus, and M. Patterson. 2002. Crosswalk Markings and the Risk of Pedestrian-Motor Vehicle Collisions in Older Pedestrians. *Journal of the American Medical Association* 288(17):2136–2143.

Krueger, R. A. 1994. *Focus Groups. Second Edition. A Practical Guide for Applied Research.* Thousand Oaks, CA: Sage Publications.

Kuhback, S. J. 1995. Communicating with Deaf Patients [letter]. *Journal of the American Medical Association* 274(10):795.

Kvalsvig, A. 2003. Ask the Elephant. *Lancet.* 362(December 20/27, 9401):2079–2080.

Lakdawalla, D. N., J. Bhattacharya, and D. P. Goldman. 2004. Are the Young Becoming More Disabled? *Health Affairs* 23(1):168–176.

Leveille, S. G., L. Fried, and J. M. Guralnik. 2002. Disabling Symptoms. What Do Older Women Report? *Journal of General Internal Medicine* 17(10):766–773.

Leveille, S. G., S. Ling, M. C. Hochberg, H. E. Resnick, K. J. Bandeen-Roche, A. Won, and J. M. Guralnik. 2001. Widespread Musculoskeletal Pain and the Progression of Disability in Older Disabled Women. *Annals of Internal Medicine* 135(12):1038–1046.

Levinson, W., and D. Roter. 1995. Physicians' Psychosocial Beliefs Correlate with Their Patient Communication Skills. *Journal of General Internal Medicine* 10(7):375–379.

Levinson, W., W. B. Stiles, T. S. Inui, and R. Engle. 1993. Physicians' Frustration in Communicating with Patients. *Medical Care* 31(4):285–295.

Linton, S. 1998. *Claiming Disability. Knowledge and Identity.* New York: New York University Press.

Logue, R. M. 2002. Self-Medication and the Elderly: How Technology Can Help. *American Journal of Nursing* 102(7):51–55.

Lollar, D. J. 2001. Public Health Trends in Disability. Past, Present, and Future. In *Handbook of Disability Studies*, edited by G. L. Albrecht, K. D. Seelman, and M. Bury, 754–771. Thousands Oaks, CA: Sage Publications.

Longmore, P. K., and L. Umansky. 2001. *The New Disability History: American Perspectives.* New York: New York University Press.

Lopez, R. 2004. Urban Sprawl and Risk for Being Overweight or Obese. *American Journal of Public Health* 94(9):1574–1579.

Lorig, K., H. Holman, D. Sobel, D. Laurent, V. González, and M. Minor. 2000. *Living a Healthy Life with Chronic Conditions. Self-Management of Heart Disease, Arthritis, Diabetes, Asthma, Bronchitis, Emphysema, and Others. Second Edition.* Boulder, CO: Bull Publishing Company.

Lorig, K., P. Ritter, A. L. Stewart, D. S. Sobel, B. W. Brown Jr., A. Bandura, V. M. González, D. D. Laurent, and H. R. Holman. 2001. Chronic Disease Self-Management Program. 2-Year Status and Health Care Utilization Outcomes. *Medical Care* 39(11):1217–1223.

Lunney, J. R., J. Lynn, D. J. Foley, S. Lipson, and J. M. Guralnik. 2003. Patterns of Functional Decline at the End of Life. *Journal of the American Medical Association* 289(18):2387–2392.

Lunney, J. R., J. Lynn, and C. Hogan. 2002. Profiles of Older Medicare Decedents. *Journal of the American Geriatrics Society* 50(6):1108–1112.

Lynn, J. 2004. *Sick to Death and Not Going to Take It Anymore!* Berkeley: University of California Press.

Lynn, J., and J. Harrold. 1999. *Handbook for Mortals. Guidance for People Facing Serious Illness.* New York: Oxford University Press.

Mace, R. L. 1998. *Removing Barriers to Health Care. A Guide for Health Professionals.* Raleigh: North Carolina State University, The Center for Universal Design.

MacKinney, T. G., D. Walters, G. L. Bird, and A. B. Nattinger. 1995. Improvements in Preventive Care and Communication with Deaf Patients. Results of a Novel Primary Health Care Program. *Journal of General Internal Medicine* 10(3):133–137.

Mahoney, K. J., L. Simon-Rusinowitz, D. M. Loughlin, S. M. Desmond, and M. R. Squillace. 2004. Determining Personal Care Consumers' Preferences for a Consumer-Directed Cash and Counseling Option: Survey from Arkansas, Florida, New Jersey, and New York Elders and Adults with Physical Disabilities. *Health Services Research* 39(3):643–663.

Mark, D. H. 2005. Deaths Attributable to Obesity. *Journal of the American Medical Association* 293(15):1918–1919.

Markakis, K. M., H. B. Beckman, A. L. Suchman, and R. M. Frankel. 2000. The Path to Professionalism: Cultivating Humanistic Values and Attitudes in Residency Training. *Academic Medicine* 75(2):141–150.

Marmor, T. R. 2000. *The Politics of Medicare. Second Edition.* New York: Aldine de Gruyter.

Marshall, C. E., D. Benton, and J. M. Brazier. 2000. Elder Abuse. Using Clinical Tools to Identify Clues of Mistreatment. *Geriatrics* 55(2):42–53.

Mashaw, J. L., and V. P. Reno, eds. 1996. *Balancing Security and Opportunity: The Challenge of Disability Income Policy. Report of the Disability Policy Panel.* Washington, DC: National Academy of Social Insurance.

Mayerson, A., and M. Diller. 2000. The Supreme Court's Nearsighted View of the ADA. In *Americans with Disabilities: Exploring Implications of the Law for Individuals and Institutions*, edited by L. P. Francis and A. Silvers, 124–125. New York: Routledge.

McCaig, L. F., and C. W. Burt. 2003. National Hospital Ambulatory Medical Care Survey: 2001 Emergency Department Summary. *Advance Data from Vital and Health Statistics.* No. 335. Hyattsville, MD: National Center for Health Statistics, 4 June.

McFarlane, J., R. B. Hughes, M. A. Nosek, J. Y. Groff, N. Swedlend, and P. Dolan Mullen. 2001. Abuse Assessment Screen-Disability (AAS-D): Measuring Frequency, Type, and Perpetrator of Abuse toward Women with Physical Disabilities. *Journal of Women's Health and Gender-Based Medicine* 10(9):861–866.

McGlynn, E. A., S. M. Asch, J. Adams, J. Keesey, J. Hicks, A. DeCristofaro, and E. A. Kerr. 2003. The Quality of Health Care Delivered to Adults in the United States. *New England Journal of Medicine* 348(26):2635–45.

McWhinney, I. 1989. The Need for a Transformed Clinical Method. In *Communicating with Medical Patients*, edited by M. Stewart and D. Roter, 25–40. Newbury Park, CA: SAGE Publications.

McWilliams, J. M., A. M. Zaslavsky, E. Meara, and J. Z. Ayanian. 2004. Health Insurance Coverage and Mortality among the Near-Elderly. *Health Affairs* 23(4):223–233.

Mechanic, D., and S. Meyer. 2000. Concepts of Trust among Patients with Serious Illness. *Social Science and Medicine* 51(5):657–668.

Medicare Payment Advisory Commission. 2003a. *Report to the Congress. Medicare Payment Policy.* Washington, DC, March.

Medicare Payment Advisory Commission. 2003b. *Report to the Congress. Variation and Innovation in Medicare.* Washington, DC, June.

Medicare Payment Advisory Commission. 2004a. *Report to the Congress. Medicare Payment Policy.* Washington, DC, March.

Medicare Payment Advisory Commission. 2004b. *Report to the Congress. New Approaches in Medicare.* Washington, DC, June.

Medicare Rights Center. 2004. *Forcing Isolation: Medicare's "In the Home" Coverage Standard for Wheelchairs.* New York: Medicare Rights Center, March.

Miller, W. R., and S. Rollnick. 1991. *Motivational Interviewing. Preparing People to Change Addictive Behaviors.* New York: Guilford Press.

Minihan, P. M., Y. S. Bradshaw, L. M. Long, W. Altman, S. Perduta-Fulginiti, J. Ector, K. L. Foran, L. Johnson, P. Kahn, and R. Sneirson. 2004. Teaching about Disability: Involving Patients with Disabilities as Medical Educators. *Disability Studies Quarterly* 24(4). Online at www.dsq-sds.org

Miranda, J., and L. A. Cooper. 2004. Disparities in Care for Depression among Primary Care Patients. *Journal of General Internal Medicine* 19(2):120–126.

Mokdad, A. H., E. S. Ford, B. A. Bowman, W. H. Dietz, F. Vinicor, V. S. Bales, and J. S. Marks. 2003. Prevalence of Obesity, Diabetes, and Obesity-Related Health Risk Factors, 2001. *Journal of the American Medical Association* 289(1):76–79.

Morris, J. 1996. *Pride Against Prejudice. Transforming Attitudes to Disability.* London: Women's Press Limited.

Murphy, R. F. 1990. *The Body Silent*. New York: W. W. Norton.

Murray-García, J. L., J. V. Selby, J. Schmittdiel, K. Grumbach, and C. P. Quesenberry, Jr. 2000. Racial and Ethnic Differences in a Patient Survey. Patients' Values, Ratings, and Reports Regarding Physician Primary Care Performance in a Large Health Maintenance Organization. *Medical Care* 38(3):300–310.

National Association of the Deaf Law Center. 2004. *ADA Questions and Answers for Health Care Providers*. www.nad.org/infocenter/infotogo/ada3qa.html, accessed May 13, 2004.

National Council on Disability. 2003. *Tennessee v. Lane: The Legal Issues and the Implications for People with Disabilities. Policy Briefing Paper*. Washington, DC: National Council on Disability, September 4.

National Institute on Aging and National Library of Medicine. 2004. *Making Your Web Site Senior Friendly. A Checklist*. www.nlm.nih.gov/pubs/checklist.pdf, accessed June 9, 2004.

National Spinal Cord Injury Statistical Center. 2001. *Spinal Cord Injury. Facts and Figures at a Glance*. Birmingham: University of Alabama. www.spinalcord.uab.edu, accessed July 17, 2003.

Nelson, E., B. Conger, R. Douglass, D. Gephart, J. Kirk, R. Page, A. Clark, K. Johnson, K. Stone, J. Wasson, and M. Zubkoff. 1983. Functional Health Status Levels of Primary Care Patients. *Journal of the American Medical Association* 249(24):3331–3338.

Newman, S. J. 1997. Housing Policy and Home-Based Care. In *Home-Based Care for a New Century*, edited by D. M. Fox and C. Raphael, 185–218. Malden, MA: Blackwell.

Nielsen, J. 2002. *Usability for Senior Citizens*. Nielsen Norman Group. April 28. www.useit.com/alertbox/20020428.html, accessed June 15, 2004.

Nightingale, F. 1863. *Notes on Hospitals. Third Edition*. London: Longman, Green, Longman, Roberts, and Green.

Northridge, M. E., E. D. Sclar, and P. Biswas. 2003. Sorting Out the Connections between the Built Environment and Health: A Conceptual Framework for Navigating Pathways and Planning Healthy Cities. *Journal of Urban Health: Bulletin of the New York Academy of Medicine* 80(4):556–568.

Nosek, M. A., R. B. Hughes, H. B. Taylor, and C. A. Howland. 2004. Violence against Women with Disabilities: The Role of Physicians in Filling the Treatment Gap. In *Welner's Guide to the Care of Women with Disabilities*, edited by S. L. Welner and F. Haseltine, 333–345. Philadelphia: Lippincott, Williams & Wilkins.

O'Brien, M. 2003. *How I Became a Human Being. Mark O'Brien with Gillian Kendall*. Madison: University of Wisconsin Press.

O'Day, B. L., M. Killeen, and L. I. Iezzoni. 2004. Improving Health Care Experiences of Persons Who Are Blind or Have Low Vision: Suggestions from Focus Groups. *American Journal of Medical Quality* 19(5):193–200.

Ogden, C. L., C. D. Fryar, M. D. Carroll, and K. M. Flegal. 2004. Mean Body Weight, Height, and Body Mass Index, United States 1960–2002. *Advance Data from Vital and Health Statistics*. No. 347. Hyattsville, MD: National Center for Health Statistics, October 27.

Oliver, M. 1996. *Understanding Disability: From Theory to Practice.* New York: St. Martin's Press.

Olkin, R. 1999. *What Psychotherapists Should Know about Disability.* New York: Guilford Press.

Olkin, R. 2004. Disability and Depression. In *Welner's Guide to the Care of Women with Disabilities,* edited by S. L. Welner and F. Haseltine, 279–299. Philadelphia: Lippincott, Williams & Wilkins.

Olmstead v. L. C. (98-536) 527 U.S. 581 (1999).

Omenn, G. S. 1999. Caring for the Community: The Role of Partnerships. *Academic Medicine* 74(7):782–789.

Oshima, S., K. L. Kirschner, A. Heinemann, and P. Semik. 1998. Assessing the Knowledge of Future Internists and Gynecologists in Caring for a Woman with Tetraplegia. *Archives of Physical Medicine and Rehabilitation* 79(10):1270–1275.

Parker, R. M., S. C. Ratzan, and N. Lurie. 2003. Health Literacy: A Policy Challenge for Advancing High-Quality Health Care. *Health Affairs* 22(4):147–153.

Pelka, F. 1997. *The ABC-CLIO Companion to the Disability Rights Movement.* Santa Barbara, CA: ABC-CLIO, Inc.

Perdue, W. C., L. A. Stone, and L. O. Gostin. 2003. The Built Environment and Its Relationship to the Public's Health: The Legal Framework. *American Journal of Public Health* 93(9):1390–1394.

Pérez-Peña, R., and G. Glickson. 2003. As Obesity Rises, Health Care Indignities Multiply. *New York Times.* November 29:A1, A13.

Perry, M., A. Dulio, and K. Hanson. 2003. *The Role of Health Coverage for People with Disabilities: Findings from 12 Focus Groups with People with Disabilities.* Menlo Park, CA: Henry J. Kaiser Family Foundation, August.

Peters, L. 1982. Women's Health Care. Approaches in Delivery to Physically Disabled Women. *Nurse Practitioner* 7(1):34–37.

Pincus, T., R. Esther, D. A. DeWalt, and L. F. Callahan. 1998. Social Conditions and Self-Management Are More Powerful Determinants of Health Than Access to Care. *Annals of Internal Medicine* 129(5):406–411.

Pope, G. C., R. P. Ellis, A. S. Ash, C.-F. Liu, J. Z. Ayanian, D. W. Bates, H. Burstin, L. I. Iezzoni, and M. J. Ingber. 2000. Principal Inpatient Diagnostic Cost Group Model for Medicare Risk Adjustment. *Health Care Financing Review* 21(3):93–18.

Potok, A. 2002. *A Matter of Dignity. Changing the World of the Disabled.* New York: Bantam Books.

President's Advisory Commission on Consumer Protection and Quality in the Health Care Industry. 1998. *Quality First: Better Health Care for All Americans.* Washington, DC: U.S. Government Printing Office.

Pucher, J., and L. Dijkstra. 2003. Promoting Safe Walking and Cycling to Improve Public Health: Lessons from the Netherlands and Germany. *American Journal of Public Health* 93(9):1509–1516.

Quint, E. H. 2004. Gynecologic Health Care for Developmentally Disabled Women. In *Welner's Guide to the Care of Women with Disabilities,* edited by S. L. Welner and F. Haseltine, 261–269. Philadelphia: Lippincott, Williams & Wilkins.

Rapp, C. E. Jr., and M. M. Torres. 2000. The Adult with Cerebral Palsy. *Archives of Family Medicine.* 9(5):466–472.

Reeve, C. 1998. *Still Me.* New York: Random House.

Reiley, P., L. I. Iezzoni, R. Phillips, R. B. Davis, L. I. Tuchin, and D. Calkins. 1996. Discharge Planning: Comparison of Patients' and Nurses' Perceptions of Patients Following Hospital Discharge. *Image* 28(2):143–147.

Reis, J. P., M. L. Breslin, L. I. Iezzoni, and K. L. Kirschner. 2004. *It Takes More Than Ramps to Solve the Crisis in Healthcare for People with Disabilities.* Chicago: Rehabilitation Institute of Chicago, September.

Reuben, D. B. 2002. Organizational Interventions to Improve Health Outcomes of Older Persons. *Medical Care* 40(5):416–428.

Riley, G. F. 2004. The Cost of Eliminating the 24-Month Medicare Waiting Period for Social Security Disabled-Worker Beneficiaries. *Medical Care* 42(4):387–94.

Riley, G. F., J. D. Lubitz, and N. Zhang. 2003. Patterns of Health Care and Disability for Medicare Beneficiaries under 65. *Inquiry* 40(1):71–83.

Rohe, D. E. 2005. Psychological Aspects of Rehabilitation. In *Physical Medicine and Rehabilitation: Principles and Practice,* edited by J. A. DeLisa, B. M. Gans, and N. E. Walsh, 1005–1024. Philadelphia: Lippincott-Raven Publishers.

Rollnick, S., P. Mason, and C. Butler. 1999. *Health Behavior Change. A Guide for Practitioners.* Edinburgh: Churchill Livingstone.

Rosenbaum, S., and J. Teitelbaum. 2004. *Olmstead* at Five: Assessing the Impact. Menlo Park, CA: Kaiser Commission on Medicaid and the Uninsured, June.

Roter, D. L., J. A. Hall, and Y. Aoki. 2002. Physician Gender Effects in Medical Communication. A Meta-Analytic Review. *Journal of the American Medical Association* 288(6):756–764.

Roter, D. L., M. Stewart, S. M. Putnam, M. Lipkin, Jr., W. Stiles, and T. S. Inui. 1997. Communication Patterns of Primary Care Physicians. *Journal of the American Medical Association* 277(4):350–356.

Roussos, S. T., and S. B. Fawcett. 2000. A Review of Collaborative Partnerships as a Strategy for Improving Community Health. *Annual Review of Public Health* 21:369–402.

Rowe, S., C. H. MacLean, and P. G. Shekelle. 2004. Preventing Visual Loss from Chronic Eye Disease in Primary Care. Scientific Review. *Journal of the American Medical Association* 291(12):1487–1496.

Runge, J. W., and T. B. Cole. 2002. Crosswalk Markings and Motor Vehicle Collisions Involving Older Pedestrians. *Journal of the American Medical Association* 288(17):2172–2174.

Saha, S., M. Komaromy, T. D. Koepsell, and A. B. Bindman. 1999. Patient-Physician Racial Concordance and the Perceived Quality and Use of Health Care. *Archives of Internal Medicine* 159(9):997–1004.

San Augustin, T. B., J. B. Atchison, and B. L. Gracer. 2004. Health Care and Deafness: Deaf Professionals Speak Out. In *Welner's Guide to the Care of Women with Disabilities,* edited by S. L. Welner and F. Haseltine, 31–44. Philadelphia: Lippincott, Williams & Wilkins.

Saxton, M. 1987. Something That Happened before I Was Born. In *With Wings,* edited by M. S. Saxton and F. Howe, 51–55. New York: Feminist Press at City University of New York.

Schaschl, S. and D. Straw. 1993. Chemical Dependency: The Avoided Issue for Persons with Physical Disabilities. In *Substance Abuse & Physical Disability,* edited by A. W. Heinemann, 165–77. New York: Haworth Press.

Scherer, M. J. 2000. *Living in the State of Stuck. How Technology Impacts the Lives of People with Disabilities, Third Edition.* Cambridge, MA: Brookline Books.

Schillinger, D., K. Grumbach, J. Piette, F. Wang, D. Osmond, C. Daher, J. Palacios, G. Diaz Sullivan, and A. B. Bindman. 2002. Association of Health Literacy with Diabetes Outcomes. *Journal of the American Medical Association* 288(4):475–482.

Schmittdiel, M., K. Grumbach, J. V. Selby, and C. P. Quesenberry, Jr. 2000. Effect of Physician and Patient Gender Concordance on Patient Satisfaction and Preventive Care Practices. *Journal of General Internal Medicine* 15(11):761–769.

Shalala, D. E. 2000. *Report to Congress. Safeguards for Individuals with Special Health Care Needs Enrolled in Medicaid Managed Care.* Washington, DC: U.S. Department of Health and Human Services, November 6.

Shapiro, J. P. 1994. *No Pity. People with Disabilities Forging a New Civil Rights Movement.* New York: Times Books.

Shattuck, F. C. 1907. Address to the Graduating Class in Medicine of the Medical Department of Yale University, June 24, 1907. *The Boston Medical and Surgical Journal.* 157(July 11):63–67. Reprinted in *The Art of Medical Care and Caring.* (No publisher or date; distributed by the Harvard Medical Alumni Association, 1982.)

Siddall, P. J., J. M. McClelland, S. B. Rutkowski, and M. J. Cousins. 2003. A Longitudinal Study of the Prevalence and Characteristics of Pain in the First 5 Years Following Spinal Cord Injury. *Pain* 103(3):249–257.

Siebens, H., K. Cairns, W. O. Schalick III, D. Fondulis, P. Corcoran, and E. Bartels. 2004. PoWER Program: People with Disabilities Educating Residents. *American Journal of Physical Medicine & Rehabilitation* 83(3):203–209.

Singer, S. J., and L. A. Bergthold. 2001. Prospects for Improved Decision Making about Medical Necessity. *Health Affairs* 20(1):200–206.

Sipski, M. L., C. Alexander, and A. Sherman. 2005. Sexuality and Disability. In *Physical Medicine and Rehabilitation Medicine: Principles and Practice,* edited by J. A. DeLisa, B. M. Gans, and N. E. Walsh, 1583–1603. Philadelphia: Lippincott-Raven Publishers.

Slack, W. V. 2004. A 67-Year-Old Man Who E-Mails His Physician. *Journal of the American Medical Association* 292(18):2255–2261.

Smith, V., K. Gilford, R. Ramesh, and V. Wachino. 2003. *Medicaid Spending Growth: A 50-State Update for Fiscal Year 2003.* Menlo Park, CA: Henry J. Kaiser Family Foundation, January.

Social Security Administration. 2003. *Disability Evaluation Under Social Security.* SSA Pub. No. 64-039. Office of Disability Programs. Washington, DC: Social Security Administration, January.

Social Security Administration. 2004. Table 33. Distribution, by Sex and Diagnostic Group, 2003. *Annual Statistical Report on the Social Security Disability Insurance Program,* 2003:92–93.

Spielberg, A. R. 1998. On Call and Online. Sociohistorical, Legal, and Ethical Implications of E-Mail for the Patient-Physician Relationship. *Journal of the American Medical Association* 280(15):1353–1359.

Spina Bifida Association of America. 2003. *Facts about Spina Bifida.* www.sbaa.org/html/sbaa_facts.html, accessed November 11, 2003.

Srinivasan, S., L. R. O'Fallon, and A. Dearry. 2003. Creating Healthy Communities, Healthy Homes, Healthy People: Initiating a Research Agenda on the Built Environment and Public Health. *American Journal of Public Health* 93(9):1446–1450.

Steinberg, A. G., L. I. Iezzoni, A. Conill, and M. Stineman. 2002. Reasonable Accommodations for Medical Faculty with Disabilities. *Journal of the American Medical Association* 288(24):3147–3154.

Stewart, M., L. Meredith, J. B. Brown, and J. Galajda. 2000. Communication between Older Patients and Their Physicians. *Clinics in Geriatric Medicine* 16(1):25–36.

Stewart, M., and D. Roter, eds. 1989. *Communicating with Medical Patients.* Newbury Park, CA: SAGE Publications.

Stone, D. A. 1984. *The Disabled State.* Philadelphia: Temple University Press.

Story, M. F., J. L. Mueller, and R. L. Mace. 1998. *The Universal Design File. Designing for People of All Ages and Abilities.* Raleigh: North Carolina State University, Center for Universal Design.

Street, R. L. Jr., E. Krupat, R. A. Bell, R. L. Kravitz, and P. Haidet. 2003. Beliefs about Control in the Physician-Patient Relationship. Effect on Communication in Medical Encounters. *Journal of General Internal Medicine* 18(8):609–616.

Sturm, R., J. S. Ringel, and T. Andreyeva. 2004. Increasing Obesity Rates and Disability Trends. *Health Affairs* 23(2):199–205.

Suchman, A., K. Markakis, H. B. Beckman, and R. Frankel. 1997. A Model of Empathetic Communication in the Medical Interview. *Journal of the American Medical Association* 277(8):678–682.

Tennessee, Petitioner v. George Lane. (02-1667) U.S. 541 (2004).

Thomas, L. 1974. *The Lives of a Cell. Notes of a Biology Watcher.* New York, NY: Viking Press.

Thomson, R. G. 1997. *Extraordinary Bodies. Figuring Physical Disability in American Culture and Literature.* New York: Columbia University Press.

Turk, M. A., C. A. Geremski, P. F. Rosenbaum, and R. J. Weber. 1997. The Health Status of Women with Cerebral Palsy. *Archives of Physical Medicine and Rehabilitation* 78(12):S-10–17.

Turk, M. A., and R. J. Weber. 2005. Congenital and Child-Onset Disabilities: Age-Related Changes and Secondary Conditions in Mobility Impairment. In *Physical Medicine and Rehabilitation: Principles and Practice,* edited by J. A. DeLisa, B. M. Gans, and N. E. Walsh, 1519–1529. Philadelphia: Lippincott-Raven Publishers.

Ulrich, R., X. Quan, C. Zimring, A. Joseph, and R. Choudhary. 2004. *The Role of the Physical Environment in the Hospital of the 21st Century: A Once-in-a-Lifetime Opportunity.* Center for Health Design Research, September. www.health-design.org/research/reports/physical_environ.php, accessed July 1, 2005.

U.S. Census Bureau. 2002a. *Property Owners and Managers Survey.* Multi-Family Properties: Handicap Accessibility, Table 18. www.census.gov/hhes/www/housing/poms/multifam/mfunit/mftab18.html, last updated August 22, 2002. Accessed June 29, 2004.

U.S. Census Bureau. 2002b. *Property Owners and Managers Survey.* Single Family Properties: Handicap Accessibility, Table 18. www.census.gov/hhes/www/housing/poms/singlefam/sfunit/sftab18.html, last updated August 22, 2002. Accessed June 29, 2004.

U.S. Census Bureau. 2003a. Characteristics of the Civilian Noninstitutionalized Population by Age, Disability Status, and Type of Disability: 2000. Table 1. www.census.gov/hhes/www/disable/disabstat2k/table1.html, accessed June 16, 2003.

U.S. Census Bureau. 2003b. Definition of Disability Items in Census 2000. www.census.gov/hhes/www/disable/disdef00.html, accessed June 14, 2003.

U.S. Department of Health and Human Services. 1988. 45 CFR Part 85. *Enforcement of Nondiscrimination on the Basis of Handicap in Programs or Activities Conducted by the Department of Health and Human Services.* Office for Civil Rights. Effective September 6, 1988. www.hhs.gov/ocr/45cfr85reg.html, accessed August 7, 2003.

U.S. Department of Health and Human Services. 2000. *Healthy People 2010. Second Edition. With Understanding and Improving Health and Objectives for Improving Health.* Two Volumes. Washington, DC: U.S. Government Printing Office, November.

U.S. Department of Health and Human Services. 2003. *Summary of the HIPAA Privacy Rule.* Office for Civil Rights. Washington, DC: May.

U.S. General Accounting Office. 1997. *Medicare Post-Acute Care. Cost Growth and Proposals to Manage It Through Prospective Payment and Other Controls.* GAO/T-HEHS-97-106. Washington, DC: April 9.

Üstün, T. B., S. Chatterji, N. Kostansjek, and J. Bickenbach. 2003. WHO's ICF and Functional Status Information in Health Records. *Health Care Financing Review* 24(3):77–88.

Villarosa, L. 2003. Barriers Toppling for Disabled Medical Students. *New York Times.* November 25:D5.

Vladeck, B. C., E. O'Brien, T. Hoyer, and S. Clauser. 1997. Confronting the Ambivalence of Disability Policy: Has Push Come to Shove? In *Disability. Challenges for Social Insurance, Health Care Financing, and Labor Market Policy,* edited by V. P. Reno, J. L. Mashaw, and B. Gradison, 83–100. Washington, DC: National Academy of Social Insurance.

Waisel, D. B. and R. D. Truog. 1995. The Cardiopulmonary Resuscitation-Not-Indicated Order: Futility Revisited. *Annals of Internal Medicine* 122(4):304–308.

Warner, M., P. M. Barnes, and L. A. Fingerhut. 2000. Injury and Poisoning Episodes and Conditions: National Health Interview Survey, 1997. *Vital and Health Statistics* 10(202).

Wartman, S. A., L. L. Morlock, F. E. Malitz, and E. Palm. 1983. Impact of Divergent Evaluations by Physicians and Patients of Patients' Complaints. *Public Health Reports* 98(2):141–145.

Waterman, A. D., G. Banet, P. E. Milligan, A. Frazier, E. Verzino, B. Walton, and B. F. Gage. 2001. Patient and Physician Satisfaction with a Telephone-Based Anticoagulation Service. *Journal of General Internal Medicine* 16(7):460–463.

Web Accessibility Initiative. 2004. *World Wide Web Consortium.* www.w3.0rg/WAI, accessed June 18, 2004.

Weil, E., M. Wachterman, E. P. McCarthy, R. B. Davis, B. O'Day, L. I. Iezzoni, and C. C. Wee. 2002. Obesity among Adults with Disabling Conditions. *Journal of the American Medical Association* 288(10):1265–268.

Welner, S. L. 1998. Caring for Women with Disabilities. In *Textbook of Women's Health,* edited by L. A. Wallis, 87–92. Philadelphia: Lippincott-Raven Publishers.

Welner, S. L. 1999. *A Provider's Guide for the Care of Women with Physical Disabilities and Chronic Medical Conditions.* Raleigh, NC: North Carolina Office on Disability and Health.

Welner, S. L., C. C. Foley, M. A. Nosek, and A. Holmes. 1999. Practical Considerations in the Performance of Physical Examinations on Women with Disabilities. *Obstetrics and Gynecology Survey* 54(7):457–462.

Welner, S. L., and B. Temple. 2004. General Health Concerns and the Physical Examination. In *Welner's Guide to the Care of Women with Disabilities,* edited by S. L. Welner and F. Haseltine, 95–108. Philadelphia: Lippincott, Williams & Wilkins.

West, J. 1991. The Social and Policy Context of the Act. In *The Americans with Disabilities Act. From Policy to Practice,* edited by J. West, 3–24. New York: Milbank Memorial Fund.

Whipple, B., and S. L. Welner. 2004. Sexuality Issues. In *Welner's Guide to the Care of Women with Disabilities,* edited by S. L. Welner and F. Haseltine, 347–355. Philadelphia: Lippincott, Williams & Wilkins.

White, C. 2003. Rehabilitation Therapy in Skilled Nursing Facilities: Effects of Medicare's New Prospective Payment System. *Health Affairs* 22(3):214–223.

Williams, B., A. Dulio, H. Claypool, M. J. Perry, and B. S. Cooper. 2004. *Waiting for Medicare: Experiences of Uninsured People with Disabilities in the Two-Year Waiting Period for Medicare.* New York: Commonwealth Fund, October.

Williams, F. H., and B. Hopkins. 2005. Nutrition in Physical Medicine and Rehabilitation. In *Physical Medicine and Rehabilitation: Principles and Practice,* edited by J. A. DeLisa, B. M. Gans, and N. E. Walsh, 1267–1287. Philadelphia: Lippincott-Raven Publishers.

Williams, G. 2001. Theorizing Disability. In *Handbook of Disability Studies,* edited by G. L. Albrecht, K. D. Seelman, and M. Bury, 123–144. Thousands Oaks, CA: Sage Publications.

Williams, M. V., T. Davis, R. M. Parker, and B. D. Weiss. 2002. The Role of Health Literacy in Patient-Physician Communication. *Family Medicine* 34(5):383–389.

Witte, T. N., and A. J. Kuzel. 2000. Elderly Deaf Patients' Health Care Experiences. *Journal of the American Board of Family Practice* 13(1):17–22.

World Health Organization. 1997. *ICIDH-2: International Classification of Impairments, Activities and Participation. A Manual of Dimensions of Disablement and Functioning. Beta-1 Draft for Field Testing.* Geneva: World Health Organization.

World Health Organization. 2001. *International Classification of Functioning, Disability and Health.* Geneva: World Health Organization.

Young, J. M. 1997. *Equality of Opportunity. The Making of the Americans with Disabilities Act.* Washington, DC: National Council on Disability.

Young, M. E., M. A. Nosek, C. Howland, G. Chanpong, and D. H. Rintala. 1997. Prevalence of Abuse of Women with Physical Disabilities. *Archives of Physical Medicine and Rehabilitation* 78(12 Supplement):S34–S38.

Zola, I. K. 1982. *Missing Pieces: A Chronicle of Living with a Disability.* Philadelphia: Temple University Press.

Index

Abernathy, Rick
  communication with clinician,
    100–101
  telephone communications, 129
abuse, vulnerability of disabled, 126–127
accessibility. *See also* health care
    facilities; healthy and accessible
    communities; independence;
    physical access; universal design
  Americans with Disabilities Act
    (ADA) regulations, 229–230
  designing health care settings,
    234–245
  design involving disabled, 236–238
  enforcement of regulations, 231–234
  making the Web, 250–251
  rules, 228–234
  suggestions for improving, 286–295
access to care. *See also* accessibility;
    Americans with Disabilities Act
    (ADA); barriers; finding care
  accommodating obesity, 89–91
  finding willing clinicians, 66–68
  patients as access advocates, 91–92
  paying enough to ensure, 57–62
accommodations. *See also* Americans
    with Disabilities Act (ADA);
    communication accommodations
  acceptability, 87–89
  auxiliary aids and services, 211
  communication, 210–214
  deaf, 15–16, 218–225
  design considerations, 167
  making, during physical exam, 87–89,
    125–127, 286–288

  mammography machine, 88–89
  medical schools, 207–208
  obesity, 89–91
  reasonable, 25, 30, 91–92, 214, 232
  requiring public, 62–64
Accreditation Council for Graduate
    Medical Education (ACGME),
    197–198
acoustics, design, 239
advocacy. *See* self-management
aging
  adults with childhood disabilities,
    68–69
  enhancing healthy, with disability,
    5–6
  patterns of functional declines, 6, 7
Alto, Joe
  access advocate, 91–92
  accessible housing, 159–160
  finding willing physicians, 66
  help that is unhelpful, 87
  high examining table, 58–60, 73
  wheelchair patient seeking care,
    58–60
American Foundation for the Blind,
    communication and mobility, 195,
    196, 216–217
American Sign Language (ASL)
  accommodating hearing needs, 218,
    220
  hiring interpreters, 62–66
  interpreters, 221–223
  language of many deaf persons, 62,
    63
  use by deaf, 15, 225

clinician peers with disabilities, 205–208
communicating patient to patient, 208–209
core competencies, 197–198
disability simulations, 201–202
effective health care, 193
elicit-provide-elicit process, 203–204
home visits, 200–201
interpersonal communication, 93, 95–97, 100–108
mutual responsibility for, 193–194
online guidelines, 255
peers with disabilities, 205–208
questions to ask, 203–205
race and ethnicity influencing, 97
recognizing barriers, 194–197
standardized patients, 199–200
training clinicians to improve, 197–202
videotaping interactions, 200
patient education, traditional and self-management, 180
patients as
access advocates, 91–92
educators of clinicians, 175–176
experts, 173–174
Patrick, Caroline
pain, 143
pregnant tetraplegic with urinary tract infections, 67–68
Paulson, Todd
examination table, 81
physical access to health care, 74–75
Pepperill, Brad
hospitalization, 102–103
miscommunication, 106
unpleasant surprises, 125
personal care assistants, 86, 127, 153–155
Peters, Eleanor
attitudes toward disability, 12–13
barrier of glass door, 3, 4
bathroom blockade, 76, 77
independent entry, 226, 227
physical barriers, 73
physical access. *See also* accessibility; access to care; accommodations; health care facilities
acceptable accommodations, 87–89
clinical facilities, 87

design basics, 238–240
inpatient challenges, 85–86
medical equipment, 240, 242–245
overweight and obese, 89–91
scale for wheelchair patients, 244
screening and services requiring, 84
Tennessee v. Lane, 232–233
physical activity, communities, 267–269
physical barriers. *See also* barriers
Americans with Disabilities Act regulations, 229–230
bathroom blockade, 77
enforcement for removing, 231–234
examining tables, 80–84
getting around health care facilities, 76, 78–80
getting in door and up/down stairs, 75–76
making health care facilities accessible, 226–228
medical equipment, 240–245
navigating unfamiliar places, 78
steps to remove, 231
physical examinations
first contacts, 118–122
getting settled in exam rooms, 121–122
making accommodations, 125–127
procedure etiquette, 123–127
receptionist's desk, 119–120
unpleasant surprises, 123–125
vulnerability to abuse by caretakers, 126–127
waiting and waiting rooms, 120–121
physicians. *See also* clinicians; finding care; interpersonal communication; medical students
Americans with Disabilities Act (ADA) requirements, 62–66
behavior during office visits, 134–135
communicating with deaf patients, 64–66
confrontation and disability determination, 24–25
core competencies, 197–198
disability definition, 17–18
finding willing, 66–68
managed care organizations, 60–62
searching for, 53–54
training, 199–202